ALLE ZEIT WACH 1842

K. Yonenobu · K. Ono · Y. Takemitsu (Eds.)

Lumbar Fusion and Stabilization

With 251 Figures

Springer-Verlag
Tokyo Berlin Heidelberg New York London
Paris Hong Kong Barcelona Budapest

Kazuo Yonenobu, M.D.
Department of Orthopaedic Surgery, Labor Welfare Corporation,
Kansai Rosai Hospital, Amagasaki, Hyogo, 660 Japan

Keiro Ono, M.D.
Dean of Medical School, Professor and Chairman, Department of Orthopaedic Surgery,
Osaka University Medical School, Osaka, 553 Japan

Yoshiharu Takemitsu, M.D.
Professor and Chairman, Department of Orthopedic Surgery,
Asahikawa Medical College, Asahikawa, Hokkaido, 078 Japan

ISBN 4-431-70116-8 Springer-Verlag Tokyo Berlin Heidelberg New York
ISBN 3-540-70116-8 Springer-Verlag Berlin Heidelberg New York Tokyo
ISBN 0-387-70116-8 Springer-Verlag New York Berlin Heidelberg Tokyo

Printed on acid-free paper

Library of Congress Cataloging-in-Publication Data
Lumbar fusion and stabilization / K. Ono, Y. Takemitsu, K. Yonenobu, (eds.). p. cm. Includes bibliographical references and index. ISBN 4-431-70116-8 (Tokyo, Berlin, Heidelberg, N.Y.). – ISBN 3-540-70116-8 (Berlin, Heidelberg, N.Y., Tokyo). – ISBN 0-387-70116-8 (N.Y., Berlin, Heidelberg, Tokyo), 1. Lumbar vertebrae – Surgery. 2. Spinal fusion. I. Ono, Keirō. II. Takemitsu, Y. (Yoshiharu), 1930– . III. Yonenobu, K. (Kazuo), 1947– . RD768.L843 1993, 617.3′75′059 – dc20, 92-46674

Typesetting, printing, and binding: Best-set Typesetter Ltd., Hong Kong

Foreword

The hour of departure of this century has brought before us innumerable questions, some of which remain to be resolved. The recent development of image technology and various therapeutic modalities emphasizes the need for orthopedists to address many problems of the lumbar spine. The role of the orthopedic surgeon in the management of lumbar disorders is yet to be ascertained. To shoulder the major responsibilities in the management of low back pain, however, we have to assess our ability to identify the causes and the underlying mechanisms of low back pain, sciatica, and intermittent claudication and to realize the limitations of therapeutic modalities in orthopedic surgery. For the surgical elimination of pain, it is essential to identify pain-eliciting lesions by means of careful history taking, physical examination, and image technology. We should be familiar with the sensitivity and specificity of each test and diagnostic modality related to the varying pathology of low back pain. With regard to pain relieving procedures, answers to certain questions should be sought and self assessment in that light should be made on each occasion. These are the questions that must be addressed: What may be the additional procedure or operative intervention that particularly guarantees pain relief and its permanent elimination in each case of low back pain, in the excision of a herniated disc, in the removal of the whole disc and in accomplishing lumbar interbody fusion, in the reduction of severe spondylolisthesis and fusion, in widening the narrow canal, and in stabilizing spinal instability accompanying painful disc, multisegmental degenerated disc with a narrow canal, and nerve tissue irritation?

Although lumbar fusion and stabilization have become more common procedures for the treatment of low back pain in routine orthopedic surgery, the identification of pain-eliciting lesions and the identification of essential surgical intervention for the elimination of pain are only occasionally reflected upon by the surgeon before these procedures are carried out. Must lumbar fusion always be indicated for disc herniation in young adults who are often required to do heavy physical work and need a life-long guarantee against pain recurrence? Must this procedure be indicated for lumbar disc degeneration with instability in elderly persons? How should one localize the dominant pain-eliciting lesion in multisegmental spondylosis with a narrow spinal canal? Should stabilization with instrumentation be added to secure pain relief in such a condition?

For successful pain eliminating surgery, the significance of technical details should never be overlooked. A master surgeon tends to adhere to routine positioning on the operation table, has well-cared for surgical instruments, and pays due regard to hemostasis. He prefers the existing reliable and well standardized instruments to the newly developed all-round ones. For the prevention of complications due to pedicle screwing, a precise knowledge of anatomy is essential, and careful rechecking of the site and the direction of screwing must be done.

Currently, for lumbar fusion, not only autogenous grafts but also allogeneic grafts and biomaterials are applicable. Materials are chosen according to their individual advantageous characteristics and availability. Allogeneic grafts are stored and delivered either in a "freeze and dry" manner or after defatting and gas sterilization. A combination of bone grafting with instrumentation shortens the period of "bed rest", enhances fusion rate, and reduces the risk of instrumentation failure.

In the middle of this century, orthopedic researchers overcame certain longstanding problems with regard to many aspects of lumbar disorders. Through the 5th International Conference on Lumbar Fusion and Stabilization, various subjects related to lumbar disorders have been studied. We hope these selected Conference papers will convey a new message of multidisciplinary expertise in current achievements and enable us to widen our perspectives of science and art in spine surgery.

Kazuo Yonenobu
Keiro Ono
Yoshiharu Takemitsu

Contents

Foreword V
List of Contributors XI

Part 1 Principles of Lumbar Fusion and Stabilization

1.1 Biomechanics of Lumbar Spine Instability
M.M. Panjabi 3
1.2 The Myth of Solid Posterior Lateral Fusion
J. Zucherman, S. Brack, K.Y. Hsu, and W. Shea 10
1.3 Radiological Evidence of Posterior Lumbar Interbody Fusion
P.M. Lin 16

Part 2 To Fuse or Not To Fuse

SECTION I DETERMINATION OF SEGMENTAL INSTABILITY

2.1 The Role of External Fixation as a Predictor of Fusion Success
D.W. Lyon, D.J. Hall, R.C. Mulholland, and J.K. Webb 25
2.2 Assessment of Segmental Spinal Instability Using Magnetic Resonance Imaging
T. Toyone, H. Moriya, H. Kitahara, K. Takahashi, M. Yamagata, M. Murakami, and Y. Takahashi 35
2.3 Intraoperative Measurement of Lumbar Spinal Stiffness
S. Ebara, M. Tanaka, Y. Morimoto, T. Harada, N. Hosono, K. Yonenobu, and K. Ono 45

SECTION II THE MERITS AND DEMERITS OF LUMBAR FUSION

2.4 The Long-Term Effect of Lumbar Spine Fusion: Deterioration of Adjacent Motion Segments
K.Y. Hsu, J. Zucherman, and A. White 54

2.5 A Critical Analysis of Motion of the Lumbar Spine Adjacent to an Interbody Fusion: A Clinical Radiological Study and Biomechanical Cadaveric Study
K.D.K. Luk, D.H.K. Chow, J.C.Y. Leong, and J. Evans 65
2.6 Anterior Interbody Fusion for Degenerative Spondylolisthesis: The Long-Term Clinical Results
K. Takahashi, H. Kitahara, M. Yamagata, M. Murakami, M. Mimura, and H. Moriya 72
2.7 Clinical Results of Lumbar Fusion for Heavy Workers with Lumbar Disk Herniation
S. Matsunaga, T. Sakou, K. Yone, E. Taketomi, T. Morimoto, and K. Ijiri 78

SECTION III MULTI-SEGMENTAL SPONDYLOSIS

2.8 Multi-Segmental Spondylosis: An Overview of Presentations at the Fifth International Conference on Lumbar Fusion and Stabilization
J. Kostuik 86
2.9 Patient Selection for Stabilization of Multisegmental Spondylosis
W. Dick, H. Widmer, and V.J. Leone 92
2.10 A Clinical Study of Degenerative Lumbar Scoliosis
M.-S. Moon, K.-S. Lee, C.-I. Lim, Y.-B. Kim, and H.-S. Lee 98
2.11 Surgical Management of Degenerative Lumbar Scoliosis
Y. Toyama 113
2.12 Treatment of Multilevel Anterior and Retrolisthesis of the Lumbosacral Spine
P. Enker, A.D. Steffee, L. Keppler, R.S. Biscup, and S.D. Miller 126
2.13 Posterior Stabilization for Lumbar Degenerative Kyphosis: In Situ Fusion in Maximum Extension on Hall's Frame
O. Nakai, I. Yamaura, Y. Kurosa, H. Komori, A. Ookawa, H. Sakai, and M. Abe 135
2.14 Operative Treatment of Lumbar Degenerative Kyphosis
Y. Takemitsu, Y. Atsuta, Y. Kamo, T. Iwahara, O. Sugawara, Y. Harada, and Y. Miyatake 150
2.15 Non-Instrumentation Stabilization/Decompression Procedure for Lumbar Spinal Stenosis: Significance of Expansive Laminoplasty
H. Tsuji, H. Matsui, M. Kanamori, N. Hirano, and Y. Katoh 160

Part 3 Stabilization Methods

3.1 How to Stabilize the Lumbar Spine: An Overview
K. Hirabayashi 169

3.2 Results of Posterior Lumbar Interbody Fusion for Lytic and Degenerative Spondylolisthesis
R.B. Cloward . . . 178
3.3 Posterior Lumbar Interbody Fusion: With and Without Pedicle Screw Fixation
S. Nakai, H. Yoshizawa, K. Kenmotsu, S. Nishimoto, and T. Morita . . . 188
3.4 Posterior Lumbar Interbody Fusion Combined Auto- and Allograft Technique
P.S. Ramani . . . 197
3.5 Posterior Lumbar Interbody Fusion with Allograft and Plates
T. Ohwada, T. Yamamoto, K. Nose, M. Inaoka, and M. Kakiuchi . . 208
3.6 Effects of Ceramic Interspinous Block on Anterior Lumbar Interbody Fusion
H. Tsuji, N. Hirano, H. Matsui, H. Ohshima, H. Ishihara, and Y. Katoh . . . 220
3.7 Boucher Screw Fixation of the Spine: A Translaminar Pedicle Screw Technique
C.E. Graham . . . 227
3.8 Reduction and Stabilization of High Grade Spondylolisthesis: A Study of 29 Patients Using a Posterior Approach
R. Roy-Camille, J.Y. Lazennec, C.H. Garreau, G. Saillant, and J.P. Benazet . . . 241
3.9 Lumbar Diskectomy, Facetectomy, and Laminectomy of L4–L5 and L5–S1 Levels: Experimental Approach and Biomechanical Consequences of Practical Application
J.Y. Lazennec, R. Desjardins, R. Roy-Camille, C.G. Laudet, A. Lazennec, and B. Roger . . . 249

Part 4 Spinal Instrumentation

SECTION I BIOMECHANICS

4.1 Biomechanical Analysis of Lumbosacral Fixation
D.H. McCord, B.W. Cunningham, Y. Shono, J.J. Myers, and P.C. McAfee . . . 259
4.2 Comparative Study of Three Pedicle Screw Devices
R. Steffen, L.-P. Nolte, and J. Krämer . . . 278
4.3 Biomechanical Study of Pedicle Screw Fixation Systems for the Lumbar Spine
M. Yamagata, H. Kitahara, S. Minami, K. Takahashi, H. Moriya, and T. Tamaki . . . 288

SECTION II PEDICLE SCREW SYSTEMS

4.4 Lumbosacral Fusion with Pedicular Screw Plating Instrumentation: 10-year Follow-up Results
R. Roy-Camille, J.-P. Desauge, and J.-P. Benazet 297
4.5 Simmons Plating System for Spinal Fusion Surgery
J.W. Simmons 303
4.6 Stabilization of Spondylolisthesis: The Hartshill System
J. Dove 312
4.7 Lumbar Spinal Stabilization by the MOSS System
M.-S. Moon, K.-S. Lee, S.-S. Kim, and D.-H. Sun 316
4.8 Internal Fixation of the Lumbar Spine: Further Clinical Experience Using Computer Assisted Design and Manufacture of a Precise System
D.C. Hemmy 332
4.9 Complications of Lumbar Spinal Surgery with Transpedicular Fixation
S.H. Davne and D.L. Myers 338

Part 5 Bank Bone and Bone Graft Substitutes

5.1 Recent Trends in the Use of Bank Bone in Spinal Surgery: Replies to Questionnaires from the United States
M. Kakiuchi and K. Ono 349
5.2 Defatted, Gas-Sterilized Bone Allograft as Bank Bone: Preparation, Safety, and Utility for Lumbar Spine Surgery
M. Kakiuchi, K. Ono, and K. Shinka 354
5.3 A Titanium Implant for Interbody Fusion in Degenerative Lumbar Disk Disease
J.W. Chang and A.C.M.C. Yau 364
5.4 Use of Hydroxyapatite Blocks in Posterior Interbody Fusion
N. Suzuki and Y. Iwamoto 371
5.5 A Carbon Fiber Implant to Aid Interbody Lumbar Fusion: 1-year Clinical Results in the First 26 Patients
J.W. Brantigan and A.D. Steffee 379

Keyword Index 397

List of Contributors

Abe, M. 135
Atsuta, Y. 150
Benazet, J.-P. 241, 297
Biscup, R.S. 126
Brack, S. 10
Brantigan, J.W. 379
Chang, J.W. 364
Chow, D.H.K. 65
Cloward, R.B. 178
Cunningham, B.W. 259
Davne, S.H. 338
Desauge, J.-P. 297
Desjardins, R. 249
Dick, W. 92
Dove, J. 312
Ebara, S. 45
Enker, P. 126
Evans, J. 65
Garreau, C.H. 241
Graham, C.E. 227
Hall, D.J. 25
Harada, T. 45
Harada, Y. 150
Hemmy, D.C. 332
Hirabayashi, K. 169
Hirano, N. 160, 220
Hosono, N. 45
Hsu, K.Y. 10, 54
Ijiri, K. 78
Inaoka, M. 208
Ishihara, H. 220
Iwahara, T. 150
Iwamoto, Y. 371
Kakiuchi, M. 208, 349, 354
Kamo, Y. 150
Kanamori, M. 160
Katoh, Y. 160, 220
Kenmotsu, K. 188
Keppler, L. 126
Kim, S.-S. 316
Kim, Y.-B. 98
Kitahara, H. 35, 72, 288
Komori, H. 135
Kostuik, J. 86
Krämer, J. 278
Kurosa, Y. 135
Laudet, C.G. 249
Lazennec, A. 249
Lazennec, J.Y. 241, 249
Lee, H.-S. 98
Lee, K.-S. 98, 316
Leone, V.J. 92
Leong, J.C.Y. 65
Lim, C.-I. 98
Lin, P.M. 16
Luk, K.D.K. 65
Lyon, D.W. 25
McAfee, P.C. 259
McCord, D.H. 259
Matsui, H. 160, 220
Matsunaga, S. 78
Miller, S.D. 126
Mimura, M. 72
Minami, S. 288

Miyatake, Y. 150
Moon, M.-S. 98, 316
Morimoto, Y. 45
Morimoto, T. 78
Morita, T. 188
Moriya, H. 35, 72, 288
Mulholland, R.C. 25
Murakami, M. 35, 72
Myers, D.L. 338
Myers, J.J. 259
Nakai, O. 135
Nakai, S. 188
Nishimoto, S. 188
Nolte, L.-P. 278
Nose, K. 208
Ohshima, H. 220
Ohwada, T. 208
Ono, K. 45, 349, 354
Ookawa, A. 135
Panjabi, M.M. 3
Ramani, P.S. 197
Roger, B. 249
Roy-Camille, R. 241, 249, 297
Saillant, G. 241
Sakai, H. 135
Sakou, T. 78
Shea, W. 10
Shinka, K. 354
Shono, Y. 259
Simmons, J.W. 303
Steffee, A.D. 126, 379
Steffen, R. 278
Sugawara, O. 150
Sun, D.-H. 316
Suzuki, N. 371
Takahashi, K. 35, 72, 288
Takahashi, Y. 35
Takemitsu, Y. 150
Taketomi, E. 78
Tamaki, T. 288
Tanaka, M. 45
Toyama, Y. 113
Toyone, T. 35
Tsuji, H. 160, 220
Webb, J.K. 25
White, A. 54
Widmer, H. 92
Yamagata, M. 35, 72, 288
Yamamoto, T. 208
Yamaura, I. 135
Yau, A.C.M.C. 364
Yone, K. 78
Yonenobu, K. 45
Yoshizawa, H. 188
Zucherman, J. 10, 54

PART 1

Principles of Lumbar Fusion and Stabilization

1.1 Biomechanics of Lumbar Spine Instability

Manohar M. Panjabi[1]

Introduction

Low back pain is the most common and costly disorder of the musculoskeletal system. The magnitude of the problem is well documented by the frequency of its occurrence. In western society, 50%–70% of the population will have low back pain once in their lifetime, and 18% of the population has low back pain at any one time. The cost of this disease for the United States has been estimated at $15–50 billion per year. Although the cause of most low back pain is not known, spinal instability is considered as one of the most important causes [1].

The purpose of this paper is to describe observations made clinically, both qualitatively and quantitatively, and biomechanical experiments that have been conducted to study the role of various spinal components in providing spinal stability. Specifically the paper examines the various attempts that have been made to objectively determine spinal instability in patients using biomechanical tools. This is followed by a look at the very important role that muscles play in providing spinal stability. Finally, knowing that healing and adaptation occur after injury, these phenomena are examined in light of findings from animal experiments.

Instability of the spine has often been equated, especially in the case of degenerative changes, to increased spinal displacement. Knutsson [2] was probably one of the first to demonstrate clinically the use of a kinematic parameter to indicate instability. This parameter was the retrodisplacement (translation) of one vertebra with respect to another when the patient was put through movement from full extension to full flexion. The displacement was documented using lateral X rays. These observations have since been confirmed in some studies, but there are also studies that have found the opposite effect. Decreased motion was found in low back pain patients as compared to

[1] Department of Orthopaedics and Rehabilitation, Yale University School of Medicine, New Haven, CT 06510, USA

the normal population [3,4]. In a younger population of athletes having low back pain, the motion was increased [3].

Other causes of instability are the injuries sustained in accidents. In these situations, besides the displacement of one vertebra with respect to another, there are other indicators of the magnitude of the trauma in the form of fractures of the vertebra. By examining the patterns of fractures, it may be possible to obtain an assessment of the magnitude of the traumatic loads involved, and therefore, the magnitude of injury to the spinal column and its consequence, i.e., instability. This approach was probably initiated by Nicoll in 1949 [5] and popularized by several people, including Holdsworth [6], Louis [7], and Denis [8]. By examining 412 X rays of patients with spinal injuries, Denis proposed a classification of the fractures of the thoracolumbar spine with the goal of determining instability. Based upon retrospective X ray examination, he proposed the division of the spinal column into three units: the anterior column, consisting of the anterior half of the vertebral body; the middle column, consisting of the vertebral body from its middle to the middle of the pedicles; and the posterior column, which included all elements posterior of the pedicle. Denis proposed that if two of the columns are destroyed or are nonfunctional, then the spine may be considered clinically unstable. Although this is presently one of the most popular classification methods for fractures of the thoracolumbar spine, it is to be noted that it is based upon a retrospective study and not a prospective study utilizing objective data sets.

The spinal column, consisting of vertebrae, is held together by disks, ligaments, and the vertebrae that articulate with each other via the facet joints. Various biomechanical experiments have focused on the determination of the effects of injuries to each of these elements on the overall effect on the stability of the spine. (In all biomechanical experiments, increased motion or flexibility is considered as a quantitative measure of instability.) These are all in vitro studies using fresh cadaveric human spine specimens. The general methodology is to study the flexibility behavior of the spine specimen before injury, and compare these results with similar results obtained after one or more sequential injuries. The measure of flexibility is most often the range of motion, although neutral zone – a measure of laxity around the neutral position, shown in Fig. 1 – has been suggested as an alternative measure of spinal instability [9]. It has been found to be a more sensitive parameter than the range of motion in biomechanically quantifying spinal injuries [10,11]. Given below are brief descriptions of selected biomechanical studies that have attempted to quantify the role of various spinal components in providing spinal stability.

The Intervertebral Disk

It has been known for a long time that the disk cannot be injured under pure compressive force [12]. Rotational torque is a more damaging load [13]. But what happens after injury? It was first believed that there was a "self-healing"

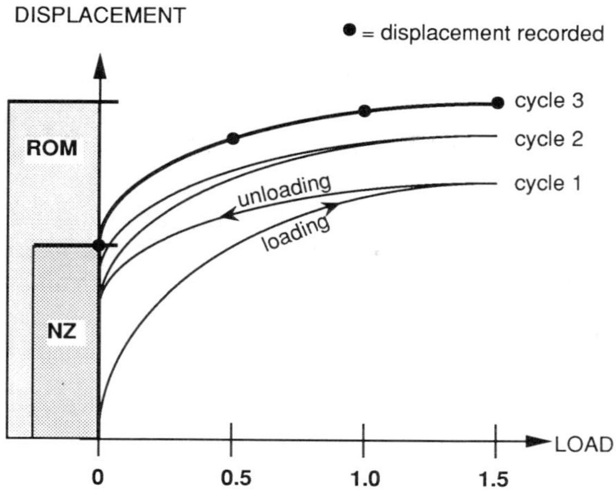

Fig. 1. The load-displacement curve of the spine is obtained by applying a load (X-axis) and measuring the resulting displacement (Y-axis). Three load/unload cycles are used to minimize the viscoelastic effects of the spine. The displacement measurements are made on the third load cycle. As the behavior of the spine is nonlinear, two parameters of displacement, i.e., neutral zone (*NZ*) and range of motion (*ROM*), are used to quantify the load-displacement curve. The neutral zone represents the laxity of the spine segment around the neutral position

phenomena when an injury is made to the disk annulus [14]. This was based on a biomechanical study of spinal segments subjected only to compression load. The study was repeated with more precise motion measurement techniques and three-dimensional load application systems, and very different results were found [15,16]. In these later studies, an injury to the disk, and especially the complete removal of the nucleus, resulted in significant changes in the three-dimensional movements of the spine. Thus, simple biomechanical studies exploring limited aspects of the spine may sometimes provide erroneous results. The spine is three-dimensional, and whenever possible, it should be so studied.

Although in 1934 Mixter and Barr showed that the low back pain was caused by disk prolapse [17], it is only recently that this mechanism has been studied and proven in a laboratory experiment. Adams and Hutton [18] conducted an experiment using fresh cadaveric lumbar spine specimens, without the posterior elements so that they could observe disk prolapse, and applied combined loads of lateral bending, hyperflexion, and a sudden axial compression force to produce disk prolapse in more than 40% of the specimens. The disk prolapse was similar to that seen clinically and more often happened in younger specimens with a viable nucleus.

The Facet Joints

The role of the facet joints in providing stability to the spine, especially in compression and torsion, has been studied by several researchers [13,19–21]. The main findings of these studies are that the load on the facets in compression is dependent upon the spinal posture, and may vary anywhere from 0%–33% of the load on the spine, depending upon the posture (greater load in extension). However, the main function for the facets in the lumbar spine seems to be to block axial rotation. In this respect, Farfan and Sullivan [13] showed that injury to the disk cannot be produced by compressive loads, but only by torsional loads. They hypothesized that, under normal conditions, the facets block the torsional motion beyond a couple of degrees to either side. However, if the facets are damaged, greater movement is allowed with the possibility of injuring the disk. Thus, facets play an important role, both by providing stability to the spine by blocking the motion, and also, indirectly, by protecting the disk, another major component of the spinal stabilizing system. The role of facets was also studied by Abumi et al. [19]. They measured three-dimensional flexibilities of the fresh cadaveric lumbar spine functional spinal units when intact and after a series of increasing transections of the facet joints. They found that the flexion motion was the first one to be affected by the injuries, while the extension and lateral bending motions were not significantly affected. The major effect on axial rotation came when one complete facet was removed. The clinical interpretation of these findings is that a facetectomy should be restricted to partial removal of the facets, 50% or less, and be symmetrical for the two facets.

Clinical Instability

The clinical instability of the spine includes more than just a mechanical derangement of the spinal column. A comprehensive definition of clinical instability has been provided that includes, besides the mechanical injuries to the spinal column, also the clinical aspects such as pain, neurological dysfunction, and deformity, both acutely and developing over time [22]. Based on these ideas, where physiological displacement was considered an important parameter to monitor, a biomechanical experiment using fresh cadaveric human spine specimens from the lumbosacral region was conducted [23]. In this experiment, sequential injuries were produced both from the front to back and from back to front. After each injury, the specimen was loaded both in flexion and then in extension, and the movements were measured. It was concluded that the spine was at the brink of mechanical instability if all of the posterior or all of the anterior elements were destroyed or were nonfunctional. The division of the anterior from the posterior elements is made by a plane parallel to the frontal plane and passing through the middle of the pedicles. This study also provided the upper limits of the normal physiological values for the translations and rotations of the functional spinal unit in the lumbar and lumbosacral regions.

Incorporating these biomechanical results of injury on the spinal column, and the neurological and pain status of the patient, a checklist was devised for the determination of clinical spinal instability of the lumbar spine [22]. Although the checklist needs to be proven by prospective controlled double-blind studies, it has provided a framework for a systematic evaluation of spinal instability in a patient by clearly differentiating the biomechanical measurements of spinal derangement from their clinical consequences, and thus, hopefully, lessening the confusion often associated with spinal instability.

Muscles Surrounding the Spinal Column

It has been shown experimentally that a whole lumbar spine specimen (L1–S1) standing erect is capable of carrying a load at L1 of only about 90 N (9 kgf) [24]. This critical value of the compressive load implies that a load greater than 90 N will buckle the spine and make it mechanically unstable. We know from daily observations that a person can carry not only his trunk weight, about 60% of the body weight, but much greater loads, say 3,000 N, even if one is not a weight lifter. The difference between an in vitro spine specimen and a living person is the muscles. The muscles play an extremely large role in providing stability to the spinal column. The consequences of the dysfunction of the muscles on the spinal stability, such as in polio, are well known.

Even though the importance of muscles in providing spinal stability is well appreciated, there are very few studies that have attempted to relate muscle dysfunction to low back problems. The major difficulty is in determining the in vivo forces that muscles generate. (Electromylographic signals do not always measure the muscle force.) As the muscles generate tensile forces between the bones to which they are attached, an in vitro simulation of the muscles was conducted to determine its effect on intact and sequentially injured spine specimens [25]. The major findings were the following: (a) the injuries destabilized the spine; (b) the application of muscle forces increased the range of motion, but decreased the neutral zone; and (c) the potential for stabilizing the spine after injury was demonstrated, if one considered neutral zone as an indicator of instability. The clinical treatment in strengthening all of the muscles surrounding the spinal column is therefore well justified.

Healing of Injuries and Adaptation

It has been shown in many in vitro experiments that an injury to the spine in the form of ligament transections, disk injury, or destruction of the facet joints causes destabilization. However, if similar injuries are produced in a living animal and are allowed to heal over a period of time, then the injuries initiate a healing process that *decreases* the spinal motion. This is based upon experiments in rabbit and canine models, that were studied for periods of up to 6 months using quantified functional X rays during the healing and adaptation period, and by biomechanical experiments on the animal corpses [26,27]. This is in contrast to the increased motion seen in the in vitro biomechanical studies [28,29]. However, the phenomena of decreased motion is not sustained throughout the healing period. Instead, an adaptive response comes into play, which results in bringing the motion back to, but not exceeding, the intact normal values. The healing/adaptation response was found to be directly related to the severity of the injury, i.e., a more severe injury resulted in a more vigorous response and greater decrease in the motion of the spine in the initial phase of healing. These studies demonstrate the potential of healing/adaptation, built within the spinal system, to respond to injury to the spinal column. This potentially stabilizing phenomena may be utilized to a greater extent in the future clinical treatments.

References

1. Nachemson A (1985) Lumbar spine instability: A critical update and symposium summary. Spine 10:290–291
2. Knutsson F (1944) The instability associated with disk degeneration in the lumbar spine. Acta Radiologica [Diagn] 25:593–609
3. Dvorak J, Panjabi MM, Novotny JE, Chang DG, Grob D (1991) Clinical validation of functional flexion/extension roentgenograms of the lumbar spine. Spine 16(8):943–950
4. Pearcy M, Portek I, Shepherd J (1985) The effect of low-back pain on lumbar spinal movements measured by three-dimensional X-ray analysis. Spine 10(2):150–153
5. Nicoll EA (1949) Fractures of the dorsolumbar spine. J Bone Joint Surg [Br] 31:376–394
6. Holdsworth FW (1962) Fractures, dislocations, and fracture/dislocations of the spine. J Bone Joint Surg [Br] 45:6–20
7. Louis R (1985) Spinal stability as defined by the three-column spine concept. Anat Clin 7:33
8. Denis F (1983) The three-column spine and its significance in the classification of acute thoracolumbar spinal injuries. Spine 8:817–831
9. Panjabi MM, Goel VK, Takata K (1982) Physiological strains in lumbar spinal ligaments. An in vitro biomechanical study. Spine 7(3):192–203
10. Oxland TR, Panjabi MM (in press) The onset and progression of spinal injury: A porcine flexion-compression trauma model. J Biomechanics
11. Panjabi MM, Duranceau JS, Oxland TR, Bowen CE (1989) Multidirectional instabilities of traumatic cervical spine injuries in a porcine model. Spine 14(10):1111–1115
12. Virgin W (1951) Experimental investigations into physical properties of the intervertebral disk. J Bone Joint Surg [Br] 33:607
13. Farfan HF, Sullivan JD (1967) The relation of facet orientation to intervertebral disk failure. Can J Surg 10:179
14. Markolf KL, Morris JM (1974) The structural components of the intervertebral disk. J Bone Joint Surg [Am] 56:675

15. Goel VK, Nishiyama K, Weinstein JN, Liu YK (1986) Mechanical properties of lumbar spinal motion segments as affected by partial disk removal. Spine 11(10):1008
16. Panjabi MM, Krag MH, Chung TQ (1984) Effects of disk injury on mechanical behavior of the human spine. Spine 9(7):707–713
17. Mixter WJ, Barr JS (1934) Ruptures of the intervertebral disk with involvement of the spinal canal. N Engl J Med 211:210
18. Adams M, Hutton W (1982) 1981 Volvo Award in Basic Science. Prolapsed intervertebral disk: a hyperflexion injury. Spine 7(3):184–191
19. Abumi K, Panjabi MM, Duranceau J, Oxland T, Crisco JJ (1990) Biomechanical evaluation of lumbar spinal stability after graded facetectomies. Spine 15(11):1142–1147
20. Nachemson A (1960) Lumbar interdiskal pressure. Acta Orthop Scand Suppl 43
21. Prasad P, King AI, Ewing CL (1974) The role of articular facets during +Gz acceleration. J Appl Mech 41:321
22. White AA, Panjabi MM (1978) Clinical biomechanics of the spine, 1st edn. Lippincott, Philadelphia
23. Posner I, White A, Edwards T, Hayes W (1982) A biomechanical analysis of the clinical stability of the lumbar and lumbosacral spine. Spine 7(4):374–389
24. Crisco JJ, Panjabi MM, Yamamoto I, Oxland TR (in press) Euler stability of the human ligamentous lumbar spine: Part II Experiment. Clin Biomechanics
25. Panjabi MM, Abumi K, Duranceau J, Oxland T (1989) Spinal stability and intersegmental muscle forces: A biomechanical model. Spine 14(2):194–200
26. Panjabi MM, Pelker R, Crisco J, Thibodeau L, Yamamoto I (1988) Biomechanics of healing of posterior cervical spinal injuries in a canine model. Spine 13(7):803–807
27. Wetzel FT, Panjabi MM, Pelker RR (1989) Temporal biomechanics of posterior cervical spine injuries in vivo in a rabbit model. J Orthop Res 7:728–731
28. Panjabi MM, White AA, Johnson RM (1975) Cervical spine mechanics as a function of transection of components. J Biomechanics 8:327–336
29. Wetzel FT, Panjabi MM, Pelker RR (1989) Biomechanics of the rabbit cervical spine as a function of component transection. J Orthop Res 7:723–727

1.2 The Myth of Solid Posterior Lateral Fusion

James Zucherman, Steven Brack, Ken Y. Hsu, and William Shea[1]

Introduction

The purpose of this investigation was to determine the incidence of false-positive and false-negative interpretations of pseudarthrosis by evaluating anteroposterior roentgenograms, lateral bending roentgenograms, and lumbar computerized tomography (CT) with multiplanar reformations (MPR) in previously fused patients.

Materials and Methods

From January 1987 to April 1989 anterior interbody lumbar fusion (AILF) was performed on a series of 78 intervertebral disks in 39 patients for failed back surgery syndrome (FBSS), ranging from two to six surgeries. All patients had undergone previous posterolateral fusion (PLF), which may or may not have had diagnostically identifiable pseudarthrosis. These patients were selected to evaluate clinical and surgical motion of each intervertebral disk space incorporated in the PLF. The only levels within the fusion reviewed were those ultimately fused by an AILF. Some levels above and below the AILF may have had a previous PLF, but were not studied because motion could not be determined without first performing an anterior lumbar diskectomy. Many of these patients underwent an anterior and posterior surgery for multiple reasons. Some patients had augmentation of the PLF and decompression of foramens or central canals before the AILF was initiated. There were 16 males and 23 females, and the patients ranged in age from 20 years to 69 years (mean age, 41 years). All but three patients had the PLF more than 1 year before undergoing the AILF. The remaining three patients had the PLF more than 9 months before the AILF.

In preoperative computer tomography (CT) scans with multiplanar reformations (MPR), lateral bending and plain anteroposterior (AP) roentgenograms

[1] St. Mary's Spine Center, 1 Shrader St., San Francisco, CA 94117, USA

were reviewed in blind fashion by WS, a coauthor and radiologist. A total of 28 patients had CT with MPR, 36 patients had sidelying lateral bending films, 30 patients had AP films, and 19 patients had all three preoperative studies performed to review for pseudarthrosis. Clinical radiographic review was performed at each motion segment of the fusion mass, so each segment could be categorized into an apparent fused segment or an apparent pseudarthritic segment. The fusion mass by CT scanning was evaluated by reviewing all films, especially curved coronal and sagittal reformations. If a pseudarthrosis was suspected on both sides of the PLF in any view, the level was recorded as the pseudarthrosis. If the pseudarthrosis was seen on only one side, then the fusion mass was considered solid. Similarly, the AP roentgenograms needed bilateral evidence of a pseudarthrosis to be considered positive for a pseudarthrosis. If a solid mass was seen unilaterally, the fusion mass was considered fused. Likewise, the bending films were also reviewed at each level and if any motion was seen, the segment was considered not fused. To review the bending films, the flexion and extension films were superimposed to identify any motion.

All patients underwent an AILF because of persistent postoperative pain. Some also required a posterior procedure before the AILF. An AILF was performed if diskography reproduced the patient's moderate to severe concordant back and/or leg pain, even if the patients appeared to have a solid fusion from clinical studies. The technique was routinely performed by us, and a vascular surgeon performed the retroperitoneal approach. A rectangular window was placed in the intervertebral disk space to prepare a bed for perforated demineralized cortical femoral ring (PDCR). Anterior diskectomy and end-plate decortication were performed, followed within the appropriate sized ring to complete the procedure. To determine motion at each intervertebral disk space, a kidney rest, elevated to a height of 12 inches, was used to increase lordosis in the lumbar spine. The kidney rest was then lowered to observe motion. An intraoperative finding of motion exceeding 2 mm, measured by calipers, was considered to be pseudarthrosis. This amount of motion corresponds to at least 3°, of intervertebral angulatory change.

Results

The distribution of fusion levels evaluated by motion at the time of the AILF are recorded in Table 1. There were 8 patients evaluated for an L3–S1 PLF, 21 patients evaluated for an L4–S1 PLF, 6 patients evaluated for an L5–S1 PLF, 1 patient for an L2–L4 PLF, 1 patient for an L3–L5 PLF, and 2 patients for an L4–L5 PLF.

We reviewed 78 levels in 39 patients to determine if any correlation could be found between the intraoperative findings of motion at each intervertebral level and the diagnostic studies (i.e., CT scan with MPR, lateral bending films, and AP films). Referring to Table 2, 54 levels were reviewed by CT scanning. There was a 42% inaccuracy rate in determining the preoperative status of the

Table 1. Distribution of fusion levels evaluated by anterior intervertebral body motion.

PLF levels	No. of patients	No. of segments
L3–S1	8	24
L4–S1	21	42
L5–S1	6	6
L3–L5	1	2
L4–L5	2	2
L2–L4	1	2
Total	39	78

Table 2. Comparing preoperative and intraoperative motion.

	Intraoperative motion (*n*)	
	+ Motion	− Motion
CT scan		
Clinically fused	17 (31%)	11 (21%)
Clinical pseudarthrosis	20 (37%)	6 (11%)
Total (54 levels)	37 (68%)	17 (32%)
Bending films		
Clinically fused	20 (30%)	13 (19%)
Clinical pseudarthrosis	30 (45%)	4 (6%)
Total (67 levels)	50 (75%)	17 (25%)
AP films		
Clinically fused	24 (40%)	9 (15%)
Clinical pseudarthrosis	20 (33%)	7 (12%)
Total (60 levels)	44 (73%)	16 (27%)

fusion mass. We found 17 levels (31%) had false-negative pseudarthrosis, and 6 levels (11%) had false-positive pseudarthrosis. Of the 54 levels, 37 levels (68%) were determined to have intraoperative motion greater than 2 mm, and 17 levels had no intraoperative motion.

The bending films showed a 36% inaccuracy rate of diagnosing a pseudarthrosis. There were 20 (30%) false-negative pseudarthroses and 4 (6%) false-positive pseudarthroses. There were 67 levels reviewed intraoperatively showing 50 levels (75%) with motion and 17 levels without motion. We reviewed 60 levels by using AP roentgenograms. There were 44 (73%) motion segments intraoperatively and 16 segments without motion. There were 24 (40%) false-negative pseudarthroses and 7 (12%) false-positive pseudoarthroses, totalling a 52% preoperative inaccuracy rate.

The fusion rates at each intervertebral level were calculated to ascertain the frequency of pseudarthrosis (Table 3). Of the 35 levels observed at the L5–S1 motion segment in surgery, 21 patients (60%) were found to have motion greater than 2 mm, and 14 patients (40%) were determined to have no motion

Table 3. Fusion observed at each level surgically.

Level	Motion seen (*n*)	Montion not seen (*n*)	No. of levels
L5–S1	21 (60%)	14 (40%)	35
L4–L5	25 (78%)	7 (22%)	32
L3–L4	10 (100%)	0	10
L3–L4	1	0	1
Total			78

or motion less than or equal to 2 mm. Reviewing the L4–5 motion segment, 25 patients (78%) of the 32 patients were found to have pseudarthrosis, and 7 patients (22%) appeared solidly fused. Of the L3–4 and L2–3 intervertebral levels, 10 patients (100%) and 1 patient, respectively, were observed to have motion greater than 2 mm.

In patients followed up for over 1 year after AILF, it was noted that three out of three who had previous solid PLF at ALIF did not improve at all. Five of 11 (45%) who had revision by ALIF and did not solidify all their fused segments improved significantly. In those who solidified all their non-fused segments, 17 of 20 (85%) improved by one or more categories from the preoperative state using excellent, good, fair and poor clinical categories. Twelve of 20 (60%) were in the good and excellent categories.

Discussion

According to Chafetz et al. [1], 30%–40% of patients will have persistent pain or recurrent pain after fusion. The frequency of patients with pain due to pseudarthrosis has yet to be determined. Frymoyer et al. [2] found a pseudarthrosis rate of 26% in a study of 96 patients with fusions and 36 patients without fusions. No significant difference between the two groups in the postoperative examination could be appreciated.

Cleveland et al. [3] found varying pseudarthrosis rates when reviewing a patient population of 594. The pseudarthrosis rates at the L5–S1, L4–S1, L3–S1 levels were 3%, 17%, and 33%, respectively, with the average being 20%. Bending biplanar radiographs were used to define the pseudarthrosis rate. In our study without the use of biplanar X rays using only the lateral bending films, the clinical pseudarthrosis rate confirmed at surgery combining all levels in our study was 45%. The surgical pseudarthrosis rates at the L5–S1, L4–L5 and L3–L4 levels were 60%, 78%, and 100%, respectively. However, our patient population was skewed because only symptomatic patients were reviewed.

The inaccuracy of diagnosis was even higher when evaluating only the AP lumbar films. The total pseudarthrosis rate was 73%, but the inaccuracy of diagnosing the pseudarthrosis was 52%, 40% false-negative and 12% false-positive. From the study by Cleveland et al. [3], the diagnostic failures were 12% with flat radiographs and clinical judgement. From a study by Dawson et al. [4], an accuracy rate of 50% was determined with full spine (AP) radiographs and 82% accuracy rate for AP, lateral, and oblique films.

Reports have stated that CT scanning with MPR provided the greatest accuracy in diagnosing pseudarthrosis. Lang et al. [5] studied 30 patients with 3-D CT scanning and 4 patients with surgical confirmation. Three patients had a pseudarthrosis repair and the fourth patient had pseudarthrosis identified by surgical identification only. The clearest display of pseudarthrosis is by CT scans using curved coronals rather than just axial CT or 3-D CT scans [6]. Laasonen and Soini [7] reviewed 48 patients with pain after fusion by evaluating the patients' CT scan. Of the 27 main lesions detected by CT, 21 were confirmed at surgery and 6 CT scans were incorrect. There was failure of fusion in 52%, and 16 of 25 (64%) cases reviewed by plain films and bending films were false-negative. However, using anterior exploration of the interspace to assess motion, the CT scans in our study were not as specific as evidenced by a 42% inaccuracy rate with 31% false-negative and 11% false-positive rates. The total pseudarthrosis rate was 67%.

There is a need to improve the diagnostic capabilities to detect pseudarthrosis; other studies are needed to increase the specificity and sensitivity. Stokes et al. [6] and Pearcy [8] have concluded that biplanar X ray increases the accuracy of diagnosis, when enhanced to AP X rays or bending X rays. An even more promising diagnostic tool is stereophotogrammetry, which entails placing metallic beads on the posterior elements at the time of surgery [9]. Our own preliminary research indicates lateral flexion/extension biplanar tomography is an accurate test for spinal motion after the fusion procedure.

In conclusion, the accuracy of evaluating FBSS patients for pseudarthrosis was extremely low, whether using CT scanning with MPR, bending films, or plain X rays, singly or in combination. In view of this, other means to accurately determine the integrity of a fusion mass must be considered. Results after AILF showed most patients with solidification of non-solid fusions were clinically improved. Those who already had solid fusions or did not consolidate usually did not improve. This implies that small amounts of anterior element motion in abnormal segments, heretofore considered by most to be of no clinical significance, are indeed frequent pain generators in FBSS.

References

1. Chafetz N, Cann CE, Morris JM, Stenbach LS, Goldberg HI (1987) Pseudarthrosis following lumbar fusion: Detection by direct coronal CT scanning. Radiology 162: 803–805
2. Frymoyer JW, Hanley EN, Howe J, Kuhlmann D, Matteri RE (1979) A comparison of radiographic findings in fusion and non-fusion patients 10 or more years following lumbar disk surgery. Spine 4:435–440

3. Cleveland M, Bosworth DM, Thompson FR (1948) Pseudarthrosis in the lumbosacral spine. J Bone Joint Surg [Am] 30:302–1312
4. Dawson EG, Clader TJ, Bassett LW (1985) A comparison of different methods used to diagnose pseudarthrosis following posterior spinal fusion for scoliosis. J Bone Joint Surg [Am] 67:1153–1159
5. Lang P, Genant HK, Chafetz N, Steiger P, Morris JM (1988) Three-dimensional computer tomography and multiplanar reformations in the assessment of pseudarthrosis in posterior lumbar fusion patients. Spine 13:69–75
6. Stokes IAF, Wilder DG, Frymoyer JW, Pope MH (1981) Assessment of patients with low-back pain by biplanar radiographic measurement of intervertebral motion. Spine 6:233–240
7. Laasonen EM, Soini J (1989) Low-back pain after lumbar fusion: Surgical and computer tomographic analysis. Spine 14:210–213
8. Pearcy M (1982) Assessment of bony union after interbody fusion of the lumbar spine using a biplanar radiographic technique. J Bone Joint Surg [Br] 64:228–232
9. Morris J, Chafetz N, Baumrind S, Genant H, Korn EL (1985) Stereophotogrammetry of the lumbar spine: A technique for the detection of pseudarthrosis. Spine 10: 368–375

1.3 Radiological Evidence of Posterior Lumbar Interbody Fusion

Paul M. Lin[1]

Introduction

The objective of posterior lumbar interbody fusion (PLIF) is bony arthrodesis or an anatomic fusion. There has been no clear acceptance concerning what roentgenologically constitutes a fusion or arthrodesis in PLIF. Conceptually, there are two objectives in PLIF. The first as proposed by Collis [1] is lumbar disk replacement by means of biocompatible bone grafting, or osteointegration. The replaced disk can maintain the height of the disk space and achieve stabilization even though the fibro-osseous matrix introduced represents a pseudarthrodesis. The second objective of PLIF is bony arthrodesis, or an anatomic fusion.

A successful arthrodesis requires:

1. Decortication of the opposing joint surfaces for early vascularization of the graft
2. Contact of the graft and the bony structure
3. Immobilization
4. Sufficient time for fusion to occur

Materials and Methods

Roentgenographs

Roentgenographic staging of PLIF is based on these primary observations: (1) surgical excision or thinning of the subchondral end-plates, (2) the presence of autogeneic cancellous bone within the disk space, which unless densely packed, is less radiopaque than cortical bone, (3) loss of graft-host interface, which may

[1] Department of Neurosurgery, Temple University Health Sciences Center, Philadelphia, Pennsylvannia, USA

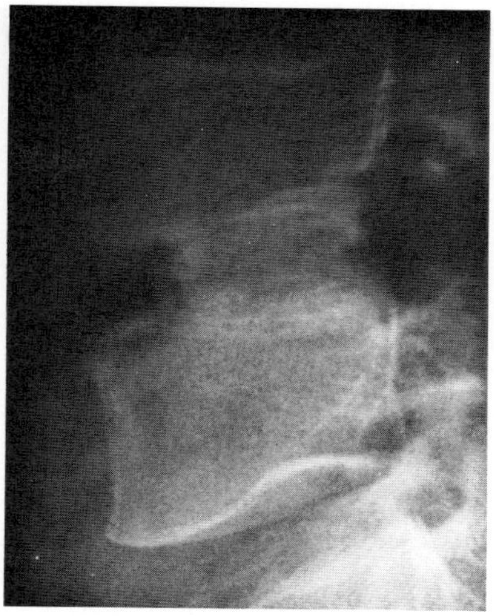

Fig. 1. Lateral radiograph of an L4–5 autograft 4 months after PLIF. Note the trabeculation pattern of the graft. This is an anatomic fusion, or an arthrodesis

be attributed to osteoblastic activity within the adjoining vertebral bodies during the stages of osteoconduction and revascularization, and (4) new bone formation with a trabecular pattern, suggesting the presence of Haversian canals. It is generally accepted that the presence of trabeculation across a graft is indicative of arthrodesis (Fig. 1).

There are six secondary roentgenographic characteristics of interbody arthrodesis. These include:

1. Absorption of the anterior intervertebral spur
2. Anterior progression of the graft within the disk space
3. Formation of a continuous posterior intervertebral cortex that includes a unified cortex of the posterior portion of the graft (Fig. 2)
4. Spontaneous facet fusion (Fig. 3)
5. Spontaneous interspinous process fusion
6. Increased bone density of the graft within the disk space at the interpedicular line, as seen on the anteroposterior (AP) view (This line represents the vertical line of stress, and the increasing bone density reflects Wolff's law that bone form follows its function)

Roentgenographically, pseudarthrodesis of PLIF appears as:

1. Progressive settlement of the disk space
2. Gradual resolution of the graft and increasing graft-host interface
3. Evidence of motion on stressed films
4. Evidence of ex vacuo phenomenon
5. Formation of anterior traction spurs
6. Evidence of progressive osteoblastic activity and sclerosis of the adjoining vertebral body beyond the expected period for arthrodesis (12 months)

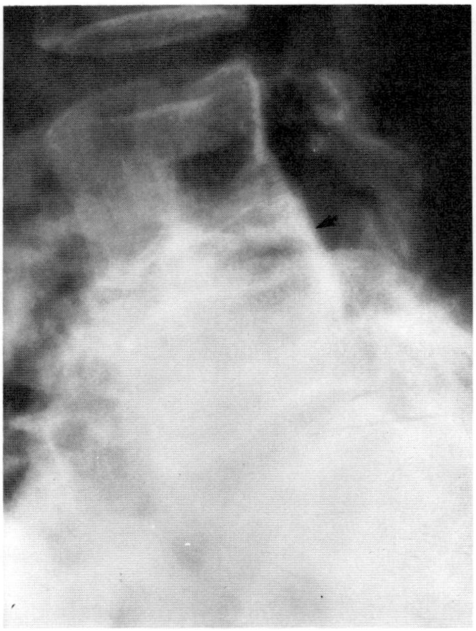
2

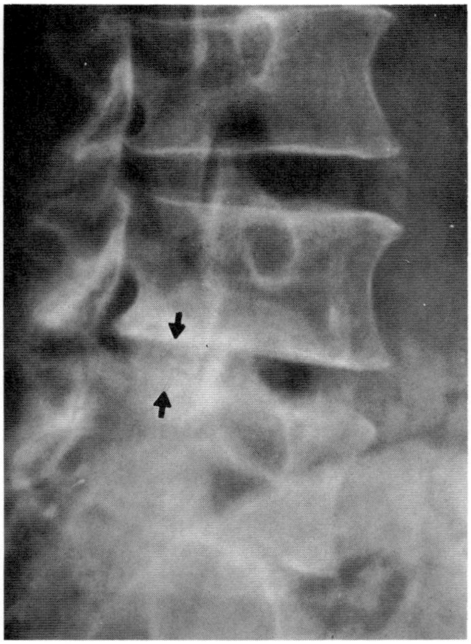
3

Fig. 2. Lateral radiograph obtained 1 year after PLIF. Note posteriorly the continuing cortical line (*arrow*) between the adjoining vertebral body and the posterior graft of the disk space

Fig. 3. Spontaneous facet fusion as seen 8 years after PLIF. *Arrows*, spontaneous facet fusion

a
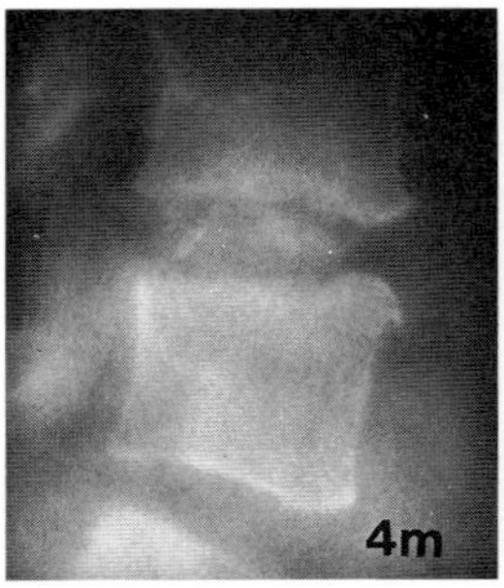

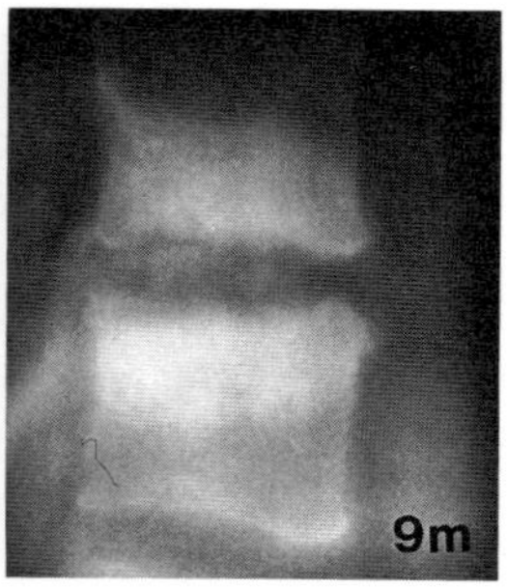

b

Fig. 4a,b. Unstable functional fibro-osseous L4–5 PLIF with autogeneic graft. Although the condition is clinically asymptomatic, it is a pseudoarthrodesis. **a** Tomogram obtained 4 months after an L4–5 PLIF showing that the disk space height has been maintained. **b** Tomogram obtained 9 months after surgery, showing that the disk space height continues to be appropriate and the anterior spur is smaller. The graft density has decreased, and the osteoblastic activity of the adjoining vertebral bodies has increased

One difference between an allograft and an autograft is that fusion takes 9–12 months with an allograft versus 3–4 months with an autograft. With an allograft the bone is dead, though it may look denser on the roentgenographic picture, and its cells are incapable of contributing to osteogenesis of the graft. The allograft serves as a lattice and is gradually replaced by creeping substitution of living bone tissue. The larger the allograft, the slower the completion of osteosynthesis by creeping substitution. With an autograft, some of the osteoprogenitor cells do remain viable and allow graft incorporation not only from the outside in but also from the inside out.

Lateral Roengenographic Tomograms

Lateral tomograms done with the polytome technique can give an excellent visualization of the fusion process of PLIF. Loss of the interface between the grafting material and the adjoining vertebral bodies is construed as evidence of early fusion. After 4 months some PLIFs (4%) may produce less evidence of fusion (Fig. 4), and some may progress to more obvious fusion [2].

Roentgenographic Stressed Films

Flexion and Extension films are frequently used to look for evidence of spinal fusion. However, this technique indicates stability only but not necessarily arthrodesis.

Radioactive Bone Scans

A positive technetium bone scan is indicative of osteoblastic activity. The absence of osteoblastic activity in the lumbar area in a bone scan done 12 months after surgery could be interpreted as a secondary sign that fusion had taken place. This is not a useful nor an accurate test for evidence of fusion in PLIF.

Magnetic Resonance Imaging

Magnetic resonance imaging (MRI) may be useful in evaluating the staging of fusion. MRI reflects more metabolic activity, especially the degree of hydration, than can be appreciated with CT or roentgenography.

Computerized Axial Tomography

Computed tomographic (CT) scanning does not show significant imaging differences during the inflammatory and osteoinductive phase of the fusion process. However, in the osteoconductive phase, new bone formation can be observed at 1–9 months. CT scans reveal that after the osteoconductive phase, the graft remodels itself and assumes the osseous bony architecture of the

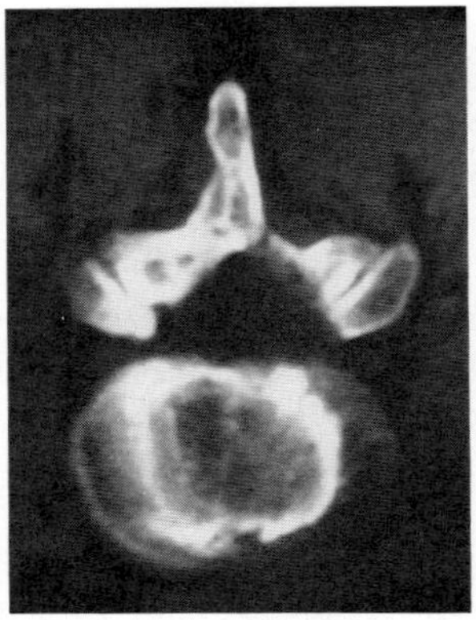

5

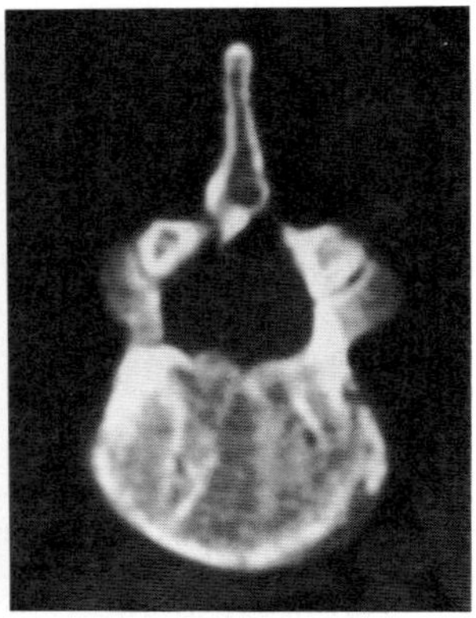

6

Fig. 5. CT scan 9 months after an L4–5 PLIF with autografts. Note the remodeling process in which the grafts assume the features of a vertebra body, a cortical ring, and a cancellous centrum

Fig. 6. Ring phenomenon 2 years after a PLIF L5–S1 using autografts. Note the advancement of the ring to the limit of the anterior limiting membrane

adjoining vertebral bodies. A cortical ring forms in the periphery of the graft and cancellous marrow forms in the center (Fig. 5). However, as time progresses, the graft may expand to the anterior limiting membrane. A double-ring phenomenon is seen when late graft progression produces a separate peripheral ring at the anterior limiting membrane (Fig. 6). The graft has not been observed to grow beyond the anatomic barrier of the anterior limiting membrane [2,3].

The presence of the ring phenomenon during the remodeling of PLIF is the most conclusive evidence of an anatomic fusion. The graft needs to occupy at least 50% of the total disk space to achieve a ring phenomenon or an arthrodesis [2].

Discussion

Experience with autogeneic grafts in PLIF suggests that optimal characteristics in bone transplantation are achieved [3–5]. Allogeneic bone grafts may be successfully used in many orthopedic applications [6,7]. Cloward reported success with allogeneic grafts in PLIF but suggested that the rate of fusion is slower than with autogeneic grafts [8].

Lateral flexion-extension films, tomography, MRI, technetium bone scans, and CT scans, including sagittal, coronal, and three-dimensional imaging, all may reflect stability of the graft in PLIF, but they do not determine the ultimate end point of an osteosynthesis, a remodeled graft that has the characteristics of a vertebral body.

References

1. Collis JS (1985) Total disk replacement: A modified PLIF. Clin Orthop 193:64
2. Lin PM, Cautilli RA, Joyce MF (1983) Posterior lumbar interbody fusion. Clin Orthop 180:154
3. Lin PM (1989) Posterior lumbar interbody fusion. In: Lin PM, Gill K (eds) Lumbar Interbody Fusion. Aspen, Rockville, Md, Chaps. 5 and 15
4. Burwell RG (1985) The function of bone marrow in the incorporation of a bone graft. Clin Orthop 200:125
5. Prolo DJ, Rodrigo JJ (1985) Contemporary bone graft physiology and surgery. Clin Orthop 200:322
6. Friedlaender GE, Mankin HL (1981) Bone banking. Current method and suggested Guidelines. In: Murray D (ed) AAOS instructional course lectures, vol 30. Mosby, St. Louis
7. Urist MR, Dawson E (1981) Intertranverse process fusion with the aid of chemosterilized autolyzed antigen-extracted allogeneic (AAA) bone. Clin Orthop 154–97
8. Cloward RB (1945) Posterior lumbar interbody fusion. Clin Orthop 193:16

PART 2

To Fuse or Not To Fuse?

SECTION I Determination of Segmental Instability

2.1 The Role of External Fixation as a Predictor of Fusion Success

David W. Lyon, David J. Hall, Robert C. Mulholland, and John K. Webb[1]

Introduction

The role of spinal fusion in the treatment of chronic low back pain is controversial [1]. There are advocates for non-operative treatment methods, while the results of surgery are often disappointing [1–9].

Spinal fusion for low back pain is based on the concept that pain arises from abnormal motion segments, and that abolition of motion should relieve the pain [10,11]. However, identification of painful motion segments remains a major problem. Plain radiographs showing degenerative changes have been shown to correlate poorly with symptoms [12,13]. The reliability of provocative diskography is disputed, and MRI, although a sensitive indicator of disk degeneration, remains non-specific [14–18]. Clearly, the outcome of surgery depends on accurate diagnosis of a surgically treatable lesion [19].

External fixation of the lumbar spine was first used to treat vertebral fractures [20]. It has been shown to be effective in relieving chronic low back pain [21], and more effective than diskography or plain radiographs as a predictor of outcome of spinal fusion [22].

The aim of this study was to identify patients who gained relief from external spinal fixation and to assess the results of subsequent fusion in this group.

Materials and Methods

Ninety-one patients with a history of chronic low back pain unresponsive to non-operative measures were assessed by external spinal fixation over a 3-year period. Most were "problem back" patients, which included those with previous failed spinal surgery, multiple-level disk disease or overt illness behaviour. All were assessed by plain radiographs, and 37 by either diskography and/or magnetic resonance imaging (MRI) (Table 1).

[1] Spinal Unit, Harlow Wood Orthopaedic Hospital, Nr. Mansfield, Nottingham, UK

Table 1. Investigations prior to fusion.

Diskography	19
MRI	12
Diskography and MRI	6

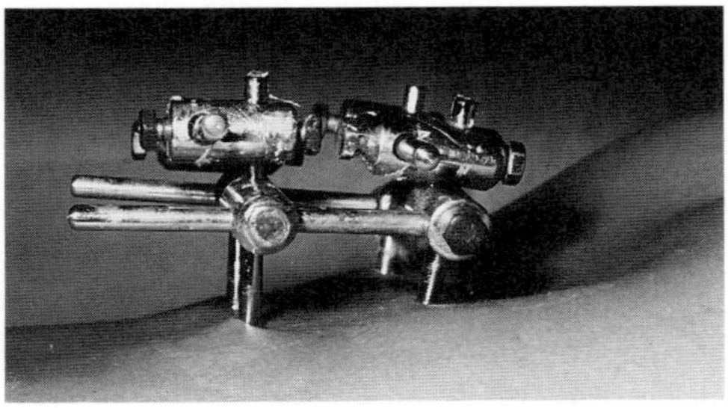

Fig. 1. The Harlow Wood external spinal fixator

The external fixator used in this study was designed and made at Harlow Wood Orthopaedic Hospital, Nottingham, UK (Fig. 1). It comprises four or more 6-mm Schanz screws attached to a purpose-built aluminium alloy frame. Longitudinal sliding rods are attached to the proximal screws by a swivel bolt which allows adjustment through 360°. The sliding rod passes through a dynamizing barrel fixed to the distal screws which allows longitudinal adjustment. Transverse stability is achieved by connecting bars between the Schanz screws held by connecting barrels with channels for the bars at 90° to each other.

The fixator is applied under fluoroscopic control with the patient under general anesthesia. After introducing the screws percutaneously to the level of the pedicle, great care is taken to make sure the screw tip does not cross the medial wall of the pedicle on the PA view until it reaches the base of the pedicle on the lateral view. This ensures the screw does not broach the pedicle during its introduction into the vertebral body. To avoid penetration of the anterior wall of the vertebral body, the screw is advanced no more than 75% of the AP diameter of the vertebra in the lateral view [23].

Patients were mobilized the day after application. Prior to discharge, adjustments were made in either compression or distraction for maximum patient comfort (Fig. 2). They were reviewed at weekly intervals for pin site care and assessment. The fixators were removed at approximately 4 weeks, although, early in the series, some were left on for up to 4 months to assist anterior interbody fusions.

The patient's response to external fixation was categorized as positive (improved) or negative (no better or worse). Patients with a positive result were offered spinal fusion. Sixty of the 91 patients underwent spinal fusion; forty of these have at least 1 year follow up, and form the basis of this review.

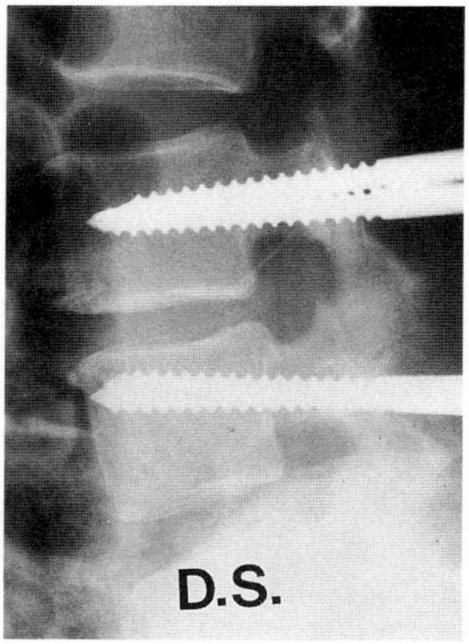

Fig. 2. A patient with the external fixator in situ

Nineteen of the forty patients had their fixator adjusted from a fixed to a dynamic configuration, in an attempt to determine any possible placebo effect of the device. They were then questioned as to their pain relief following the "adjustments."

Thirty-five patients were reviewed and examined independently; three responded to a questionnaire and two were assessed by case note review only. Each patient was asked to categorize their pain relief as follows:

1. Greater than 75% improved
2. 25%–75% improved
3. Less than 25% improved
4. Worse

Their compensation status was assessed, and they were asked if they considered the operation worthwhile and if they would undergo it again. All patients, except two, answered the Oswestry Low Back Pain Disability Questionnaire [24].

The clinical result at follow up was categorized as:

- GOOD Greater than 75% pain relief
  Operation worthwhile, would have it again Oswestry score 0%–40%
- FAIR 25%–75% pain relief
  Operation worthwhile, would have it again
  Oswestry score 40%–60%
- POOR Less than 25% pain relief or worse
  Operation not worthwhile, would not have it again
  Oswestry score 60%–100%

Plain radiographs at least 1 year after surgery were examined by two independent observers, and the fusion categorized into two groups: group a, fused; group b, probably not fused or unsure.

Results

Forty patients with a positive result from external fixation were reviewed at least 1 year following spinal fusion. There were 18 males and 22 females. Ages ranged from 21 to 62 years (mean, 40 years). Follow up ranged from 12 to 39 months (mean, 24 months).

At presentation, low back pain was the dominant symptom in all but five patients, with a duration from 2 to 40 years (mean, 11 years). Twenty-three patients had no compensation claim, 13 had a claim that was resolved, and 4 were pending. Fourteen patients had undergone no previous lumbar spine operations, while 26 had undergone between one and five procedures (mean, 1.8).

The number of levels externally fixed were: one level in 6, two levels in 24 and three levels in 10. Most patients underwent two-level posterolateral fusions with pedicle screw fixation (Table 2). Three patients had two motion segments immobilized using six screws, with alternate dynamization, to determine which was the symptomatic level.

They subsequently underwent fusion of only one motion segment, accounting for the discrepancy in levels externally fixed and subsequent levels fused.

Twenty-seven patients experienced a significant symptomatic improvement with external fixation, while 13 noticed only slight improvement. There were 25

Table 2. Type of fusion performed.

Number of levels fused	Anterior	Pedicle screw fixation	AO trans-facetal screws
One	2	5	2
Two	5	18	–
Three	4	4	–

Table 3. Complications of external fixation.

Complication	Number
Pin tract infection	9
Pin loosening	6
Radicular pain	10

Table 4. Complications of spinal fusion related to result of fusion.

Complication	Result
Hematoma (re-explored)	Good
Radicular pain (screw repositioned)	Good
Fusion re-explored	Fair
Neuroma at graft site	Poor
Radicular pain	Poor
Deep infection	Poor
Metal removal	Poor

complications of external fixation in 24 patients (Table 3). Most were relatively minor and settled soon after removal of the external fixator. Radicular pain prompted repositioning of screws or removal of the offending screw and this was accompanied by rapid pain relief in all but three cases – they had persistent radicular pain at review. There were seven significant complications of fusion excluding failure to fuse (Table 4). The infection settled following removal of the internal fixation; one patient with radicular pain found relief after re-siting the sacral screw, but another has persistent root pain despite removing the screws.

Five patients required further procedures in an attempt to secure a sound fusion. Two three-level anterior fusions were subsequently supplemented with posterolateral fusions using pedicle screw fixation, one requiring a second attempt at posterolateral fusion. One is rated a good result and one poor, despite both appearing solid fusions on the radiographs. Two patients with two-level anterior fusions had two-level posterolateral fusions with pedicle screw fixation. Both rated an overall poor result, despite satisfactory radiological fusion. One patient with lumbosacral posterolateral fusion underwent a subsequent anterior fusion, and rates poor, despite satisfactory anterior and posterior fusion radiologically.

Overall, there were ten good results following fusion, ten fair and 20 poor. The results have been analyzed in relation to a number of factors as follows.

Number of Previous Operations

Patients with a satisfactory result (good or fair) had undergone one-third the number of previous operations compared to those with an unsatisfactory (poor)

Table 5. Result of fusion related to previous surgery.

Result	Previous operations
Good (10)	6
Fair (10)	7
Poor (20)	39

Table 6. Result of fusion related to number of levels fused.

Level	Good	Fair	Poor
One	2	4	1
Two	4	6	15
Three	4	0	4

Table 7. Result of fusion related to result of external fixation.

Result of external fixation	Result of fusion	
	Satisfactory	Unsatisfactory
Significant relief (27)	13	14
Slight relief (13)	7	6

result (Table 5). This association is statistically significant using the Kruskal-Wallis test ($P = 0.007$).

Number of Levels Fused

Multiple level fusion did not produce inferior results as compared to single level fusions (Table 6).

Result of External Fixation

The patients are evenly distributed between the satisfactory and unsatisfactory categories, regardless of whether they had significant or slight symptomatic relief with external fixation (Table 7).

The result of adjusting the fixator from a fixed to a dynamic mode in 19 patients was analyzed. Six patients with increased pain, with the fixator loose, had a satisfactory result of fusion; three patients with decreased pain, with the fixator loose, had poor results of fusion. Three patients had a poor fusion result despite having increased pain when the fixator was loose. In seven patients, it was difficult to assess the results of adjusting the fixator.

Complications

There were twice the number of significant complications in the unsatisfactory group compared to the satisfactory group, but the numbers were too small to determine statistical significance (Table 8). Minor, transitory complications of external fixation were excluded.

Table 8. Result of fusion related to significant complications.

Result of fusion	Complications	
	External fixation	Fusion
Good (10)	0	2
Fair (10)	0	1
Poor (20)	3	4

Table 9. Result of fusion related to the radiological assessment of fusion.

Result	Fused	Not fused
Good (10)	10	0
Fair (10)	7	2
Poor (20)	9	9

Radiological Assessment of Fusion

Table 9 shows the relationship between clinical results of fusion and radiological appearance of fusion. There was a statistically significant association between satisfactory results and presence of a fusion (17 of 19 fused) using the Fisher Exact Test ($P = 0.02$). This is in contrast to the association between unsatisfactory results and presence of fusion: 9 of 18 fused. Three radiographs were not available for review.

Discussion

The socioeconomic effect of back pain on Western society has been shown to be enormous [25,26]. Successful treatment of chronic low back pain is difficult with wide variation in results of both conservative and operative treatments [27–31]. Fusion for back pain is based on considerable successful experience with fusion of painful joints in the peripheral skeleton, but the results are generally inferior. Techniques to identify symptomatic abnormal motion segments are unfortunately unreliable.

External fixation of the spine is designed to simulate the effect of fusion, particularly when the fusion technique includes transpedicular fixation. It is a technically demanding procedure with a definite learning curve, and there is a high incidence of minor complications such as pin tract infection (38%), and more worrying complications such as nerve root irritation (25%).

Careful selection of patients for spinal fusion, and accurate identification of painful motion segments, is crucial, since a poor result of surgery can be devastating. It is therefore justified to submit patients to an invasive selection process involving a general anesthetic and known complications if it can be shown to significantly improve the results of fusion surgery. The overall result of fusion in this biased sample of "problem back" patients was a 50% satisfactory outcome. This compares favourably with the quoted incidence of improvement following multiple spinal operations (one-third improved after a third operation [7,32]), although it is not significantly superior to the placebo response (normally about 30% or stronger after major intervention [26]).

A number of factors have been considered to be important if a good result from fusion is to be achieved, including correct patient selection, correct level, presence of a fusion and absence of complications [33]. This study shows that satisfactory results correlate significantly with the presence of a fusion, as judged by plain radiographs. Previous studies have shown an unreliable correlation between radiological fusion and outcome [3,32]. This study suggests that if a fusion is achieved over the painful levels, as determined by external fixation, then satisfactory results can be expected provided complications can be avoided.

Several fusion techniques were employed in this study, and 4 of 11 anterior fusions required further posterior procedures. Considering the association between satisfactory results and presence of a fusion, it may be that a more reliable fusion technique would produce better results.

It is probable that a painful lumbar segment is sensitive not only to movement, but to loading, and hence disk pressure changes. Pain on diskography is associated with a change in disk pressure rather than segmental movement. It is therefore likely that a fusion must not only stop movement, to relieve pain, but must also offload the disk sufficiently to stop any pressure change when the spine is loaded. If one accepts this concept, it is likely that many fusions (especially posterolateral fusions) are sufficient to stop movement, but are still flexible enough to permit continued load bearing by the painful segment.

A major problem has been assessing the patients' response to external fixation – the major criteria in assessment is relief of pain, which remains subjective. Patients in this study were in the "problem back" category and difficult to assess. Many regarded surgery as their last hope for relief of pain, and may therefore have exaggerated their response to external fixation in order to "qualify" for a spinal fusion. In order to detect this situation, 19 patients underwent "adjustment" of the fixator to a dynamic mode, but the response was difficult to interpret. Pain relief from external fixation has been shown to continue after removal of the device [21], which places further doubt on the validity of assessing the placebo effect by this technique. However, the very dramatic relief seen in some patients, associated with marked functional improvement, despite the presence of the external fixator, was so impressive that it lends strong support to the view that adequate fixation of a painful segment is pain relieving.

Ideally, to determine the usefulness of external fixation as a predictor of spinal fusion, all patients should go on to fusion surgery regardless of their response to external fixation – we are beginning a further prospective trial in which all patients assessed by external fixation will be offered spinal fusion.

Esses et al. [22] claimed a strong association between pain relief from external fixation and positive outcome of subsequent fusion, but only two patients with no pain relief from external fixation were fused. Although these two patients had a negative outcome following fusion, it remains unknown whether the other six patients in their study with a negative result of external fixation would benefit from fusion.

The role of external fixation in assessing the "problem back" case for spinal fusion remains difficult to evaluate. From this study, it would seem that if good relief of symptoms is achieved by external fixation, and subsequently a solid fusion is obtained, then a good result can be expected. However, perhaps the most important aspect of this study is the probability that the poor results of spinal fusion are due to failure to achieve a truly load sparing fusion.

References

1. Nachemson A, Bigos SJ (1984) The low back. In: Cruess RL, Rennie WRJ (eds) Orthopaedics. Livingston, New York, 877–879
2. Ehni G (1981) The role of spine fusion: Question 9. Spine 6:308–310
3. Flynn JC, Hoque MD (1979) Anterior fusion of the lumbar spine. J Bone Joint Surg [Am] 61:1143–1150
4. Frymoyer JW (1981) The role of spine fusion: Question 1. Spine 6:284–290
5. Lehmann TR, Spratt KF, Tozzi JE, Weinstein JN, Reinarz SJ, El-Khourg GY, Colby H (1987) Long-term follow up of lower lumbar fusion patients. Spine 12: 97–104
6. Nachemson A (1976) A critical look at conservative treatment for low back pain. In: Jayson M (ed) The lumbar spine and low back pain. Pitmann, London
7. Stauffer RN, Coventry MB (1972) Anterior interbody spine fusion. J Bone Joint Surg [Am] 54:756–768
8. Tunturi T, Kataja M, Keski-Misula L, Lapinsuo M, Lepisto P, Paakkala T, Patiala H, Rokkanen P (1979) Posterior fusion of the lumbosacral spine. Acta Orthop Scand 50:415–425
9. Zucherman JJ, Hsu K, White A, Wynne G (1988) Early results of spinal fusion using a variable spine plating system. Spine 13:570–579
10. Dupuis PR, Yong-Hing K, Cassidy D, Kirkaldy-Willis WH (1985) Radiologic diagnosis of degenerative lumbar spinal instability. Spine 10:262–276
11. Morgan FP, King T (1957) Primary instability of lumbar vertebrae as a common cause of low back pain. J Bone Joint Surg [Br] 39:6–22
12. Frymoyer JW, Newberg A, Pope MH, Wilder DG, Clements J, MacPherson B (1984) Spine radiographs in patients with low-back pain: An epidemiological study in men. J Bone Joint Surg [Am] 66:1048–1055
13. Torgeson WR, Dotler WE (1976) Comparative roentgenographic study of the asymptomatic and symptomatic lumbar spine. J Bone Joint Surg [Am] 58:850–853
14. Gibson MJ, Buckley J, Mawhinney R et al. (1986) Magnetic resonance imaging and diskography in the diagnosis of disk degeneration. A comparative study of 50 disks. J Bone Joint Surg [Br] 68:369–373
15. Holt Jr EP (1968) The question of lumbar diskography. J Bone Joint Surg [Am] 50:720–726

16. Linson MA, Crowe CH (1990) Comparison of magnetic resonance imaging and lumbar diskography in the diagnosis of disk degeneration. Clin Orthop 250:160–163
17. Nachemson A (1989) Editorial comment. Lumbar Diskography – Where are we today? Spine 14:555–557
18. Weinstein J, Claverie W, Gibson S (1988) The pain of diskography. Spine 13: 1343–1348
19. Waddell G, Morris EW, Di Paola MP, Bircher M, Finlayson D (1986) A concept of illness tested as an improved basis for surgical decisions in low-back disorders. Spine 11:712–719
20. Magerl FP (1984) Stabilization of the lower thoracic and lumbar spine with external skeletal fixation. Clin Orthop 189:125–141
21. Olerud S, Sjostrom L, Karlstrom G, Hamberg M (1986) Spontaneous effect of increased stability of the lower lumbar spine in cases of severe chronic back pain. Clin Orthop 203:67–74
22. Esses SI, Botsford DJ, Kostuik JP (1989) The role of external spinal skeletal fixation in the assessment of low-back disorders. Spine 14:594–600
23. Whitecloud TS, Skalley TC, Cook SD, Morgan EL (1989) Roentgenographic measurement of pedicle screw penetration. Clin Orthop 245:57–68
24. Fairbank JCT, Couper J, Davies JB, O'Brien JP (1980) The Oswestry low back pain disability questionnaire. Physiotherapy 66:271–273
25. Kelsey JL (1980) Epidemiology and impact of low back pain. Spine 5:133–142
26. Waddell G (1982) An approach to backache. Brit J Hosp Med September:187–219
27. Freebody D, Bendall R, Taylor RD (1971) Anterior transperitoneal lumbar fusion. J Bone Joint Surg [Br] 53:617–627
28. Lehmann TR, La Rocca HJ (1981) Repeat lumbar surgery: A review of patients with failure from previous lumbar surgery treated by spinal canal exploration and lumbar spinal fusion. Spine 6:615–619
29. Taylor TKF (1970) Anterior interbody fusion in the management of disorders of the lumbar spine. Proceedings of the Combined Meeting of Orthopaedic Associations. J Bone Joint Surg [Br] 52:784
30. Waddell G (1987) Failures of disk surgery and repeat surgery. Acta Orthop Belg 53:300–302
31. Waddell G, Kummel EG, Lotto WN, Graham JD, Hall H, McCulloch JA (1979) Failed lumbar disk surgery and repeat surgery following industrial injuries. J Bone Joint Surg [Am] 61:201–207
32. Stauffer RN, Coventry MB (1972) Posterolateral lumbar spine fusion. J Bone Joint Surg [Am] 54:1195–1204
33. Crock HV (1976) Observations on the management of failed spinal operations. J Bone Joint Surg [Br] 58:193–199

2.2 Assessment of Segmental Spinal Instability Using Magnetic Resonance Imaging

Tomoaki Toyone, Hideshige Moriya, Hiroshi Kitahara, Kazuhisa Takahashi, Masatsune Yamagata, Masazumi Murakami, and Yuzuru Takahashi[1]

Introduction

Defining motion segment instability has not always been possible with conventional dynamic radiographs and measuring techniques. It is known that the biomechanical stress on the vertebral bodies which is associated with degenerative disk disease can cause a variety of pathological changes in the marrow. Therefore, we used magnetic resonance (MR) to detect focal alterations in bone marrow signal intensity adjacent to the end-plates in patients with degenerative disks to assess segmental spinal instability.

Materials and Methods

MR studies of the lumbar spine were retrospectively evaluated in 308 sequential patients with degenerative disk disease who presented to the Department of Orthopaedic Surgery at Chiba University from April 1990 to September 1991. The presence of disk degeneration was identified when there was decreased signal intensity of the nucleus/inner annulus complex on T2-weighted images [1]. A total of 924 disk levels (L3/4–L5/S1) were analyzed and disk degeneration was noted in 502 of 924 disk interspaces (Table 1). The study included 60 patients (19%) with end-plate and associated marrow changes; 28 male and 32 female patients who ranged in age from 13 to 70 years (mean age: 52 years). Clinical evaluation was done according to the score rating system of the Japanese Orthopaedic Association [2] (JOA score: Table 2). Low back pain and lower extremity pain were defined to be present in patients with a score of 1 point or less. Lateral flexion-extension roentgenograms were obtained from patients in the lateral decubitus position. Radiographic lumbar spinal instability was judged to be positive when either the back of the disk opened up in flexion

[1] Department of Orthopaedic Surgery, School of Medicine, Chiba University, 1-8-1 Inohana, Chuo-ku, Chiba, 260 Japan

Table 1. Details of patients with degenerative disks and vertebral body marrow changes noted on MR imaging.

	Age (years)						
	0–19	20–29	30–39	40–49	50–59	60–69	70–
Number of patients	36	54	50	90	46	24	10
Number of degenerative disks (L3/4–L5/S1)	46	73	72	146	91	50	30
End-plate and associated marrow changes	4	1	7	20	12	13	3

Table 2. Score rating system of the Japanese Orthopaedic Association.

	Points
A. Low back pain	
a. None	3
b. Occasional mild pain	2
c. Frequent mild or occasional severe pain	1
d. Frequent or continuous severe pain	0
B. Lower extremity pain and/or tingling	
a. None	3
b. Occasional slight symptoms	2
c. Frequent slight or occasional severe symptoms	1
d. Frequent or continuous severe symptoms	0

(kyphotic angle at one segment of more than 5°) or dynamic anteroposterior translational sliding was greater than 3.0 mm from flexion to extension [3]. Finally, the histology of seven specimens obtained during surgery was investigated.

The MR studies were performed using a 0.5-T superconductive system (MRT50; Toshiba, Tokyo). Spin-echo pulse sequences were obtained in the sagittal plane with either a 400/30 (T1-weighted) sequence and a 2000/80 (T2-weighted) sequence. Five- to ten-millimeter-thick multiple images were obtained using two or four excitations and a 256 × 256 matrix.

Results

Magnetic resonance imaging with short TR/TE pulse sequences (T1-weighted images) gave the best results. The two basic patterns of marrow changes on the T1-weighted images were investigated in this study (Fig. 1a,b). These changes were seen at 67 of 502 levels in patients with evidence of degenerative disks. The incidence was especially high in patients with spondylolisthesis: 26 of 41 patients who had spondylolisthesis showed the lesion. The patients were divided into two groups: the high signal group who showed increased signal a 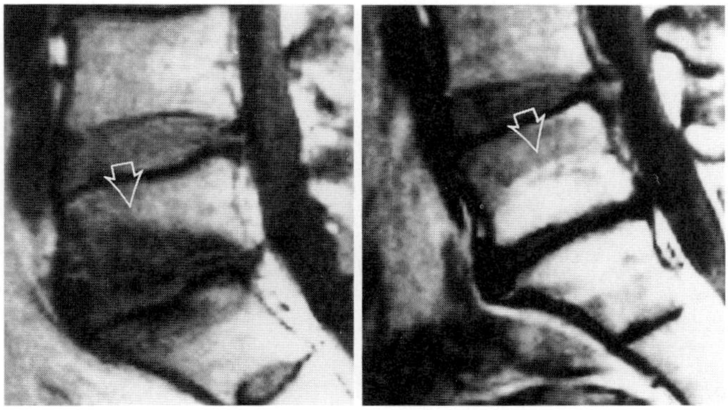 b

Fig. 1a,b. Two basic patterns of end-plate and associated marrow changes on T1-weighted images. **a** Low signal intensity. **b** High signal intensity. The *arrows* indicate the margin of the marrow changes

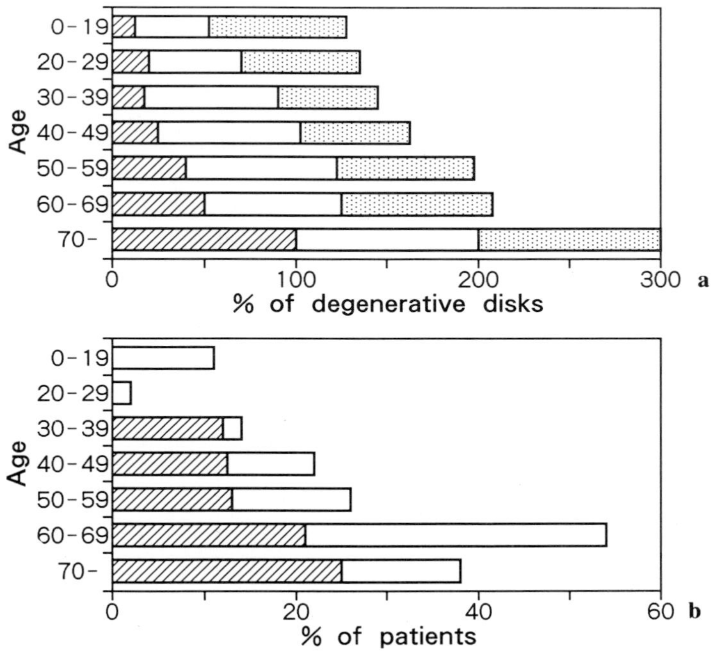

Fig. 2. a The incidence and distribution of disk degeneration in individual patient by level and age. *Hatched area*, L3–L4; *white area*, L4–L5; *dotted area*, L5–S1. **b** The incidence and distribution of end-plate and associated vertebral body marrow changes by age. *Hatched area*, high signal intensity on T1-weighted image; *white area*, low signal intensity on T1-weighted image

intensity on the T1-weighted spin-echo images, and the low signal group who showed decreased signal intensity. Both groups contained 30 patients. All 5 patients under 30 years old who had spondylolisthesis were in the low signal group (Fig. 2a,b).

The incidence of low back pain was 17% (5 patients) in the high signal group (Fig. 3a). On the other hand, of the 30 patients with a decreased signal intensity (low signal group), 26 (87%) complained of low back pain. Regarding complaints of lower extremity pain, there was no difference between the high signal group (25 patients, 83%) and the low signal group (26 patients, 87%). The incidence of objective findings was not significantly different in the two groups.

Conventional radiographs (lateral flexion-extension roentgenograms) demonstrated instability in 21 (70%) of the patients in the low signal group (Fig. 3b). The dynamic anteroposterior translational sliding was positive in 7

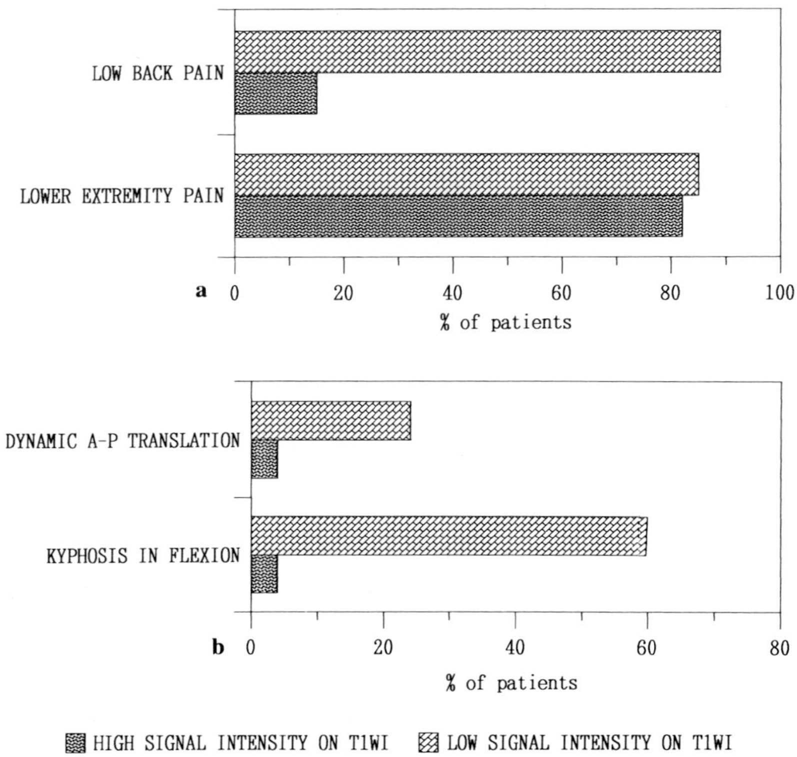

Fig. 3. **a** Comparison of clinical findings in the two groups. **b** Comparison of segmental instability demonstrated on conventional lateral flexion-extension roentgenograms in the two groups. *Hatched area*, high signal intensity; *dotted area*, low signal intensity

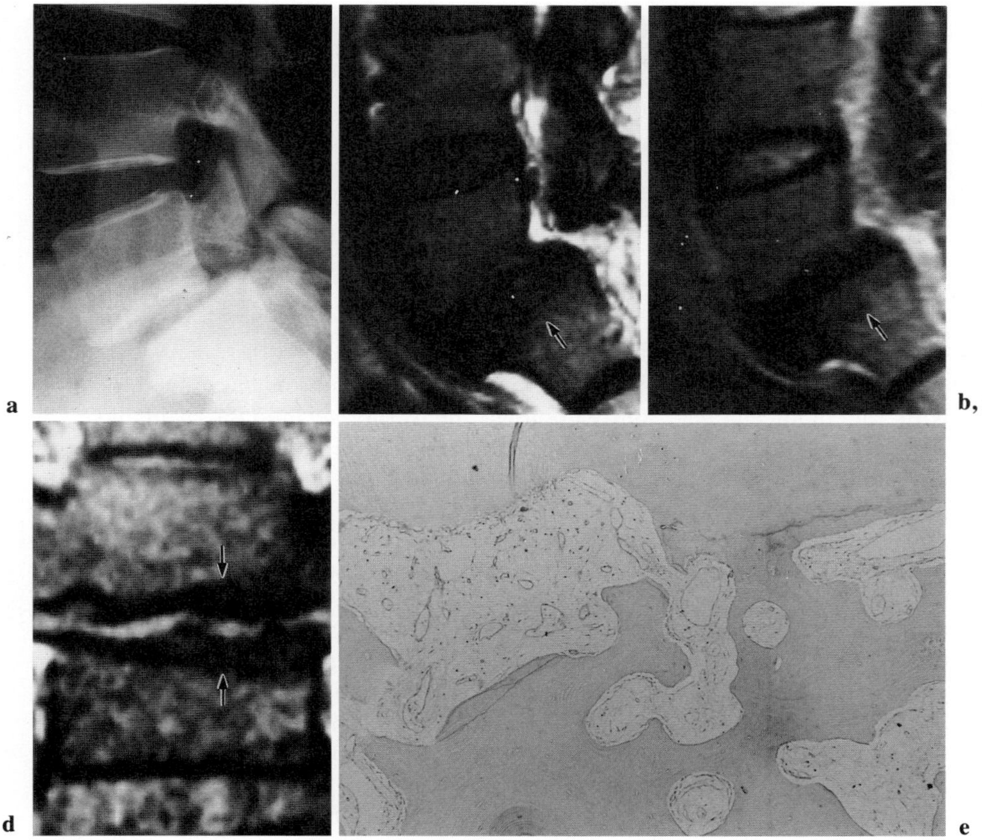

Fig. 4a–e. A 26-year-old female with spondylolisthesis. **a** Plain lateral roentgenogram. **b** T1-weighted sagittal section. The signal intensity at the adjacent portion of the S-1 vertebral body at L5–S1 has decreased. **c** T2-weighted sagittal section. There is a slightly decreased signal intensity of the adjacent portion of the S-1 vertebral body at L5–S1. **d** T1-weighted coronal section. The low signal intensity of the marrow within the disk space at the L5–S1 level is demonstrated. **e** Histologic specimen. Disruption of the end-plate and vascularized fibrous tissues within the adjacent marrow were demonstrated (H&E ×100)

(23%) of the patients in the low signal group. Eighteen of these patients (60%) had a positive segmental kyphosis in flexion. Only two patients (6%) in the high signal group had any demonstrable evidence of instability.

The high signal group demonstrated a high signal intensity on the T1-weighted images and an isointense or moderately increased intensity on the T2-weighted images. Histological sections through the lesions at the high signal intensity areas revealed disrupted vertebral end-plates and marrow elements replaced by fat. The low signal group had a low signal intensity on the T1-weighted images and either an increased or decreased intensity on the T2-weighted images. Histological sections through the lesion at low signal intensity areas revealed injured end-plates and vascularized fibrous tissue surrounding markedly thickened bony trabeculae (Fig. 4a–e). These changes did not correlate well with vertebral sclerosis seen using plain radiographs and computed tomography.

Discussion

A definition of motion segmental instability has not always been possible with the biomechanical and radiologic measuring techniques available. The American Academy of Orthopaedic Surgeons has defined segmental instability as "an abnormal response to applied loads characterized by motion in the motor segment beyond normal constraints."

In 1944, Knuttson first used lateral flexion-extension radiographic examination to detect lumbar vertebral instability [4]. He stated that anteroposterior translational sliding could be observed before any radiographic findings of disk narrowing, sclerosis, or marginal osteophytes. Since then, the amount of data from clinical and cadaveric studies has been generated on normal and abnormal motion. However, the normal motion of the lumbar spine has not yet been defined precisely. In 1989, Hayes et al. questioned the reliability of flexion-extension bending films as a primary determinant of lumbar segmental instability. They reported a wide range of motion and there was often significant overlap between asymptomatic and symptomatic patients [5]. In 1990, Boden and Wiesel proposed that the assessment of flexion-extension radiography be done by calculating dynamic motion rather than static vertebral positions [3]. We used this method in our study. Despite the use of such improved dynamic radiographs and measuring techniques, it was difficult to define criteria for segmental spinal instability. Because of this problem, we considered alternative approaches. Biomechanical stress on the vertebral bodies which is associated with degenerative disk disease causes a variety of pathological changes in the marrow. Since magnetic resonance imaging is an excellent method for detecting bone marrow abnormalities, we hypothesized that MR might be useful in detecting biomechanical stress.

In 1987, Roos et al. described three basic patterns of marrow changes adjacent to the intervertebral disks in 29 patients with degenerative disk disease [6]. Modic et al. identified three types of signal intensity changes and he stated some patients with type 1 changes (decreased signal intensity on the T1-weighted spin-echo images and increased signal intensity on the T2-weighted images) subsequently developed type 2 changes (increased signal intensity on the T1-weighted images and isointense or slightly increased signal intensity on the T2-weighted images) [7]. In 1990, Lang et al. studied 33 postfusion patients, and demonstrated a high signal intensity on the T1-weighted images of the patients with a solid fusion [8].

In the present study, we have attempted to correlate any changes in the marrow in the presence of degenerative disk disease with clinical symptoms and segmental instability. Magnetic resonance imaging with short TR/TE pulse sequences (T1-weighted images) gave the best results. Therefore the two basic patterns of the end-plate and associated marrow changes on the T1-weighted

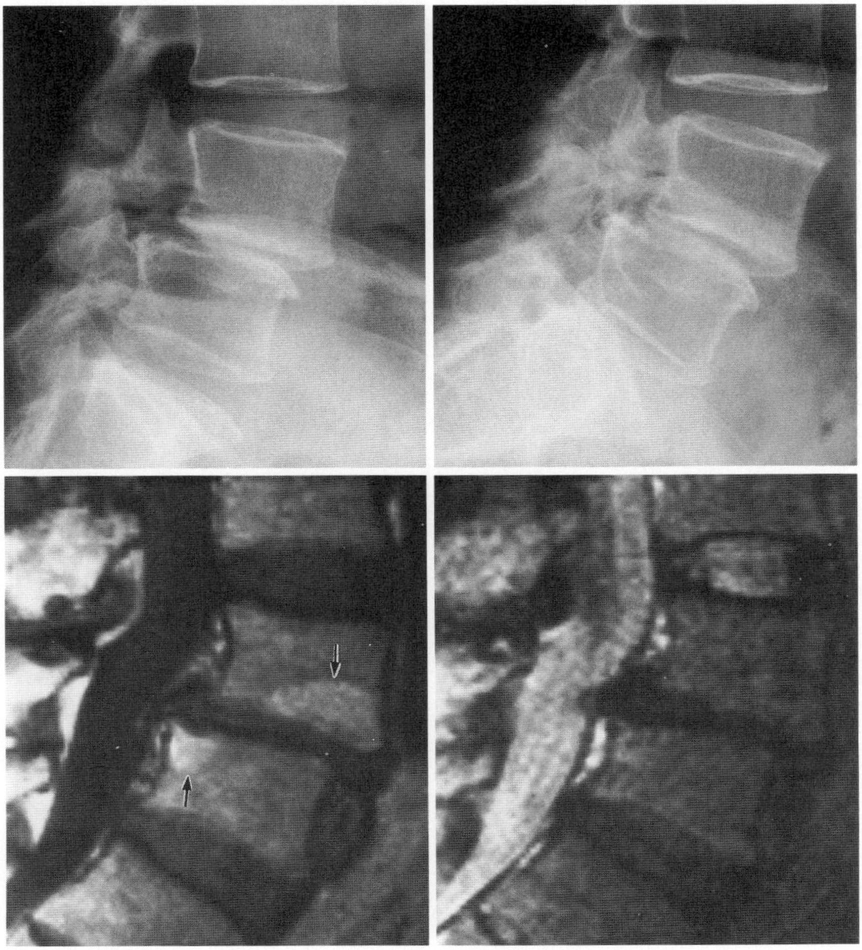

a

b

Fig. 5a,b. A 46-year-old woman with spondylolisthesis whose complaints of low back pain spontaneously resolved after a long history of such pain. **a** Plain lateral flexion-extension roentgenogram which does not demonstrate any evidence of instability. **b** T1-weighted sagittal image showing a high signal intensity of the adjacent anterior portion of L4 and posterior portion of L5 vertebral body at L4–L5 (*arrows*)

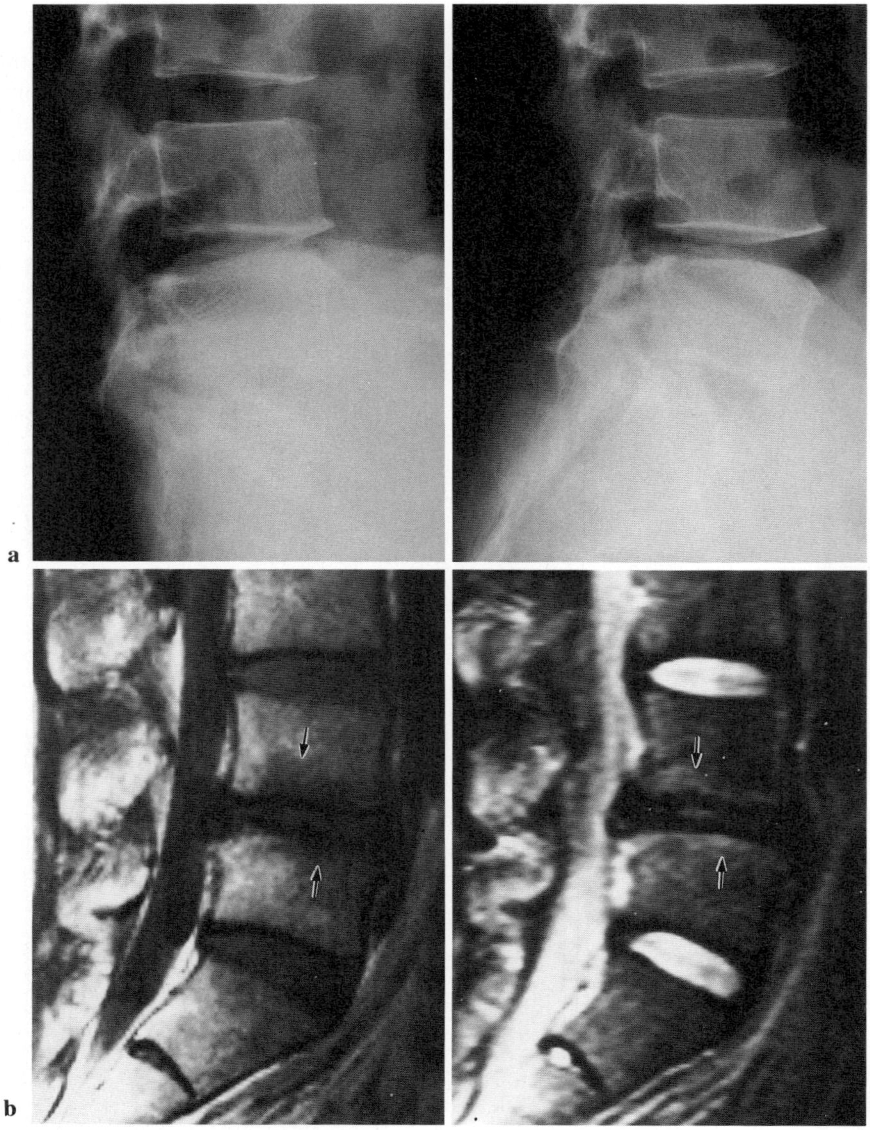

Fig. 6a,b. A 32-year-old man presented with a complaint of severe low back pain. **a** Lateral flexion-extension roentgenogram. The back of the disk opens up in flexion at L4–L5. Segmental instability is judged to be positive. **b** T1-weighted sagittal image reveals low signal intensity within the vertebral body marrow at the adjacent portions of the L4–L5 disk space (*arrows*). On the T2-weighted sagittal image, the linear lesion of increased signal intensity of the adjacent portion of end-plate and associated marrow is noted (*arrows*)

images were investigated in this study. These changes correlated with the presence of low back pain and segmental instability. White et al. studied sclerosis of the lumbar spine and its association with low back pain [9]. To our knowledge, no previous study investigating the vertebral body marrow changes noted on MR imaging and its association with low back pain has been published.

Some limitations were present in this investigation. Although it was designed to define lumbar instability by using a new approach, the results correlated with segmental instability determined by conventional radiographic measurements. Some patients were examined when they had severe low back pain which may restrict flexion and extension.

The increased signal intensity on the T1-weighted spin-echo images reflected a significantly more stable stage of degenerative disk disease than a decreased signal intensity on the T1-weighted images. This change is commonly observed in patients with late stage degenerative disk disease whose complaints of low back pain spontaneously resolve after a long history of such pain (Fig. 5a,b). This stage is a "restabilization phase," according to the concept introduced by Kirkaldy-Willis and Farfan [10]. It is also seen that successful solid fusions are associated with a high incidence of this change in the marrow adjacent to the fused degenerative disks.

Low signal intensity on the T1-weighted images are commonly seen in the marrow adjacent to disk spaces affected with active degeneration and segmental instability (Fig. 6a,b). These marrow changes are significant in some cases, and physical signs are suggestive of instability, though these changes have not been correlated with any type of dynamic radiographic measurement.

We hypothesized on the pathogenesis of these marrow changes. Intervertebral disks are well known avascular body structures, so their nutrition is derived mainly from the diffusion of nutrients across the end-plates [11]. Injury to the vertebral end-plate will lead to inflammation in conjunction with the reparative process. Vascularization may promote an autoimmune mechanism to disk material which is recognized as foreign [12]. This autoimmune response leads to chronic inflammation of the marrow and sclerosis of the end-plate. Following this response, there is marrow degeneration with fatty replacement.

In this study, the vertebral body marrow changes noted on MR imaging correlated with low back pain and instability. Increased signal intensity on the T1-weighted spin-echo images reflected a relatively stable stage of degenerative disk disease. MR imaging is useful for assessing segmental spinal instability and may be helpful in deciding whether fusion surgery is indicated.

References

1. Gibson MJ, Buckley J, Mawhinney R, Mulholland RC, Worthington BS (1986) Magnetic resonance imaging and discography in the diagnosis of disc degeneration: A comparative study of 50 disks. J Bone Joint Surg [Br] 68:369–373

2. Izumida S, Inoue S (1986) Assessment of treatment for low back pain (in Japanese). J Jpn Orthop Assoc 60:391–394
3. Boden SD, Wiesel SW (1990) Lumbosacral segmental motion in normal individuals. Have we been measuring instability properly? Spine 15:571–575
4. Knutsson F (1944) The instability associated with disk degeneration in the lumbar spine. Acta Radiol 25:593–609
5. Hayes MA, Howard TC, Gruel CR, Kopta JA (1989) Roentgenographic evaluation of lumbar spine flexion-extension in asymptomatic individuals. Spine 14: 327–331
6. Roos A, Kressel H, Spritzer C, Dalinka M (1987) MR imaging of marrow changes adjacent to end-plates in degenerative lumbar disk disease. AJR 149:531–534
7. Modic MT, Steinberg PM, Ross JS, Masaryk TJ, Carter JR (1988) Degenerative disk disease: Assessment of changes in vertebral body marrow with MR imaging. Radiology 166:193–199
8. Lang P, Chafetz N, Genant HK, Morris JM (1990) Lumbar spinal fusion. Assessment of functional stability with magnetic resonance imaging. Spine 15:581–588
9. White AA, McBride ME, Wiltse LL, Jupiter JB (1986) The management of patients with back pain and idiopathic vertebral sclerosis. Spine 11:607–616
10. Kirkaldy-Willis WH, Farfan HF (1982) Instability of the lumbar spine. Clin Orthop 165:110–123
11. Kraemer J, Kolditz D, Gowin R (1985) Water and electrolyte content of human intervertebral disks under variable load. Spine 10:69–72
12. Gertzbein SD (1977) Degenerative disk disease of the lumbar spine: Immunological implications. Clin Orthop 129:68–71

2.3 Intraoperative Measurement of Lumbar Spinal Stiffness

Sohei Ebara[1], Masao Tanaka[2], Yoshiharu Morimoto[2], Takeo Harada[1], Noboru Hosono[1], Kazuo Yonenobu[1], and Keiro Ono[1]

Introduction

Spinal instability has been assessed according to certain physiological or radiographic abnormalities of the spine [1–5]. A quantitative assessment of spinal instability is, however, essential for justification of lumbar fusion or stabilization and this has actually been conducted by few researchers [6] (D.C. Holmes, M.D. Brown, E.C. Eckstein, et al. 1989, In Vitro and In Vivo Measurement of Lumbar Spine Motion Segment Unit Stiffness; unpublished work, University of Miami School of Medicine). We attempted to develop a method of measuring spinal instability that could be carried out during lumbar spine surgery [7–10]. This method enabled us to measure the alterations of lumbar spinal instability in each step of surgical decompression, stabilization, or bone grafting. The final aim of this research was to establish an objective criterion for fusion and stabilization [6,11–14].

Methods

We measured the tensile stiffness of a motion segment (vertebra-disk-vertebra) with a spinal distractor during spinal decompression surgery in order to quantify spinal instability. Stiffness [15] was calculated from the relation of load and displacement between two adjacent spinous processes where a vertebral spreader was suspended. This study defined the stiffness as the curve produced during a cyclic loading from 0 to 100 N, and as the tangent stiffness at the middle range of loading (Fig. 1). We subjected a spinal motion segment to five cyclic sessions of loading to 100 N at a speed of 20 mm/s as constant as possible, and recorded a hysteresis loop of the last cycle.

---

[1] Department of Orthopaedic Surgery, Osaka University Medical School, Fukushima, Fukushima-ku, Osaka, 553 Japan
[2] Department of Engineering Science, Osaka University Engineering Science School, Machikaneyama, Toyonaka, Osaka, Japan

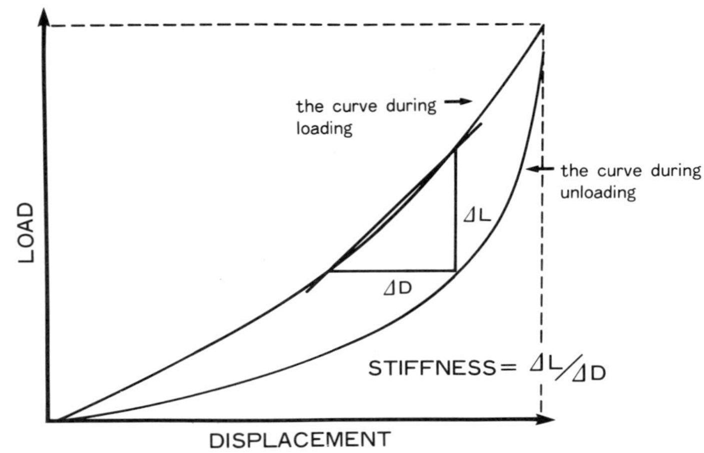

Fig. 1. Stiffness was calculated from the relation of load (*L*) and displacement (*D*) between two adjacent spinous processes where a vertebral spreader was suspended. This study defined the stiffness as the curve produced during a cyclic loading from 0 to 100 N. The stiffness was defined as the tangent stiffness at the middle range of loading

The lumbar spinal spreader (lamina spreader, 02-161-00, Mizuho Co., Tokyo, Japan) is a device for measurement of stiffness of a spinal motion segment. It is equipped with two pieces of measurement apparatus, one of which is a load strain gauge (KFC-5-Cl-1, Kyowa Co., Tokyo, Japan) attached to the distal legs of the spreader in order to measure the load during distraction of two spinous processes (Fig. 2). The other is a displacement transducer (Type DT-F, Kyowa Co., Tokyo, Japan) attached between the two proximal legs of the spreader in order to measure the displacement between the two adjacent spinous processes (Fig. 2). Electrical changes are amplified (DPM-600, Kyowa Co., Tokyo, Japan) and then plotted on an X-Y recorder as a true load and displacement by calibration (Fig. 2). The patients remained in a prone position on a Hall frame during the measurement, as in the usual position for lumbar spine surgery.

Materials

We performed the measurement on 28 motion segments in a total of 14 patients, consisting of 11 males and 3 females. There were 17 segments with lumbar spondylotic changes, 5 with lumbar disk herniation, 3 with degenerative spondylolisthesis, and 3 with normal disks. The age range was 22–65 years, the average being 61.2 years. Surgery involved either partial laminectomy and facetectomy with or without Luque fixation, or partial laminectomy and

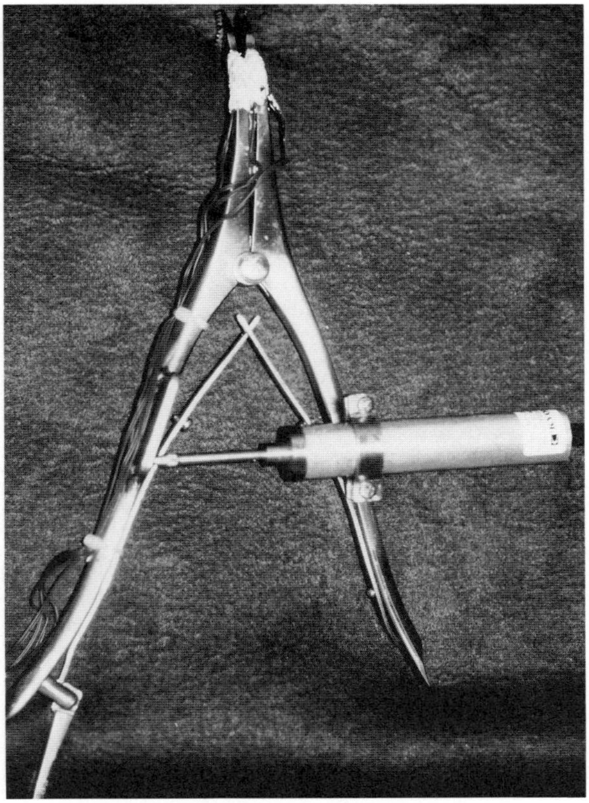

a

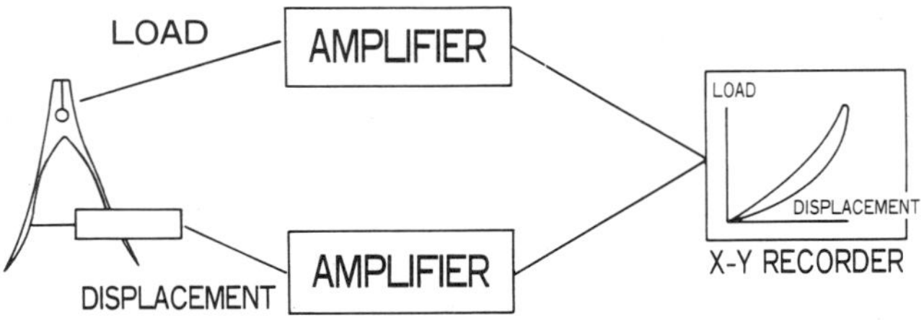

b

Fig. 2a,b. The lumbar spinal spreader. **a** (Lamina spreader, 02-161-00, Mizuho Co., Tokyo) is a device for measurement of stiffness of a spinal motion segment. It is equipped with two pieces of measurement apparatus. **b** One of which is a load strain gauge (KFC-5-Cl-1, Kyowa Co., Tokyo) attached to the distal legs of the spreader in order to measure the load during distraction of two spinous processes. The other is a displacement transducer (Type DT-F, Kyowa Co., Tokyo) attached between the two legs of the spreader in order to measure the displacement between two adjacent spinous processes. Electrical changes are amplified and then plotted on an X-Y recorder as a true load and displacement by calibration

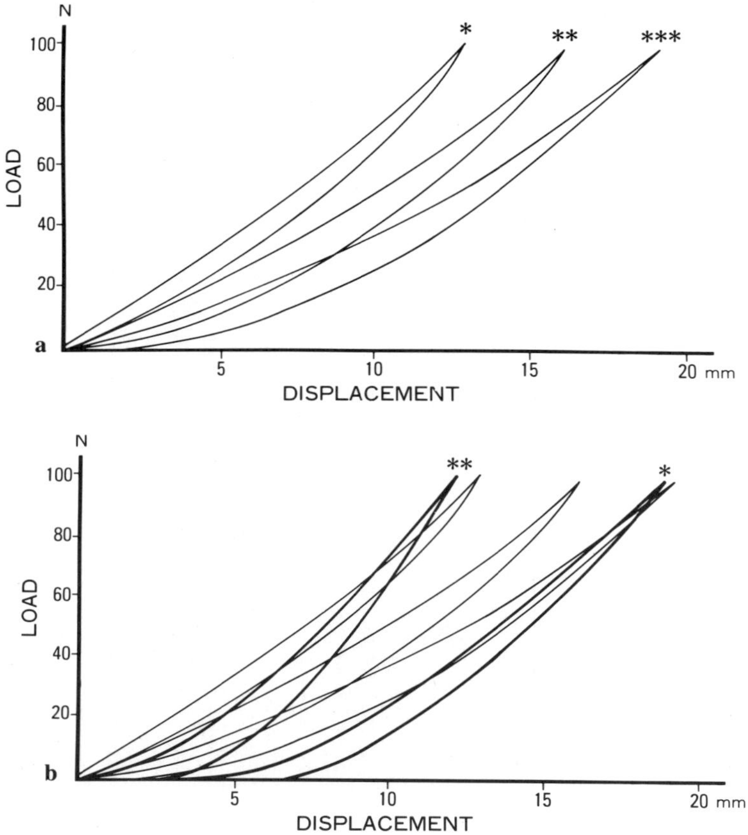

Fig. 3a,b. The case of a 45-year-old male patient who had been suffering from L3/4, L4/5 and L5/S spondylosis. MRI showed a severe degree of degeneration of the L3/4 disk. **a** When the supra- and interspinous ligaments were resected, stiffness of the motion segment (L3/4) calculated from the hysteresis loop was 6.9 N/mm (*). The stiffness reduced to 5.9 N/mm (86% of the initial stiffness) when partial laminectomy and facetectomy were completed (**). After diskectomy, the stiffness decreased further to 4.4 N/mm (64% of the initial stiffness) (***). **b** After iliac bone graft was inserted to the intervertebral space, the stiffness increased to 7.4 N/mm (107% of the initial stiffness) (*). After Luque fixation stiffness further increased to 9.3 N/mm (135% compared with the initial stiffness) (**)

diskectomy with posterior interbody fusion by iliac bone graft [16] accompanied with or without Luque fixation.

Magnetic resonance imaging (MRI) was employed for 24 motion segments in 12 patients to estimate the disk degeneration. The disk levels were considered as normal where the supra- and interspinous ligaments were resected in order to pass Luque wires above and below the operated disk levels. When a patient's MRI signals were within normal range, the patient was used as a normal control.

Results

The measurement produced load-displacement curves of a high reproducibility showing hysteresis loops in every case.

Figure 3 shows the case of a 45-year-old male patient who had been suffering from L3/4, L4/5, and L5/S spondylosis. MRI shows a severe degree of degeneration of the L3/4 disk. In this case, when the supra- and interspinous ligaments were resected, stiffness of the motion segment (L3/4) calculated from the hysteresis loop was 6.9 N/mm. The stiffness reduced to 5.9 N/mm (86% of the initial stiffness) when partial laminectomy and facetectomy were completed. After diskectomy, the stiffness decreased further to 4.4 N/mm (64% of the initial stiffness). After iliac bone graft was inserted to the intervertebral space, the stiffness increased to 7.4 N/mm (107% of the initial stiffness). Stiff-

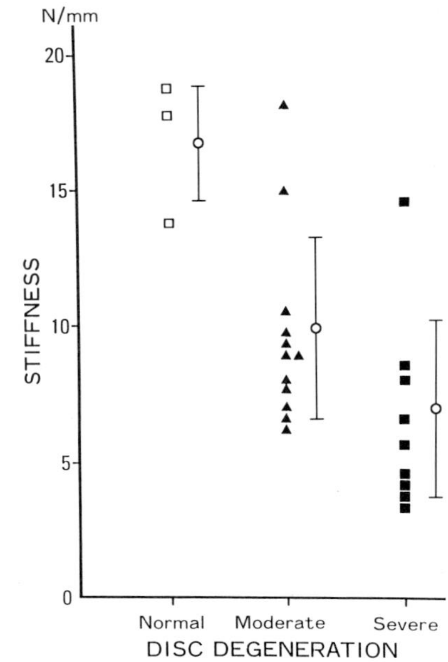

Fig. 4. Stiffness of the spinal motion segments decreased as disk degeneration developed. The average stiffness of the spinal motion segments were 16.6 N/mm, 10.0 N/mm, and 6.8 N/mm in the normal, moderate, and severe forms, respectively. The *open squares*, *solid triangles*, and *solid squares* stand for the MRI findings of normal, moderate, and severe degeneration of the disk, respectively

ness further increased to 9.3 N/mm after Luque fixation (135% compared with the initial stiffness).

The spinal motion segments were separated into three grades based on the disk degeneration defined by MRI according to Thompson et al. [17]. Normal denotes grade I of Thompson's grading; moderate, grade II and III; and severe, grade IV and V, respectively.

Stiffness of the spinal motion segments decreased as disk degeneration developed. The average stiffness of the spinal motion segments were 16.6 N/mm, 10.0 N/mm, and 6.8 N/mm in the normal, moderate, and severe forms respectively (Fig. 4).

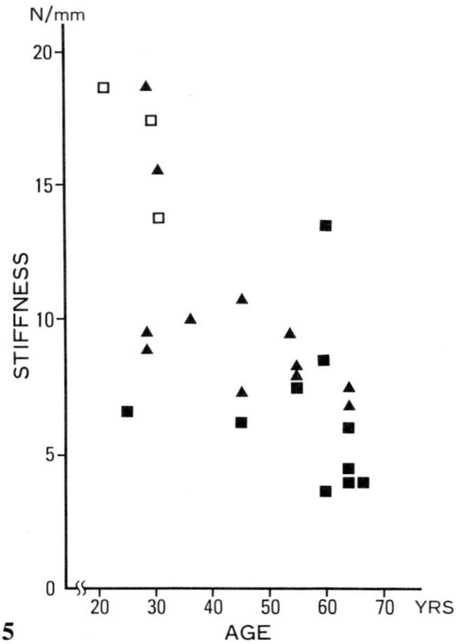

5

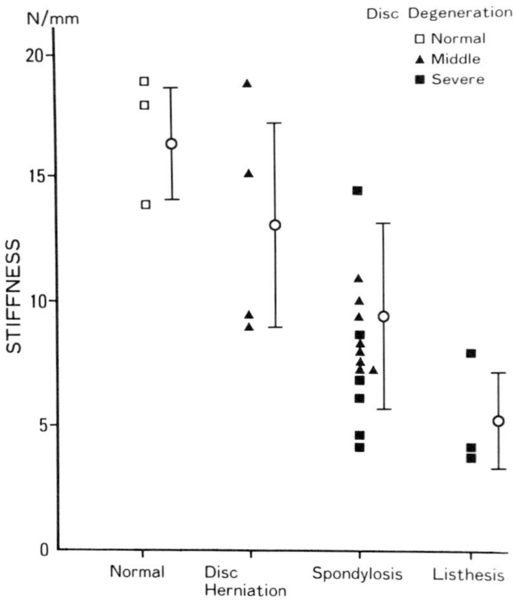

6

Fig. 5. The variation of stiffness relating to both aging and disk degeneration. Stiffness of the motion segment showed marked decrease with age. The *open squares*, *solid triangles*, and *solid squares* stand for the MRI finding of normal, moderate, and severe degeneration of the disk respectively

Fig. 6. The relation of stiffness and disease. Degenerative spondylolisthetic cases showed the lowest stiffness, with an average of 5.4 N/mm. The average stiffness of spondylotic cases was 8.1 N/mm. The average stiffness of the spinal motion segments of herniated disk cases was 13.1 N/mm and as compared with listhetic cases, this was comparatively high. Stiffness of the motion segments presenting normal MRI was 16.6 N/mm and proved to be higher than the affected ones. The *open squares*, *solid triangles*, and *solid squares* stand for the MRI finding of normal, moderate, and severe degeneration of the disk, respectively

Figure 5 indicates the variation of stiffness relating to both aging and disk degeneration. Stiffness of the motion segment showed marked decrease with age.

Figure 6 indicates the relation of stiffness with disease. In particular, degenerative spondylolisthetic cases showed the lowest stiffness, with an average of 5.4 N/mm. The average stiffness of spondylotic cases was 8.1 N/mm. However, the average stiffness of the spinal motion segments of herniated disk cases was 13.1 N/mm and as compared with listhetic cases, this was comparatively high. Stiffness of the motion segments presenting normal MRI was 16.6 N/mm and proved to be higher than the affected ones.

Stiffness of the motion segment decreased stepwise as the anatomical structures were removed for decompression. Figure 7 indicates the change of stiffness in each case treated by partial laminectomy and facetectomy, diskectomy, iliac bone graft inseting, and Luque instrumentation. Stiffness of motion segments proved to reduce to 84% after partial laminectomy and facetectomy, and then to 65% after diskectomy on the average, when the stiffness of the motion segment before decompression was assumed as 100%. It increased to 133% and to 184% after interbody insertion of iliac bone graft and then Luque fixation.

a

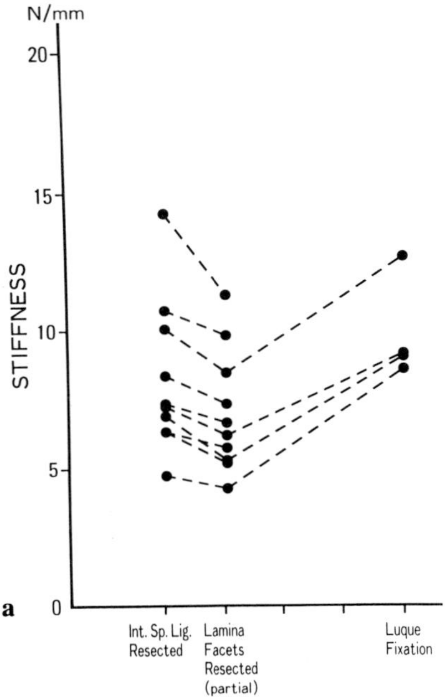

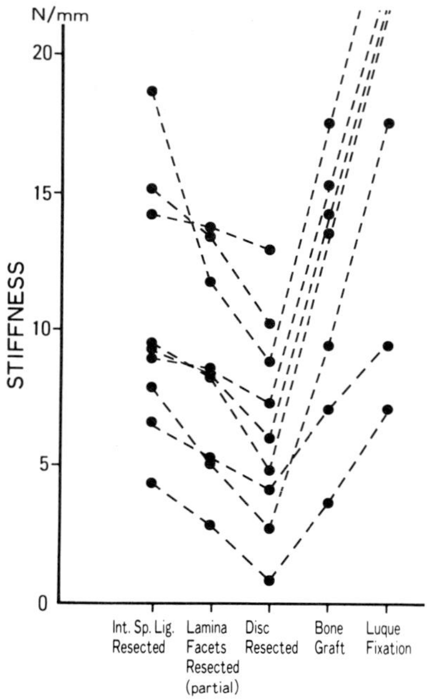

b

Fig. 7a,b. The change of stiffness in each case treated by partial laminectomy and facetectomy, diskectomy, iliac bone graft insertion, and Luque instrumentation. Stiffness of the motion segment decreased stepwise as the anatomical structures were removed for decompression

Discussion

"Spinal instability" is still controversial and subjective in its definition [4,5, 18,19]. Loss of stiffness is one of the rational approaches for instability [4]. Stiffness is the ratio of load applied to the structure and the displacement that occurs. According to this intraoperative measurement, it is possible to apply a load directly to a certain spinal motion segment in order to estimate its stiffness. As can be seen in the present study, stiffness of spinal motion segments reduced in accordance with progression of disk degeneration. We would quantitatively define instability of the spinal motion segment of concern, if we were able to establish a normal range of stiffness of the motion segment of respective areas of the spine in various age groups.

It is also possible to quantify a stepwise reduction of the stiffness of a particular motion segment during partial laminectomy or facetectomy, as has been mentioned above. The fate of the motion segment assuming reduced stiffness can be anticipated through this in order to judge the need for stabilization or fusion during surgery in the future.

Acknowledgment. This study was supported by a grant from the Ministry of Education, Science and Culture, Grant-in-Aid for Scientific Research (A) 02404059. The authors deeply thank for his valuable suggestions and cooperation the late Mr. Yasuyuki Seguchi (Professor and Chairman of the Department of Engineering Science, Osaka University Engineering Science School).

References

1. Denis F (1984) Spinal instability as defined by the three-column spine concept in acute spinal trauma. Clin Orthop 189:65–76
2. Kirkaldy-Willis W, Farfan HF (1982) Instability of the lumbar spine. Clin Orthop 165:110–123
3. Pearcy M, Shepherd J (1985) Is there instability in spondylolisthesis? Spine 10: 175–177
4. Pope MH, Panjabi MM (1985) Biomechanical definitions of spinal instability. Spine 10:255–256
5. White AA, Southwick WO, Panjabi MM (1976) Clinical instability in the lower cervical spine. A review of past and current concepts. Spine 1:15–27
6. Brown MD, Holmes DC, Cammisa FP (1991) Intraoperative measurement of lumbar spine motion segment unit stiffness: Clinical significance. Presented at the 58th annual meeting of AAOS, Anaheim, March 7–11
7. Ebara S, Yonenobu K, Fujiwara K, Hosono N, Ono K (1989) An experiment of intraoperative measurement of lumbar spinal instability. Presented at the annual meeting of the 18th meeting of Japan Spine Research Society, Osaka, June 18–19
8. Ebara S, Hosono N, Yonenobu K, Ono K (1990) Intraoperative measurement of lumbar spinal instability. J Jpn Orthop Assoc 64:347

9. Ebara S, Hosono N, Yonenobu K, Ono K (1990) Intraoperative measurement of lumbar spinal instability. Presented at the annual meeting of the SICOT 90, Montreal, September 9–13
10. Ebara S, Hosono N, Harada T, Ono K (1991) Intraoperative measurement of lumbar spinal instability. Presented at the 18th annual meeting of ISSLS, Heidelberg, May 12
11. Feffer HL, Wiesel SW, Cuckler JM, Rothman RH (1985) Degenerative spondylosis. To fuse or not to fuse. Spine 10:287–289
12. Frymoyer JW, Selbey DK (1985) Segmental instability. Rationale for treatment. Spine 10:280–286
13. Olerud F, Sjostron L, Karlstrom G, Hamberg M (1986) Spontaneous effects of increased stability of the lower lumbar spine in cases of severe chronic back pain. Clin Orthop 203:67–74
14. Tibrewal SB, Pearcy MJ, Portek I, Spivey J (1985) A prospective study of lumbar spinal movements before and after discectomy using biplanar radiography. Correlation of clinical and radiographic findings. Spine 10:455–460
15. Timoshenko S (1955) Strength of materials. Part 1: Elementary theory and problems. D Van Nostrand, New York
16. Cloward RB (1963) Lesions of the intervertebral disks and their treatment by interbody fusion methods. The painful disk. Clin Orthop 27:51–77
17. Thompson JP, Pearce RH, Schechter MT, Adams ME, Tsang IKY, Bishop PB (1990) Preliminary evaluation of a scheme for grading the gross morphology of the human intervertebral disk. Spine 15:411–415
18. Farfan HF, Gracovetsky S (1984) The nature of instability. Spine 9:714–719
19. Nachemson A (1985) Lumbar spine instability. A critical update and symposium summary. Spine 10:290–291

SECTION II The Merits and Demerits of Lumbar Fusion

2.4 The Long-Term Effect of Lumbar Spine Fusion: Deterioration of Adjacent Motion Segments

Ken Y. Hsu, James Zucherman, and Arthur White[1]

Introduction

The long-term effect of spinal fusion on adjacent motion segments is a common concern [1–10], but there have been no large, well documented series in which normal motion segments adjacent to lumbar fusions have undergone deterioration. It is still not known at what frequency normal lumbar segments deteriorate when fusion is performed adjacent to them. There are no studies in the literature that have evaluated such segments with verification of normalcy prior to adjacent fusions.

Patients and Methods

Of the patients who were treated for severe deterioration of the motion segment adjacent to lumbar fusion at St. Mary's Hospital in San Francisco, 30 patients met the following criteria:

1. Good or excellent results lasting 16 months or more following fusion, where:
   a. Excellent results entailed complete resolution of prior symptoms.
   b. Good results indicated marked improvement with occasional pain or occasional use of pain medications, and no functional limitations.
2. Increasing clinical deterioration after 16 months or more without evidence of pseudarthrosis. The new symptoms were due to the following at the adjacent unfused level:
   a. Significant disk herniation or degeneration.
   b. Central, lateral recess or foraminal stenosis.

[1] St. Mary's Spine Center, 1 Shrader St., San Francisco, CA 94117, USA

   c. Segmental instability manifested as spondylolisthesis or retrolisthesis.
3. Normal radiographs, myelograms, diskograms, or CT scans of this adjacent unfused level prior to fusion.
   a. Significant disk herniations of at least 4 mm documented on CT scans or myelograms. Disk degeneration was shown by loss of at least 50% of disk height on radiographs or significant painful degeneration on diskograms.
   b. Stenosis, considered to be significant if narrowing of the central canal, lateral recess or neural foramen was greater than 50% of the prefusion state (on the axial view of a CT scan for central and lateral stenosis, and lateral reconstruction view for foraminal stenosis).
   c. Segmental instability, manifested as spondylolisthesis or retrolisthesis (subluxation) of more than 5 mm on lateral radiographs, with or without flexion-extension views.

Patients with congenital stenosis or scoliosis were not included.

Results

The 30 patients included 18 females and 12 males, ranging in age from 31 to 64 years with a mean of 51 years at the time of treatment for the problem adjacent to the fusion. The initial lumbar fusions were performed for the following pathologies: 21 cases of disk herniation, 6 of spondylolisthesis, and 3 of lateral recess and/or foraminal stenosis.

The period of good or excellent results following the spinal fusions ranged from 16 months to 28 years with a mean of 8.1 years. There were two cases of L5–S1 fusions with good results, lasting 6 and 7 years respectively. There were 25 cases of L4–S1 fusion that had good or excellent results, lasting from 16 months to 28 years with a mean of 8.6 years. In addition, 3 L3–S1 fusions showed good or excellent results of 2, 4, and 7 years respectively, with a mean of 4.3 years.

The pathological changes occurring at the motion segment adjacent to the fusions usually consisted of a combination of disk degeneration, herniation, facet arthropathy, infolding of thickened ligamentum flavum, and central, lateral recess or foraminal stenosis. However, disk herniation or degeneration predominated in 14 patients. Figures 1–4 show CT scan study of a male patient who developed a disk extrusion above the L4–S1 fusion. Note the normal CT scan of the same disk prior to the fusion 5 years earlier. In 12 patients, central, lateral recess or foraminal stenosis were the primary cause of severe symptoms. In 3 patients, there was spondylolisthesis with 7-mm, 8-mm, and 10-mm subluxations respectively on lateral radiographs (Figs. 5–7). Retrolisthesis of 7 mm of L3 on L4–S1 fusion was also found in 1 patient. Figures 8–12 show the sequential radiographs of a woman who had a successful L4–S1 fusion. However, narrowing of L3–4 disk space was noted 15 years following the fusion. This was followed by further disk narrowing and degenerative

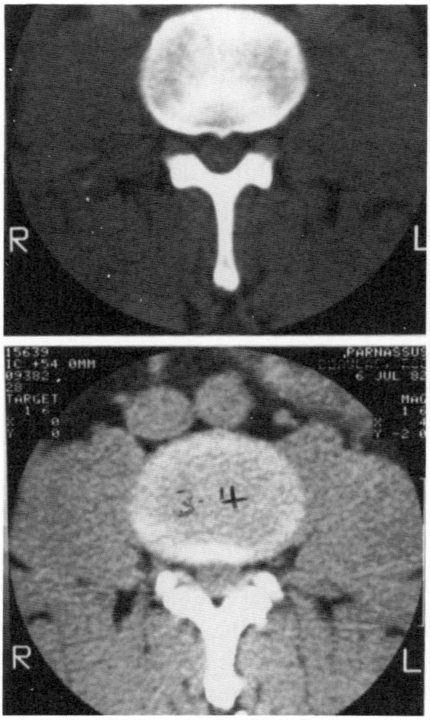

1

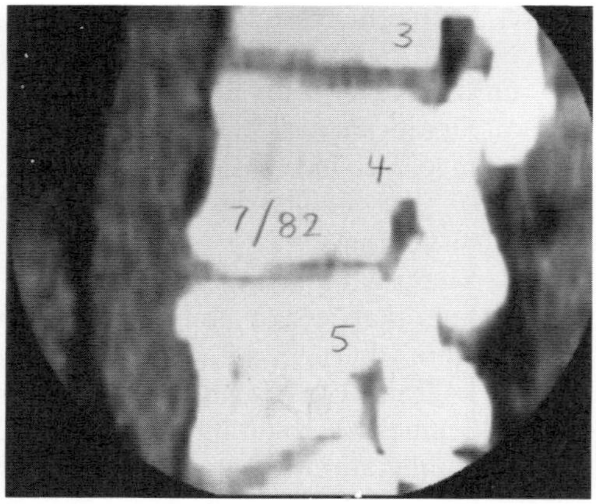

2

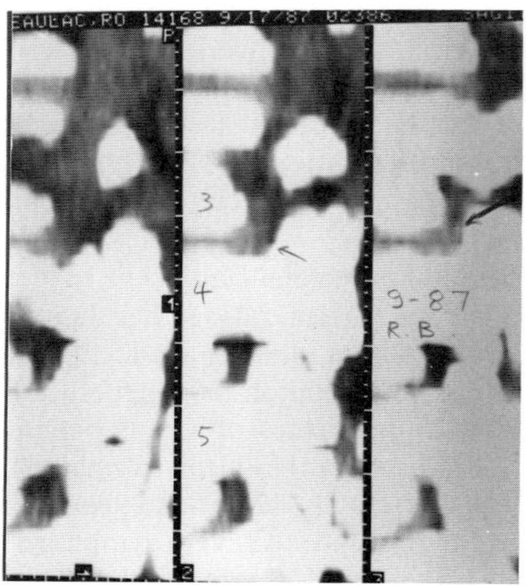

3

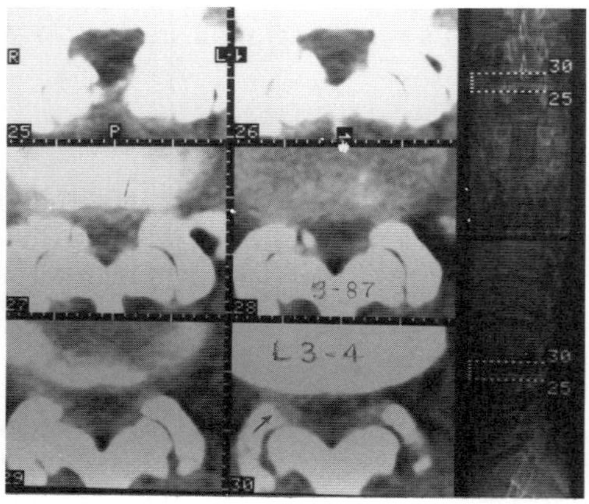

4

Fig. 1. Axial view of the normal L3–4 disk before fusion

Fig. 2. Lateral reconstruction of a CT scan showing the normal L3–4 disk and neural foramen before fusion

Fig. 3. Lateral reconstruction of a CT scan 5 years after fusion showing extrusion of the L3–4 disk. Note the L3–4 neural foramen being filled by disk material (*arrows*). *White areas*, disk material

Fig. 4. Axial views of L3–4 disk herniation and extrusion 5 years after fusion of L4–S1

Fig. 5. A 64-year-old woman who underwent L4–S1 posterolateral fusion for spondylolisthesis of L4 on L5 in 1983. Preoperative lateral radiograph showing the L3–4 disk to be of normal height in 1980

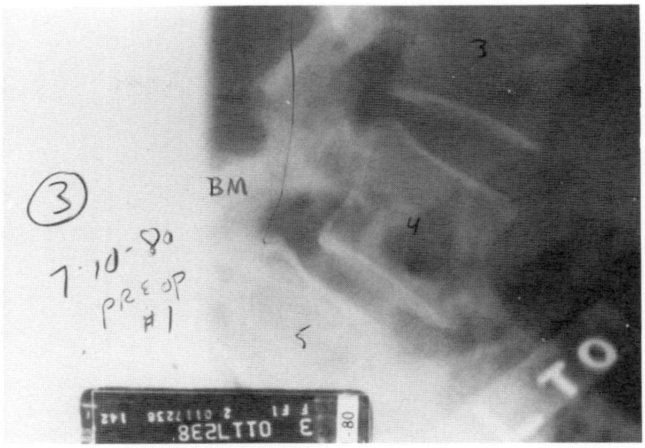

5

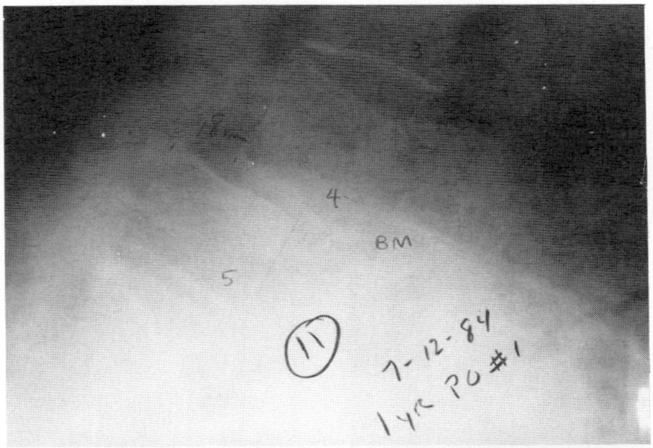

6

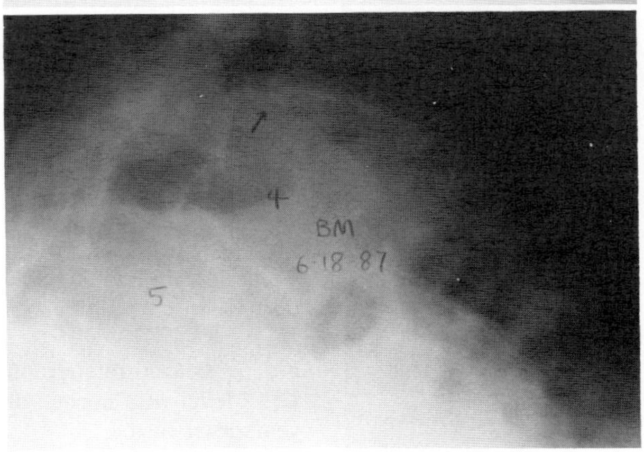

7

Fig. 6. One-year post-fusion radiograph of the same patient shown in Fig. 5. Some narrowing of the L3–4 disk space in 1984 can be seen

Fig. 7. Four-year post fusion radiograph of the same patient showing further disk narrowing and anterior subluxation of L3 on L4

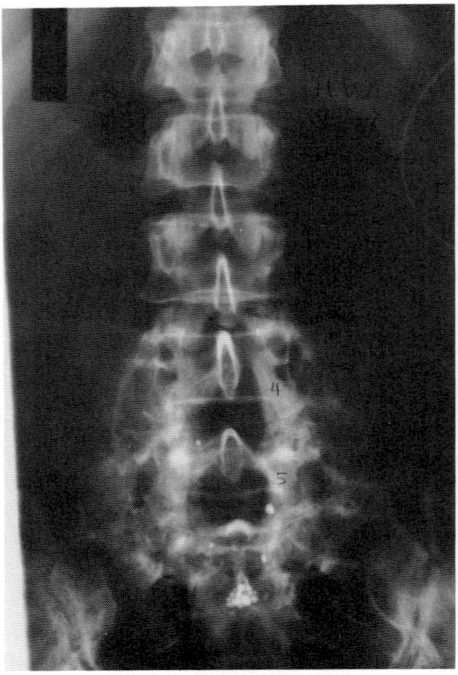

8

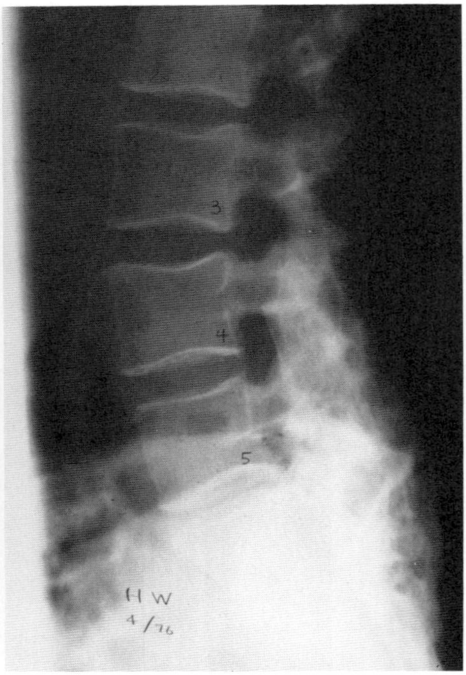

9

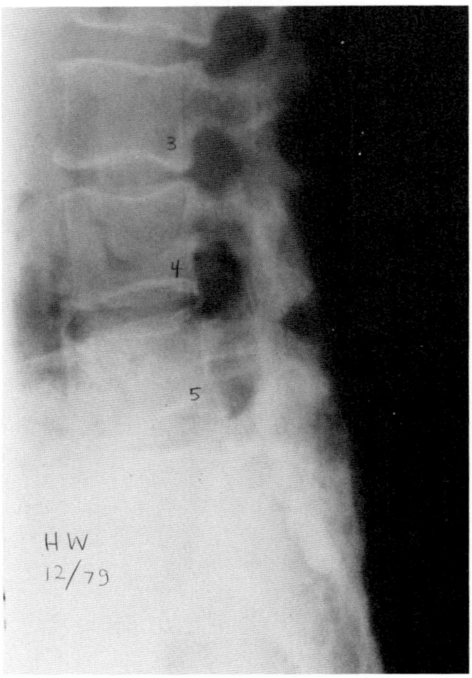

10

Fig. 8. AP radiograph of a 53-year-old woman who had a successful L4–S1 posterolateral fusion in 1964

Fig. 9. Lateral radiograph showing the L3–4 level with normal disk height, 12 years after fusion

Fig. 10. Lateral radiograph showing narrowing of the L3–4 disk 15 years after fusion

11
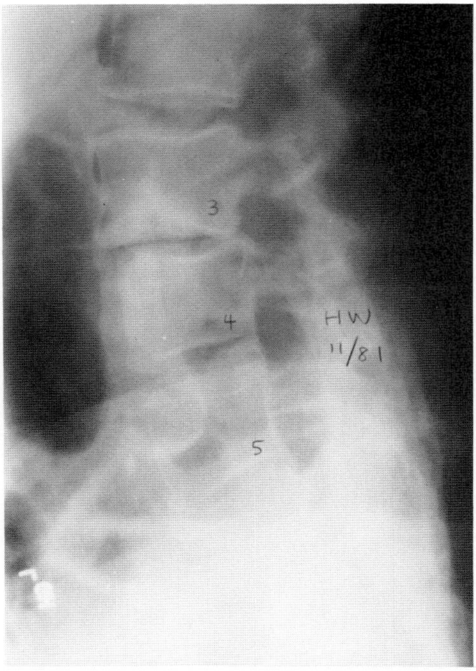

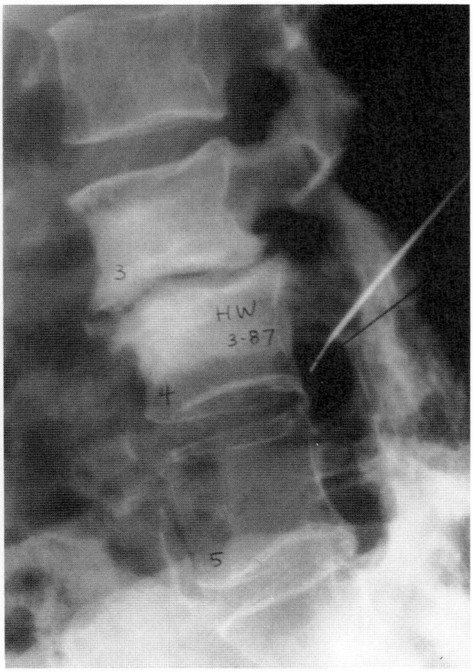

12

Fig. 11. Lateral radiograph showing further narrowing and anterior subluxation of L3 on L4, 17 years after fusion

Fig. 12. Lateral radiograph showing severe deterioration of the L3–4 segment above the fusion, 23 years following fusion

spondylolisthesis later. Figure 13 is a myelogram demonstrating central stenosis. This patient underwent surgical decompression of central, lateral recess and foraminal stenosis as well as L3–L4 fusion 23 years after the L4–S1 fusion.

In cases where stenosis was predominant, severe symptoms started between 5 and 28 years after fusion, with a mean of 11.6 years. The stenoses were all associated with disk degeneration, herniation, and facet arthropathy. In general, patients with disk degeneration or herniation presented earlier: between 16 months and 8 years after fusion, with a mean of 4.3 years.

Thirteen fusions were performed with internal fixation using Knodt rods, Harrington rods or variable screw placement (VSP) plates. Their good or excellent results ranged from 16 months to 9 years, with a mean of 5.3 years. There were nine Knodt rod fusions (Fig. 14) and two Harrington rod fusions. Two patients underwent internal fixation with VSP plates and pedicle screws (Figs. 15 to 18). In 17 cases of posterior or posterolateral fusion, metal rods or plates were not used. Their good or excellent results ranged from 2 to 28 years, with a mean of 9.9 years, before failure of the adjacent motion segment.

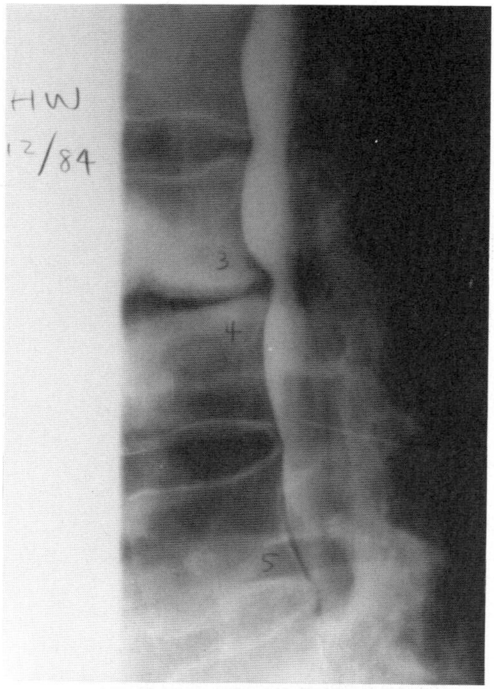

Fig. 13. Lateral view myelogram demonstrating central stenosis

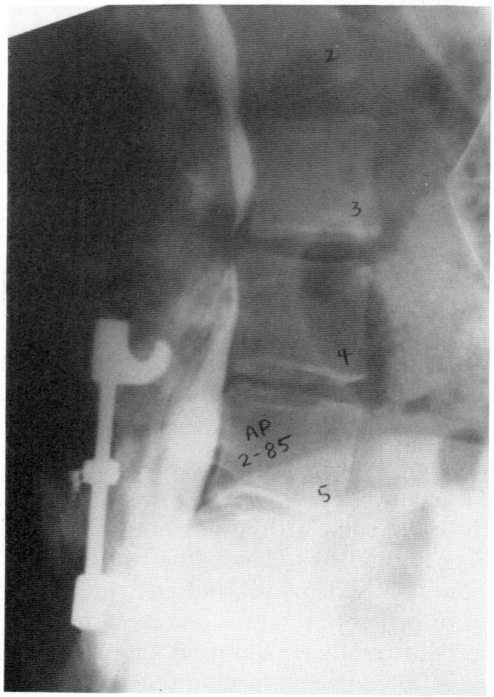

Fig. 14. Lateral view myelogram demonstrating severe central stenosis at the L3–4 level above an L4–S1 Knodt rod fusion in a 43-year-old woman, 7 years after fusion. This patient did well following her fusion in 1977, and was able to work full-time for 6 years, until January 1985

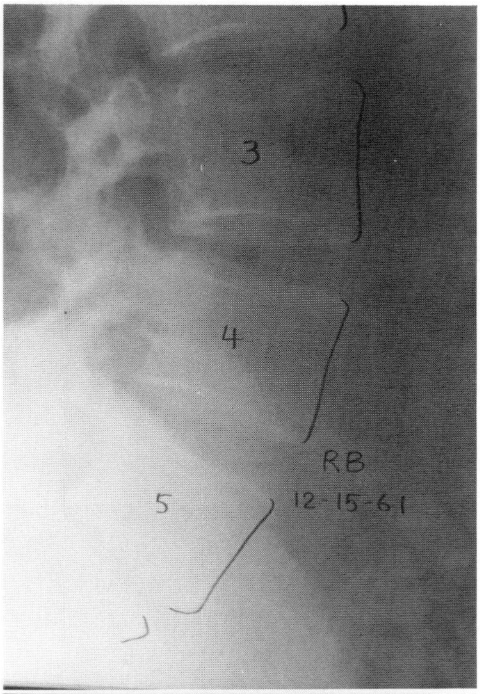

Fig. 15. A 63-year-old woman who presented in 1961 (age 38 years) with low back pain. Note narrowing of the L5–S1 disk space

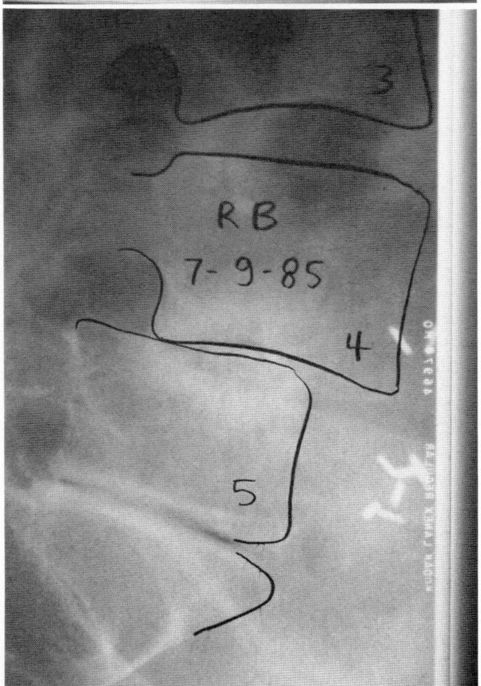

Fig. 16. Preoperative radiograph showing the L3–4 level with normal disk height in the same patient as shown in Fig. 15

17
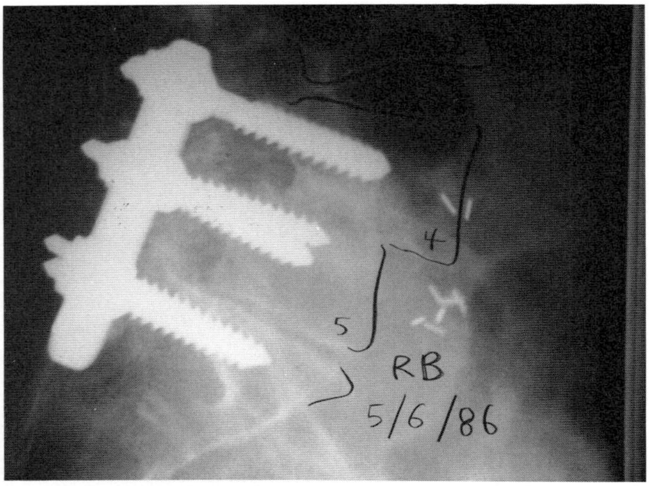

18
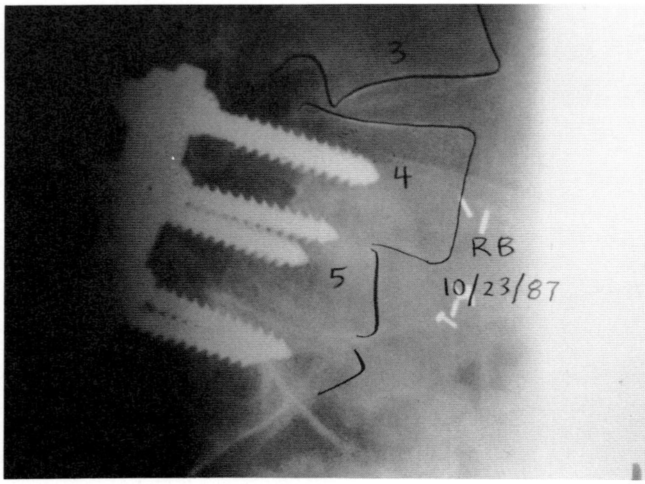

Fig. 17. Lateral radiograph 6 months following L4–S1 fusion using VSP plates and pedicle screws in the same patient. The radiograph was obtained in the neutral position

Fig. 18. Lateral radiograph showing anterior subluxation of L3 on L4 2 years after fusion in the same patient. The radiograph was obtained in the neutral position without flexion or extension of the spine

Discussion

We have presented details of patients with deterioration of the motion segments adjacent to lumbar spine fusions. Thirty of these clearly developed progressive clinical disease after a long symptom-free interval of 16 months or more.

They eventually developed severe clinical deterioration due to significant disk degeneration, herniation, degenerative stenosis, segmental instability, spondylolisthesis or retrolisthesis at the motion segment adjacent to the fused levels. Normality of these prefusion levels was documented by radiographs, diskograms, or CT scans in all 30 cases. The above clinical data reinforces the concern about increased mechanical stress at motion segments immediately adjacent to fusions. It has been stated by Wiltse that lumbar fusion adjacent to abnormal segments causes rapid deterioration and symptoms (Wiltse L, personal communication, 1987).

The effect of posterior or posterior lateral lumbar fusion on adjacent free segments is probably somewhat different from the effect of interbody fusion on adjacent motion segments. According to Lee and Langrana [6], all types of spinal fusion result in cephalad movement of the center of rotation of the adjacent free segments, with posterior fusion showing a tendency towards a shift in the center of rotation to the posterior fusion mass, and anterior interbody fusion a tendency towards an anterior shift. They felt that posterior fusions exerted increased stress on the facet joints and anterior fusions increased shear stress and compression stress on the disk. Although posterior and posterolateral fusions were performed in all of our 30 cases, there was no particular predilection for facet arthropathy.

In this series, all the patients with stenosis had disk degeneration. Brodsky reported a predominance of stenosis in the breakdown above his fusions [1]. The increased frequency of degenerative disk change in our cases is likely due to its earlier appearance relative to stenosis. If enough time elapsed, stenosis would probably result as an end stage of degenerative instability in all cases. This finding is consistent with the pathophysiology of the motion segment described by Kirkaldy-Willis et al. [11]. Damage to a disk or posterior joint from increased stress concentration in the disk predisposes it to annular tears which coalesce to produce disk herniation and more severe deterioration. This then effects the other members of the "three joint complex" which are intimately linked. Later, the interplay among the changes in the three joint complex lead to stenosis and/or subluxation.

The difference between one- and two-level fusion was not significant. However, the difference between two- and three-level fusion was marked, but not significant, due to the small sample size. Transfer of stress of the level above a three-level fusion is expected to be greater. As more levels are fused, fewer free motion segments remain to share the load. The longer lever arm produces a greater stress riser at the first mobile segment and in many cases the lumbar lordosis is largely gone, resulting in hyperextension of the first mobile segment.

There were significant differences in results between the fusions performed with metal fixation and fusions done without ($t \pm 2.818$, $P < 0.02$). Good or excellent results lasting a mean of 5.3 years were noted in those with metal fixation, and a mean of 9.9 years was found in those without. Rigidity conferred by the metallic implants increases stress risers in the adjacent motion segments. This effect is expected to be proportional to the rigidity of the system. This was exemplified by the two patients who underwent fusion using VSP plates, a more rigid system. The transition between the instrumented level and the adjacent unfused level was abrupt. Distraction effected by the Knodt and Harrington rods causes loss of lumbar lordosis and may be responsible for increased stresses to the adjacent motion segment by altering stress distribution and biomechanics.

Close scrutiny of levels adjacent to proposed spine fusion is in order, especially when rigid fixation is planned. We recommend diskogram or saline acceptance tests of adjacent levels before all fusions to prevent ending a fusion adjacent to a degenerated, potentially painful segment. MRI scans are useful to determine the normality of the adjacent motion segment, but they are not totally accurate (Zucherman JF, Hsu KY, personal communication, 1987). Removal of rigid metal fixation after solid bone fusion has occured in order to diminish adjacent segment stress is a logical consideration in that there is some "give" to most posterior bone fusions (Selby D, Zucherman JF, personal communication, 1987).

References

1. Brodsky AE (1976) Post-laminectomy and post-fusion stenosis of the lumbar spine. Clin Orthop 115:130
2. Cochran T, Irstam L, Nachemson A (1983) Long-term anatomic and functional changes in patients with adolescent idiopathic scoliosis treated by Harrington rod fusion. Spine 8:576–584
3. DePalma AF, Rothman RH (1969) Surgery of the lumbar spine. Clin Orthop 63:162–170
4. Frymoyer JW, Hanley EN, How J, Kuhlman D, Matteri RE (1979) A comparison of radiographic findings in fusion and non-fusion patients 10 or more years following lumbar disk surgery. Spine 4:435–440
5. Ginsburg HH, Goldstein LA, Robinson SC, Haake PW, Devanny JR, Chan DPK, Suk S (1979) Back pain in postoperative idiopathic scoliosis – Long-term follow-up study. Spine 4:518
6. Lee CK, Langrana NA (1984) Lumbosacral spinal fusion – A biomechanical study. Spine 9:574–581
7. Lehmann TR, Spratt KF, Tozzi JE, Weinstein JN, Reinarz SJ, El-Khoury GY, Colby H (1987) Long-term follow up of lower lumbar fusion patients. Spine 12:97–104
8. Quinnell RC, Stockdale HR (1981) Some experimental observations of the influence of a single lumbar floating fusion on the remaining lumbar spine. Spine 6:263–267
9. Unander-Scharin L (1950) On low back pain. With special reference to the value of operative treatment with fusion. Acta Orthop Scan [Suppl] 5
10. Unander-Scharin L (1951) Spinal fusion in low back pain. Acta Orthop Scand 20:335–341
11. Kirkaldy-Willis WH, Wedge JH, Yong-Hing K, Reilly J (1978) Pathology and pathogenesis of lumbar spondylosis and stenosis. Spine 3:319–328

2.5 A Critical Analysis of Motion of the Lumbar Spine Adjacent to an Interbody Fusion: A Clinical Radiological Study and Biomechanical Cadaveric Study

K.D.K. Luk, D.H.K. Chow, J.C.Y. Leong, and J. Evans[1]

Introduction

Fusion of different lengths of the spine is indicated in various conditions. The redistribution of stress among the unfused segments has been correlated with and blamed for subsequent degeneration. In the literature, the incidence of clinically significant degeneration after various types of spinal fusions remains controversial. Some authors believe that it is uncommon, however others have reported a near 15% incidence of significant symptoms with some requiring reoperations [1,2]. Radiologically, however, there is a concensus that accelerated degeneration has been observed especially in the level immediately above the fusion mass. This is particularly true after long fusions with instrumentation [3]. Logically one would also expect that the amount of extra stress should relate directly to the stiffness of the fusion mass. Biomechanical studies in vitro have shown that the stiffness of the fusion mass is maximum after anterior interbody fusion and less so after posterior fusions [4]. One would therefore expect to see earlier degeneration in patients with the former type of fusions. This is a report of a retrospective clinical radiological analysis of the segmental mobility of the lumbar spine after short segment anterior interbody fusion and a biomechanical study on the lumbar spinal mobility using human cadaveric specimens before and after simulated anterior interbody fusions. This study also attempts to identify other factors that may contribute to degeneration of the unfused segments.

[1] Department of Orthopaedic Surgery, University of Hong Kong, 5F Professorial Block, Queen Mary Hospital, Hong Kong

Materials and Methods

Clinical Radiological

Thirty normal volunteers who had no history of back discomfort were used as controls. The mean age was 37.2 years. Lateral radiographs of the lumbar spine in maximum flexion and extension in the side-lying position were taken in a standardized fashion. The intersegmental mobility of each disk space of the lumbar spine from L2 and below were measured with the Cobb method using a computer digitizer.

A total of 111 consecutive patients who had one-level L4–L5 or two-level L4–S1 anterior interbody fusions performed in this department for degenerated disk disease were reviewed. Of these patients, 53 who showed definite radiological union at the last follow-up and had sufficient flexion/extension radiographs taken serially were included. All these patients were clinically asymptomatic at the final follow-up, they were actively employed, and had satisfactory range of spinal movement clinically. Thirty-two patients had one-level L4–L5 fusion and 21 patients had two-level L4–S1 fusions. The average follow-up of the first group was 4 years and the second group was 6.5 years. The mean age at operation was 37.5 years. The radiographs were measured similarly. Intra- and interobserver errors and also error during the digitization process were estimated and were found to be not statistically significant.

Biomechanical Cadaveric Study

Six fresh cadaveric lumbar spine specimens including L1 to S3 with the adjacent ilium were harvested. They were stored at −25°C until use. Each specimen was mounted onto a test apparatus specially designed and constructed for loading the specimen into flexion and extension. The sacrum and the adjoining ilium was fixed to a base box and the top of the L1 was attached to a loading cap

Table 1. Mean segmental mobility (clinical radiological).

	Mean segmental mobility (°)		
	Normal	L4–5 fusion	L4–S1 fusion
L2–3	10.6	8.6	9.2
L3–4	12.7	9.9	11.6
L4–5	13.9	1.7	1.2
L5–S1	16.7	10.9	0.7
ROM	53.8	31.2	22.6
% L2–3	19.5	27.0	41.7
% L3–4	23.5	33.6	54.1
% L4–5	26.1	4.5	3.3
% L5–S1	30.9	34.9	0.8

with the L3–L4 disk being leveled to the horizontal. A preload of 30% of the cadaver body weight was used. The specimen was then put through 30° of flexion and 20° of extension balanced by a pair of cables attached to the top loading plate simulating the erector spinae muscles in vivo. Reflective markers were attached to each vertebra and the intersegmental mobility in the sagittal plane was monitored with a three-dimensional motion analysis system (Elite, Bioengineering Technology and Systems, Milan, Italy).

The test was first performed with the intact specimen and then repeated after simulated L4–L5 or L4–S1 anterior interbody fusions with bone cement and wiring.

Results

Clinical Radiological

From the radiological study, the mean total range of movement of the lumbar spine from L2 to S1 was found to be reduced from 53.8° to 31.2° after a single-level L4–L5 fusion. This was further reduced to 22.6° after a double-level L4–S1 fusion (Table 1). The mean absolute mobility of each unfused disk space was significantly reduced compared with the normal controls (Fig. 1). The mobility at the level immediately above the fusion was less after single-level than after double-level fusions. The normal pattern of increasing segmental mobility from cephalad to caudal however remained normal.

When the mobility of each individual segment was expressed as a percentage of the total lumbar mobility, it was found that after L4–L5 or L4–S1 fusions there was a higher increase in percentage mobility in the segment immediately above the fusion mass (Fig. 2). Again, this increase is smaller after 1 level fusion than after 2 level fusion.

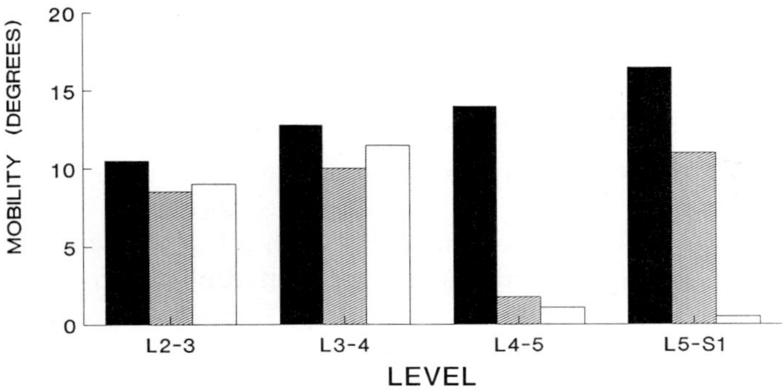

Fig. 1. Absolute intersegmental mobilities (clinical radiological). *Black area*, normal; *hatched area*, L4–L5 fusion; *dotted area*, L4–S1 fusion. $P < 0.05$

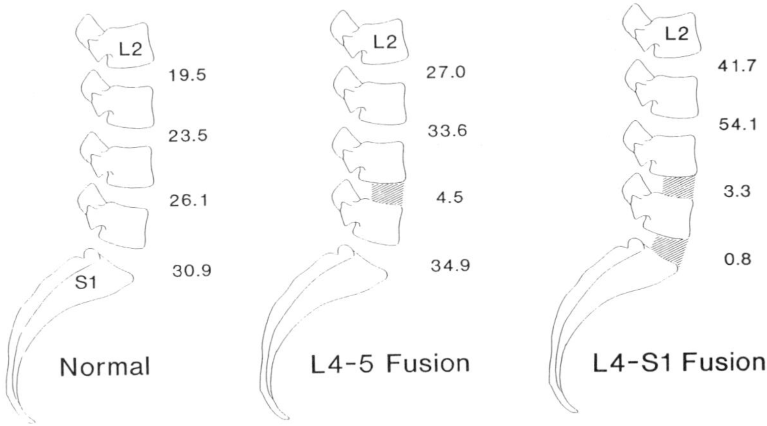

Fig. 2. Percentage segmental mobility (clinical radiological). $P < 0.05$

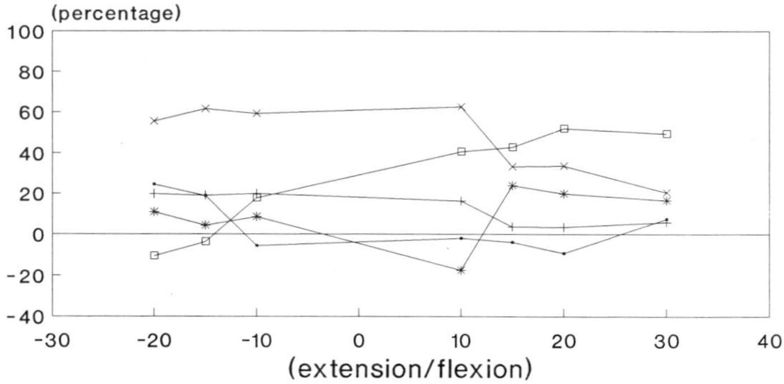

Fig. 3. Distribution of percentage deformation (biomechanical). *Solid square*, L1-L2; *vertical line*, L2–L3; *asterisk*, L3–L4; *open square*, L4–L5; *cross* L5-S1

Biomechanical Cadaveric Study

Consistent results were obtained from biomechanical testings performed on 6 cadaveric specimens.

In the intact specimen, it was found that both the absolute and percentage mobility of the spinal segments increased from cephalad to caudal as was similarly found in the clinical radiological study. The percentage mobility of the L4–L5 increased from extension to flexion and that of the L5–S1 decreased from extension to flexion. The percentage mobility of the other segments remained almost constant in different ranges of lumbar flexion and extension (Fig. 3).

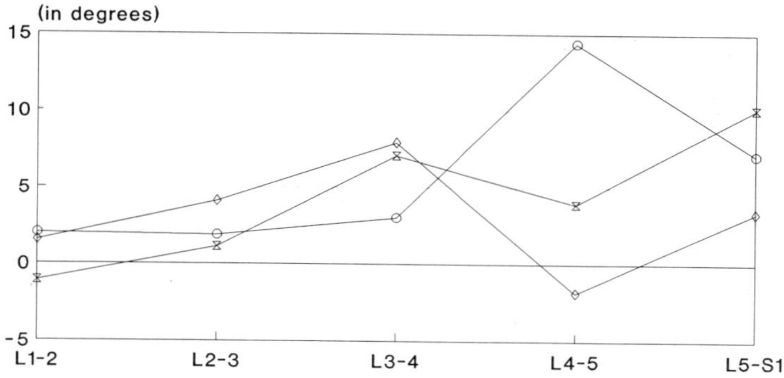

Fig. 4. Neutral to full flexion (biomechanical). *Circle*, intact; *double triangle*, L4–L5 fusion; *diamond*, L4–S1 fusion

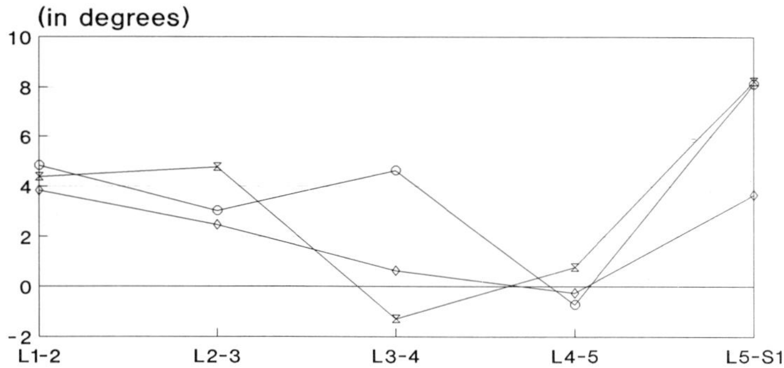

Fig. 5. Neutral to full extension (biomechanical). *Circle*, intact; *double triangle*, L4–L5 fusion; *diamond*, L4–S1 fusion

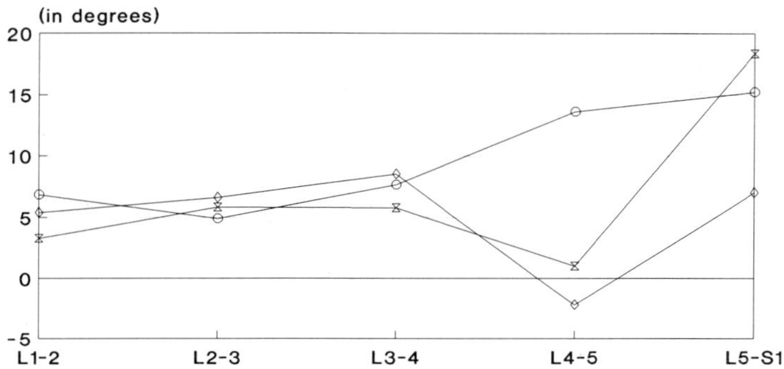

Fig. 6. Full extension to full flexion (biomechanical). *Circle*, intact; *double triangle*, L4–L5 fusion; *diamond*, L4–S1 fusion

After a simulated one-level L4–L5 fusion, there was a distinct loss of mobility at the fusion level (Figs. 4, 5). Proximal to the fusion, there was no significant change in the flexion or extension mobility of the L12 and L23 disk spaces. At the L3–L4 disk space just proximal to the fusion, there was increased flexion but decreased extension range with a resultant unchanged total mobility. Distal to the fusion at the L5–S1 space, there was increased flexion range but no change in the extension range. The total mobility at this space was thus increased (Fig. 6).

After a simulated two-level L4–S1 fusion, there was again distinct loss of mobility at the fusion level. At the L1–L2 and L2–L3 spaces, there was increased flexion but unchanged extension mobility (Figs. 4, 5). At the juxta-fusion L3–L4 space there was increased flexion but decreased extension mobility with a resultant increased total mobility (Fig. 6).

The segmental hypomobility observed in the in vivo study was not detected in the in vitro experiment.

Discussion

It is generally believed that fusion of part of the spine would throw extra stress onto the unfused segments. The longer and stiffer the fusion mass, the worse the situation would be and the earlier degeneration would set in at the unfused segments. Previous analytical study [5] has shown that there is a definite redistribution of mobility in the lumbar spine after short segmental fusions. The level immediately proximal to the fusion would take up most of the extra percentage mobility and this correlated well with the clinical observation that maximum degeneration is found at these levels. However, from a long-term study on patients who had short anterior interbody fusions followed up for 12.7 years, although Leong et al. [6] have found that disk degeneration was present in 52.5% of the patients, it was also noted that the degenerative changes were worse after single-level fusions than after double-level fusions. They could not find a satisfactory explanation for this and concluded that anterior interbody fusion is unlikely to have enhanced the degeneration.

From the present cadaveric biomechanical study simulating the situation immediately following an interbody fusion, it is found that the normal pattern of increasing segmental mobility from cephalad to caudal is preserved after surgery. After a one-level "floating" L4–L5 fusion, only the levels immediately above and below the fusion have shown changes in mobility. Both levels showed an increase in flexion mobilities but more importantly, there is a decrease in the extension mobility at the L34–L4 level. This pattern of increased flexion mobility is also seen in all the unfused levels after an "anchoring" L4–S1 fusion. Also, the decrease in extension mobility is only found at the C3–L4 level. It is obvious that at the levels immediately above the fusion mass in both L4–L5 or L4–S1 fusions, the total arc of movement has shifted towards the flexion side and the relative loss of extension mobility is more severe after one-level than two-level fusions. One may argue that this is related to the posture of the fusion segment whether it has been fused in either too much lordosis or kyphosis. This is unlikely to be true since the fusion procedures in this study were performed with the spinal specimen being fixed on a rigid frame making sure that the fusion was done in the neutral position preserving the normal natural lordosis of the specimen.

From the clinical radiological analysis, we have confirmed the redistribution of mobility in the lumbar spine after short segmental anterior interbody fusion. We agreed that the level immediately above the fusion mass would take up more of the percentage mobility. The most interested finding, however, is the diminished absolute mobility of all the unfused segments when compared with the normal controls. It appears that the lumbar spines do become significantly less mobile even after a single-level fusion at 4–6 years after surgery and that the unfused segments have not been able to compensate by becoming more "hypermobile." It is also apparent that the "hypomobility" at the level immediately proximal to the fusion mass is more severe after single- than double-level fusions. Since this study is not a longitudinal study, we are not able to demonstrate the pattern of progression during the follow-up period.

When one correlates the present findings with the clinically observed maximal disk degeneration at the level immediately above a fusion mass [3] and that it is worse after single-level than double-level fusions [6], it leads one to postulate that immediately after a short anterior interbody fusion, a decrease in the extension mobility may be responsible for the accelerated degeneration. This degeneration will subsequently present clinically as "hypomobility" of the unfused segments as demonstrated in our clinical radiological study. As to the pathophysiology of how a decrease in extension mobility of an intervertebral disk should lead to disk degeneration, it remains to be proven.

References

1. Strayer L, Risser J, Waugh T (1968) Results of spinal fusion for scoliosis twenty-five years or more after surgery. Read at the Annual Meeting of the Scoliosis Research Society, Houston, Texas, September
2. Van Grouw A Jr, Nadel CI, Weierman RJ, Lowell HA (1976) Long-term follow-up of patients with idiopathic scoliosis treated surgically. A preliminary subjective study. Clin Orthop 117:197–201
3. Hsu KY, Zucherman J, White A, Reynolds J, Goldthwaite N (1988) Deterioration of motion segments adjacent to lumbar spine fusions. Ortho Transact (J Bone Joint Surg) 12:605–606
4. Lee CK, Langrana NA (1984) Lumbosacral spinal fusion. A biomechanical study. Spine 9:574–581
5. Lee CK (1988) Accelerated degeneration of the segment adjacent to a lumbar fusion. Spine 13:375–377
6. Leong JCY, Chun SY, Grange WJ, Fang D (1983) Long-term results of lumbar intervertebral disk prolapse. Spine 8:793–799

2.6 Anterior Interbody Fusion for Degenerative Spondylolisthesis: The Long-Term Clinical Results

Kazuhisa Takahashi, Hiroshi Kitahara, Masatsune Yamagata, Masazumi Murakami, Masaya Mimura, and Hideshige Moriya[1]

Introduction

Since 1958, we have performed anterior interbody fusion to treat patients with degenerative spondylolisthesis [1,2]. We report the long-term postoperative courses of the patients.

Materials and Methods

A total of 43 patients, 37 females and 6 males, underwent anterior decompression and interbody fusion for degenerative spondylolisthesis between February 1958 and October 1990. All the operations were performed with basically the same technique of transperitoneal (n = 25) or retroperitoneal (n = 18) anterior diskectomy and interbody fusion [3]. This treatment was not indicated for spinal canal stenosis with multilevel involvement or severe central stenosis. The average age of patients was 51.6 years (range, 34–74 years), and the average length of follow-up was 13.9 years (range, 1–32.5 years). Vertebral level of slippage and level of anterior interbody fusion are shown in Table 1.

Clinical evaluation was done using the rating system of the Japanese Orthopaedic Association (JOA score) [4]. A full JOA score is 29 points based on three subjective symptoms (9 points), three clinical signs (6 points), and seven activities of daily living (14 points). Patients with JOA scores of 25 points or more were rated as "satisfactory," while those with scores of 24 points or less were rated as "unsatisfactory." A survival curve was obtained from the postoperative period during which the patient was judged to be "satisfactory" [5]. Patients who died or were lost to follow-up exited the life table at the date of their last evaluation.

[1] Department of Orthopaedic Surgery, School of Medicine, Chiba University, 1-8-1 Inohana, Chuo-ku, Chiba, 260 Japan

Table 1. Vertebral level of slippage and level of surgical treatment.

Slippage \ Surgery	(n)	L3–4	L3–4 L4–5	L4–5	L4–5 L5–S	L5–S
L3	(4)	3	1			
L3 + L4	(1)		1(1)			
L4	(34)			28	6(3)	
L4 + L5	(2)				2	
L5	(2)					2

Figures in parentheses represent cases of pseudarthrosis

To evaluate the influence of age at surgery on the postoperative course, we divided the subjects into four age groups: Group I, patients in their thirties (mean age at surgery, 36.5 years); Group II, patients in their forties (mean age at surgery, 45.1 years); Group III, patients in their fifties (mean age at surgery, 54.5 years), and Group IV, patients of 60 years old or more (mean age at surgery, 65.4 years).

Results

Complete bony union was obtained in all patients undergoing single-level fusion. Pseudarthrosis was recognized in four of ten patients with two-level fusion (Table 1). The average degree of slippage was reduced from 15.9% to 6.9%.

The average JOA score for the 42 patients at the time of final examination was 7.3 ± 1.7 (81% of the normal value) for subjective symptoms, 5.4 ± 0.9 (90%) for clinical signs, 12.2 ± 1.9 (87%) for activities of daily living, and 25.0 ± 4.0 (86%) for the total score.

Intermittent claudication was noted by 36 of the 43 patients preoperatively; it disappeared in all but 4 patients during the follow-up period. Gait disturbances were relieved completely in 2 of these 4 patients after surgery, but reappeared 10 and 19 years postoperatively, respectively. The other 2 patients had severe spinal stenosis. Revision surgery was performed through a posterior approach in 1 patient with multilevel involvement.

Overall survivorship results show 73% of the patients had satisfactory results for 10 years after anterior interbody fusion was performed, 55% for 20 years, and 28% for 30 years (Fig. 1).

As shown in Fig. 2, all Group I patients maintained satisfactory results for 22 years after surgery. Results were also satisfactory in 80% of Group II patients for 14 years, and 84% of Group III patients for 10 years. Results were satisfactory in only five of the eight patients in Group IV immediately after surgery.

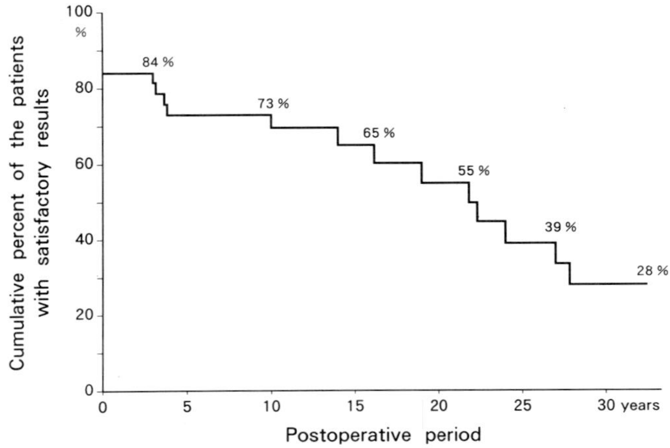

Fig. 1. Kaplan-Meier curve of overall cumulative percentage of patients with satisfactory results

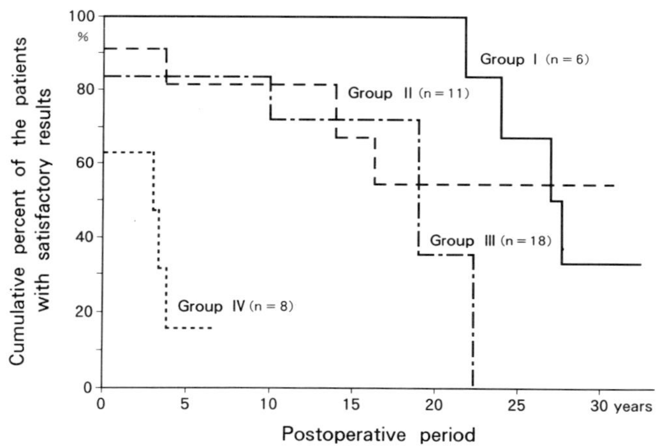

Fig. 2. Kaplan-Meier curve of the cumulative percentage of patients with satisfactory results classified by age at time of surgery

Case Reports

Case 1. A 71-year-old woman presented with degenerative spondylolisthesis of the fourth lumbar vertebra. She had undergone anterior interbody fusion in 1959, when she was 39 years old. The patient reported an unremarkable course for 32 years. Her JOA score at final examination was 27 points (Fig. 3).

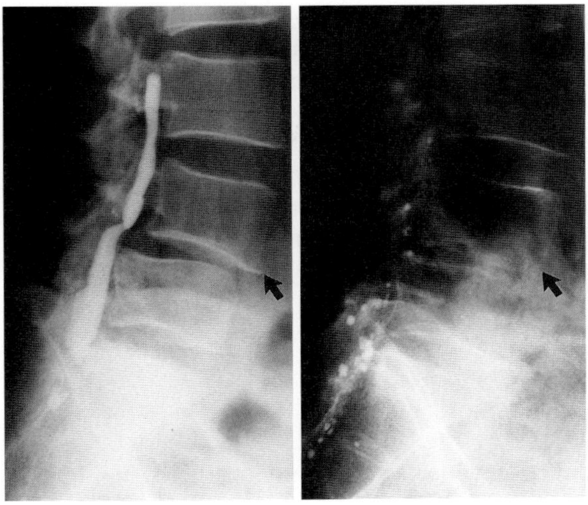

a b

Fig. 3a,b. Case 1. **a** Preoperative myelogram of a 71-year-old woman with degenerative spondylolisthesis of the fourth lumbar vertebra (*arrows*). **b** Plain roentgenogram taken 32 years after initial surgery

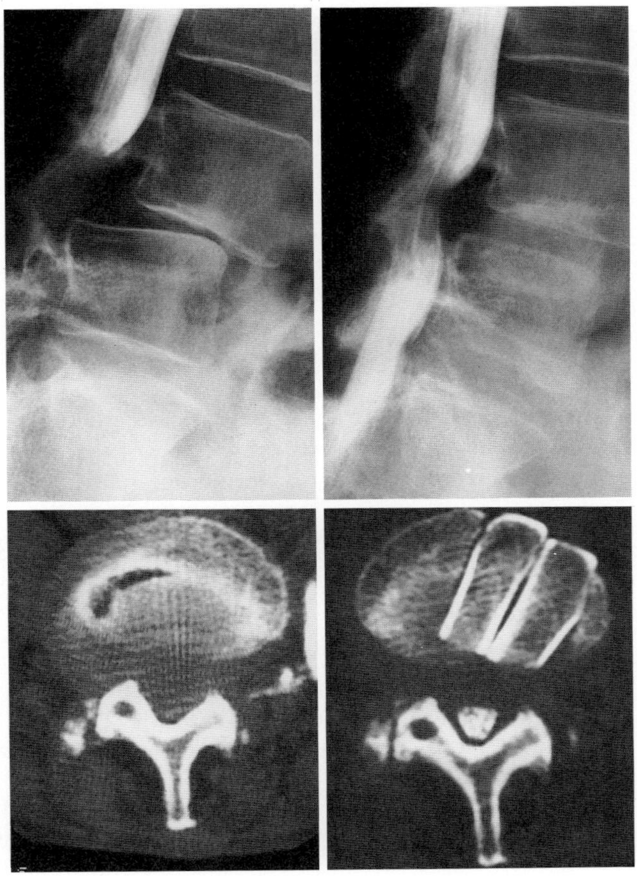

a b

Fig. 4a,b. Case 2. **a** Preoperative myelogram and computed tomographic myelogram of a 50-year-old woman with degenerative spondylolisthesis of the fourth lumbar vertebra. **b** Postoperative myelogram and computed tomographic myelogram in the same patient

Case 2. A 50-year-old woman with systemic lupus erythematosus and degenerative spondylolisthesis of the fourth lumbar vertebra had a 7-year history of low back pain and numbness of the lower extremities bilaterally. Ambulation was limited to 10 m at time of admission. Neurologic examination revealed involvement of the fifth lumbar roots bilaterally. Flexion-extension radiographs disclosed significant instability at the level of slippage. Figure 4 shows pre- and postoperative myelograms and computed tomographic myelograms. Postoperatively, complete blockage of the subarachnoid space was relieved, and the patient's intermittent claudication disappeared. The JOA score increased from 13 to 24 points.

Discussion

Since degenerative spondylolisthesis has been classified as a type of lumbar spinal canal stenosis, surgery generally has been performed using a posterior approach. However, the stenosis is mainly due to structural changes at a single level caused by forward slippage of a lumbar vertebra with an intact neural arch. In addition, patients can have dynamic instability at the level of slippage [6]. Herkowitz and Kurz [7] reported that concomitant intertransverse-process arthrodesis provided better results than decompressive laminectomy alone, proving the importance of stabilization in the treatment of degenerative spondylolisthesis.

The benefit of an anterior approach is attainment of neural decompression and stabilization of unstable segments simultaneously without any damage to the neural tissues in the canal or back muscles. This procedure is not indicated for patients with multilevel involvement or patients with severe stenosis. At present we do not use this procedure in patients with perineal symptoms or signs.

This study suggests that, in general, patients of up to about 60–65 years old can expect satisfactory results irrespective of their age at surgery. Deterioration of the JOA score probably is due to age-related phenomena, such as general weakness.

Anterior decompression and interbody fusion is a treatment that can provide good long-term results for patients with degenerative spondylolisthesis.

References

1. Inoue S, Watanabe T, Goto S, Takahashi K, Takata K, Sho E (1988) Degenerative spondylolisthesis, pathophysiology and results of anterior interbody fusion. Clin Orthop 227:90–98
2. Takahashi K, Kitahara H, Yamagata M, Murakami M, Takata K, Miyamoto K, Mimura M, Takahashi Y, Moriya H (1990) Long-term results of anterior interbody fusion for treatment of degenerative spondylolisthesis. Spine 15:1211–1215

3. McCulloch JA, Inoue S, Moriya H, Takahashi K, Takata K (1990) Surgical indications and techniques. In: Weinstein JN, Wiesel SW (eds) The lumbar spine. Saunders, Philadelphia pp 407–414
4. Izumida S, Inoue S (1986) Assessment of treatment for low back pain (in Japanese). J Jpn Orthop Assoc 60:391–394
5. Kaplan EL, Meier P (1958) Nonparametric estimation from incomplete observations. J Am Stat Assoc 53:457–481
6. Mimura M (1990) Rotational instability of the lumbar spine, a three-dimensional motion study using bi-plane X-ray analysis system (in Japanese). J Jpn Orthop Assoc 64:546–559
7. Herkowitz HN, Kurz LT (1991) Degenerative lumbar spondylolisthesis with spinal stenosis. J Bone Joint Surg [Am] 73:802–808

2.7 Clinical Results of Lumbar Fusion for Heavy Workers with Lumbar Disk Herniation

Shunji Matsunaga, Takashi Sakou, Kazunori Yone, Eiji Taketomi, Tamotsu Morimoto, and Kosei Ijiri[1]

Introduction

Diskectomy has been the most frequently used surgical treatment for lumbar disk herniation. Although this operation has achieved good results in many cases, it has been reported that about 10%–20% of all cases require reoperation [1–5].

In past assessments of the operative results for patients with lumbar disk herniation, patients with various activity levels were collectively evaluated. [1,6,7]. For this reason, differences in the activity levels among individual cases affected the assessment of operative results and made it impossible to compare the operative results among different studies.

It is still controversial whether or not lumbar fusion should be combined with diskectomy [2,6–9]. With heavy workers, the most important decision in the surgical treatment of this disease is whether or not fusion of the lumbar spine should be combined with diskectomy. Dvorak et al. have reported that conventional diskectomy alone does not provide satisfactory treatment for these workers [1]. Therefore, we recently analyzed whether, and to what extent, the combination of lumbar fusion with diskectomy would allow heavy workers to return to their original occupations.

Materials and Methods

We studied 40 patients with lumbar disk herniation who underwent diskectomy combined with lumbar fusion. Posterolateral fusion with a Knodt rod was done in 37 patients and anterior fusion with a Kaneda device was done in 3 patients. Complete bone union was achieved in all cases. Of these 40 patients, 10 received fusion of the lumbar spine during the primary operation. The remain-

[1] The Department of Orthopaedic Surgery, Faculty of Medicine, Kagoshima University, 8-35-1 Sakuragaoka, Kagoshima, 890 Japan

ing 30 underwent conventional diskectomy alone during the primary operation and later required one or more reoperations because of poor results. These 30 patients [multiply operated back (MOB) patients] were given fusion of the lumbar spine during reoperation.

The site of herniation was the L4–L5 space in 31 patients, L5–S1 in 10 patients, and L3–L4 in 1 patient. Herniation of multiple intervertebral spaces was observed in 2 patients. The level of lumbar fusion was L4 through S1 in 31 patients, L3 through S1 in 5, and L3 through L5 in 1. Anterior fusion of L5–S1 was performed in 3 patients and the same fusion of L4–5 in 1. Although adjacent segments had no abnormalities causing lumbago before surgery, L5–S1 disks that concentrated the mechanical stress were also fused to prevent postoperative problems – instability, recurrence of herniation, degenerative change, and so on. The postoperative follow-up period ranged from 1 to 12 years, with a mean period of 5 years.

The patients included 31 males and 9 females. Their ages at operation ranged from 21 to 61 years with a mean age of 36.9 years. The patients were divided into heavy and light work groups. The heavy work group included patients engaged in agriculture, fishing, construction and other manual labor. The heavy work group consisted of 24 patients. The light work group consisted of 16 patients engaged in office work and housekeeping.

Although the most frequent preoperative symptom was lumbago in both the primary operation group and the MOB group, there was no evidence of degenerative spondylotic changes and instability during clinical and roentgenographical examination. In addition, sciatica and sensory disturbances were also noted. Muscle weakness and bladder dysfunction were rare (Fig. 1).

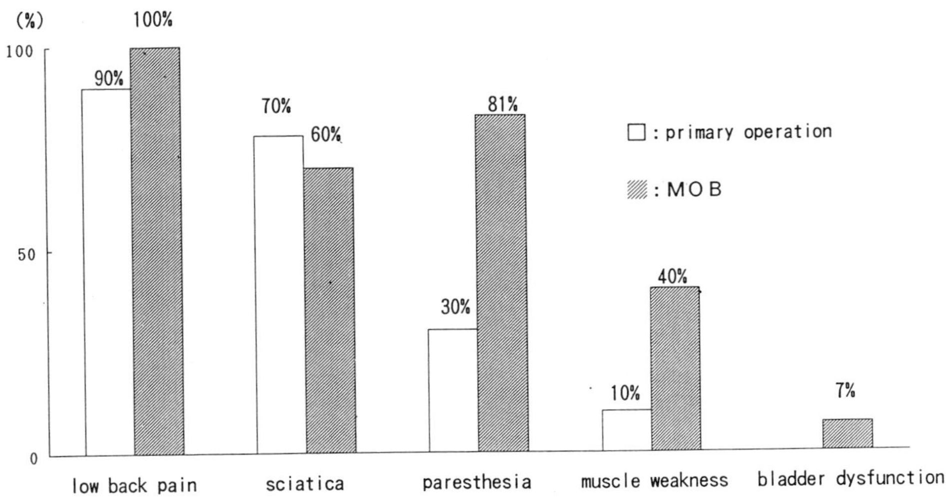

Fig. 1. Subjective symptoms before operation

To compare the outcome of lumbar fusion and diskectomy to diskectomy only, 19 patients who engaged in heavy work and underwent only the conventional diskectomy in our clinic were also studied.

The parameters examined include the degree of improvement in clinical symptoms, the percentage of patients who were able to return to their original occupations, and factors which affected the operative results. Radiographical assessments of the degeneration of the adjacent motion segment was also done. Narrowing of the intervertebral space and instability was examined. Instability was assessed in accordance with the criteria of Nachemson [10]. Patients were also examined for the presence or absence of psychological abnormalities using the Maudsley Personality Inventory [11].

Results

Improvements in lumbago were graded on a four-grade scale: excellent, when lumbago completely disappeared and no further medication was required; good, when there were occasional complaints of lumbago and medication was required; fair, when there were frequent complaints of lumbago; and poor, when there was no change or when the lumbago became worse. In the primary operation group, 90% of all cases were rated as excellent or good. In the MOB group, 71% showed some improvement.

To assess the rate of return to work, patients were graded on a four-grade scale: excellent, when the patient returned to his previous occupation without disability; good, when the patient resumed work with slightly reduced activity; fair, when the patient had to switch to light work because of disability; and poor, when the patient could not resume work and continued to receive treatment. In the primary operation group, all heavy workers returned to their original work levels. In the MOB group, 60% resumed heavy work. In contrast, only 53% (10/19) were able to return to heavy work after conventional diskectomy (Fig. 2).

When the relationship between return to original occupation and age was analyzed, return to heavy and light work was found to be more frequent among younger patients (Fig. 3).

In the analysis of the relationship between return to the patient's original occupation and the presence or absence of psychological abnormalities, all heavy workers with psychological abnormalities and 60% of light workers with psychological abnormalities were rated as fair or poor (Fig. 4). This result suggests that psychological factors also greatly affect the postoperative resumption of the previous occupation.

The incidence of narrowing of the adjacent intervertebral spaces and the incidence of instability were not high, being 5% and 10%, respectively. However, these incidences increased with time, indicating the necessity of long-term follow-up.

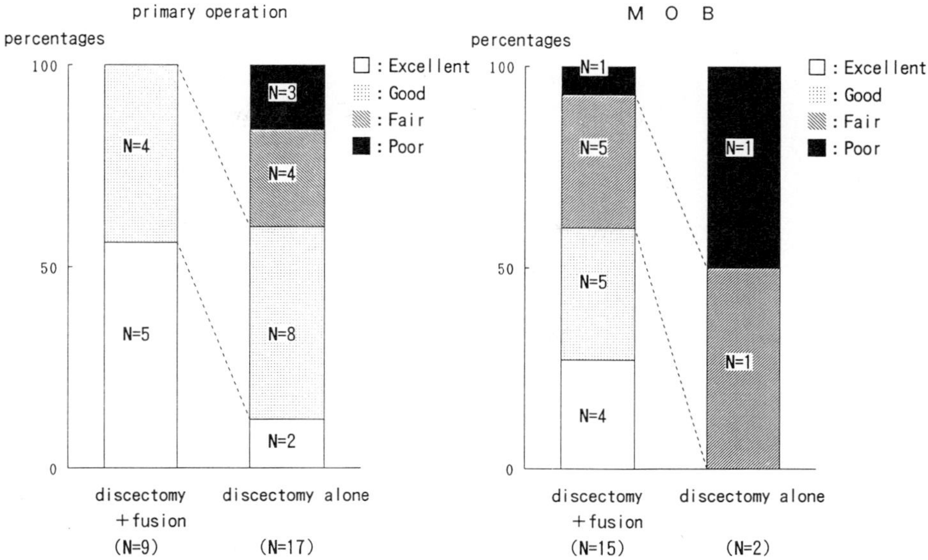

Fig. 2. Rate of return to heavy work

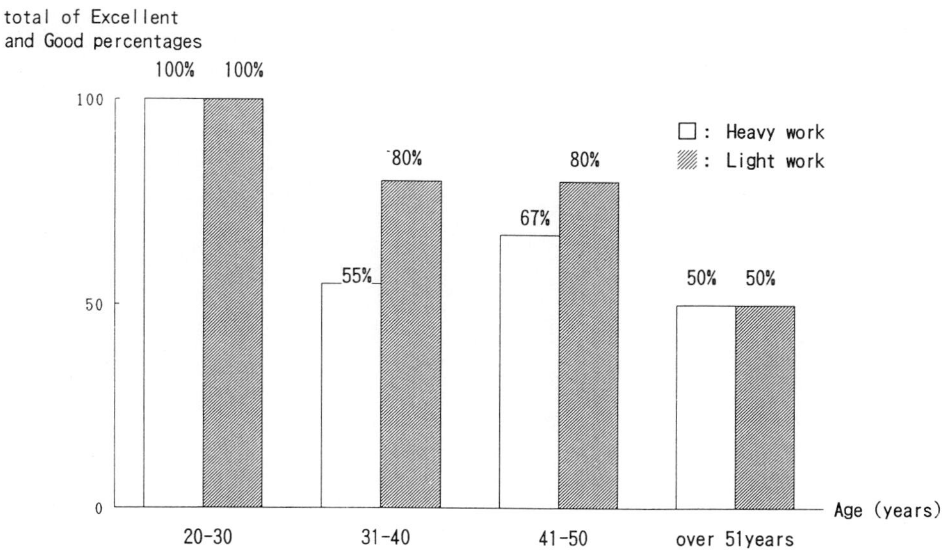

Fig. 3. Relationship between return to original work and age

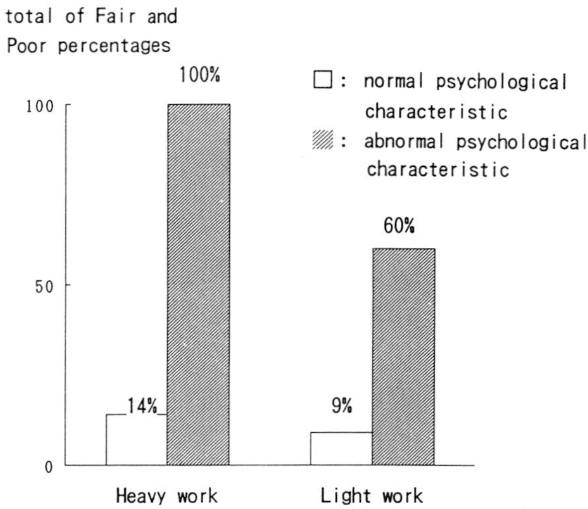

Fig. 4. Relationship between return to original work and psychological abnormalities

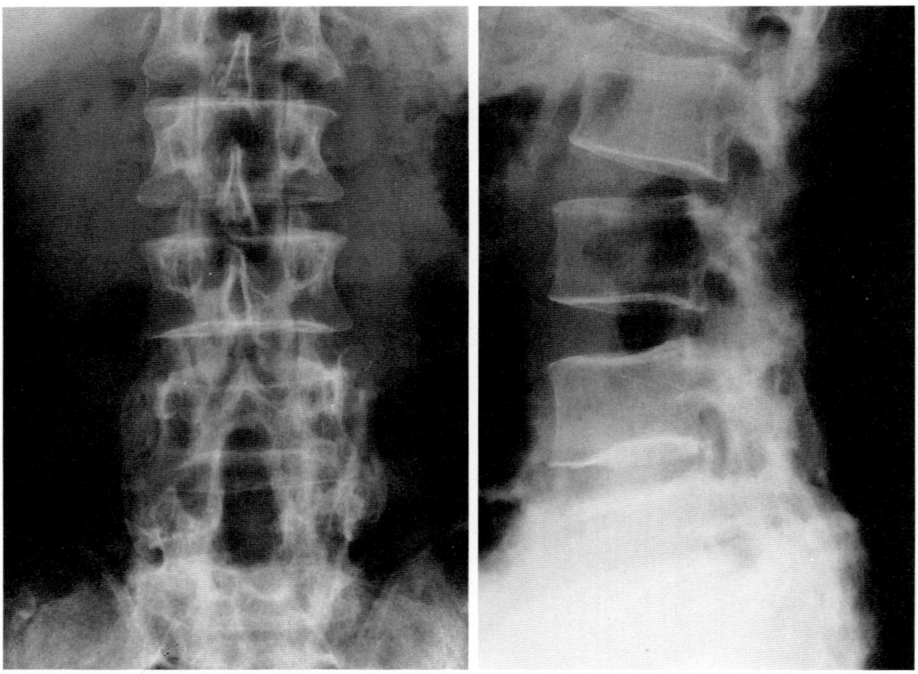

Fig. 5. 37-year-old farmer in the MOB group. Final X-ray after 5 years

Case Report

A 37-year-old farmer in the MOB group. This patient underwent laminectomy of the fifth lumbar vertebra and posterolateral fusion of L4–S1. One year after his operation, the patient returned to his original occupation. Postoperative X-ray revealed good bone union and well preserved physiological lordosis of the lumbar spine 5 years after surgery. No degeneration of the adjacent motion segment was recognized (Fig. 5).

Discussion

Whether or not to fuse the lumbar spine in association with disk excision still remains a controversial issue. The results of disk excision alone versus disk excision with primary fusion has been compared by many investigators [2,6–9]. The long-term study by Frymoyer et al. demonstrates a high percentage of unsatisfactory results in patients who had had either simple disk excision, or disk excision combined with spinal fusion [2]. Each of these studies demonstrated a slight but statistically insignificant benefit from combined fusion and disk excision.

One of the most important factors affecting the operative results in lumbar disk herniation is the patient's activity level. Frymoyer et al. summarized that patients engaged in heavy manual labor had significantly more postoperative back pain than patients performing light jobs, whether they underwent spinal fusion or not [2]. In patients who had initial spinal fusion, the most common source of failure is pseudarthrosis. However, since the study by Frymoyer et al., the improvement of internal fixation devices provides a higher rate of fusion. Therefore, the clinical results of lumbar fusion in patients engaged in heavy manual labor should be reconfirmed. The solid fusion may provide satisfactory results for patients engaged in heavy manual labor. Our findings of excellent results in patients engaged in heavy manual labor confirmed the effectiveness of lumbar fusion.

We disagree with Vaughan et al., who recommend routine fusion on all primary L4-L5 disk excisions to protect late segmental instability after disk excision alone [9]. In determining the indication of lumbar fusion in cases of lumbar disk herniation, we have to consider the patient's activity level, age, muscle power, degree of spinal degeneration, and psychological factors. Although lumbar fusion should be done in all MOB patients [12,13], whether or not to fuse the lumbar spine in primary cases should be decided after careful consideration of these factors.

Psychological characteristics of the patients have considerable relevance to the outcome [1]. It is well established from the study by Wiltse and Roshio that patients with personality correlates of hysteria, depression, hypochondriasis, and somatization have poorer outcome than those who do not have these personality traits [14]. The data presented here are similar to that study. Psychological factors need to be considered in selecting therapy.

Lehmann et al. recently presented a retrospective review of the incidence of pathologic conditions of the free motion segment adjacent to the lumbosacral fusion and concluded that accelerated degeneration at the free segment above the lumbosacral fusion is found on roentgenographic evaluation but is seldom associated with serious clinical symptoms [15]. On the other hand, Lee reported that the pathologic conditions at the adjacent segment may produce significant clinical problems [16]. Application of a rigid internal fixation system is predicted to produce additional amounts of stress concentration at the adjacent segment by increased stiffness of the fused segment and by posterior displacement of the center of rotation at the adjacent segment. In this study, although the incidence of degenerative change of the adjacent motion segment was 10%, no new symptoms arising from the adjacent segment developed within the average 5-year follow-up. We need more long-term follow-up study about the pathological change of the adjacent unfused segments.

Conclusions

1. We applied lumbar fusion along with diskectomy to patients with lumbar disk herniation and surveyed their return to work.
2. Return to the original heavy work load was possible for all patients in the initial operation group and for 60% in the MOB group.
3. Operative results seemed to be affected not only by the patient's age and muscle power but also by psychological factors.
4. Patients who engaged in heavy work can more effectively return to work through the combination of diskectomy and lumbar fusion.

References

1. Dvorak J, Gouchart W, Valach L (1988) The outcome of surgery for lumbar disc herniation. I. A 4–17 years' follow-up with emphasis on somatic aspects. Spine 13:1418
2. Frymoyer JW, Hanley E, Howe J, Kuhlmann D, Matteri R (1978) Disc excision and spine fusion in the management of lumbar disc disease: A minimum ten years follow-up. Spine 3:361
3. Hurme M, Alaranta T, Torma T, Einolas S (1983) Operated lumbar disc herniation: Epidemiological aspects. Ann Chir Gynaecol 72:33
4. Nashold BS, Blaine S (1971) Lumbar disc disease: a twenty year clinical follow-up study. Mosby, St. Louis
5. Naylor A (1974) Late results of laminectomy for lumbar disc prolapse: A review of ten to twenty-five years. J Bone Joint Surg [Br] 56:17
6. Barr JS, Kubik GS, Molloy MK (1967) Evaluation of end results in treatment of ruptured lumbar intervertebral disc with protrusion of nucleus polposus. Surg Gynecol Obstet 125:250

7. Young HH, Love GJ (1959) End results of removal protruded lumbar intervertebral discs with and without fusion. Am Acad Orthop Surg Instruct Course Lect 16:213
8. Nachlas IW (1952) End-result study of treatment of herniated nucleus polposus by excision with fusion and without fusion. J Bone Joint Surg [Am] 34:981
9. Vaughan PA, Malcolm BW, Maistrelli GL (1988) Results of L4–L5 disc excision alone versus disc excision and fusion. Spine 13:690
10. Nachemson A (1981) The role of spine fusion. Spine 6:306
11. Jensen AR (1958) The Maudsley personality inventory. Acta Psychol 14:314
12. Wiesel SW (1985) The multiply operated lumbar spine. Am Acad Orthop Surg Instruct Course Lect 34:68
13. Yashiro K, Hokari Y, Katsumi Y (1991) Necessity of the spinal fusion in salvage operation for the operated lumbar disc herniation (in Japanese). Orthop Surg 42:1495
14. Wiltse LL, Roshio PD (1975) Preoperative psychological tests as predictors of success of chemonucleolysis in the treatment of low-back syndrome. J Bone Joint Surg [Am] 57:478
15. Lehmann TR, Spratt KF, Tozzi JE, Weinstein JN, Reinarz ST, El-Khoury GY, Colby H (1987) Long-term follow-up of lower lumbar fusion patients. Spine 12:97
16. Lee CK (1988) Accelerated degeneration of the segment adjacent to a lumbar fusion. Spine 13:375

2.8 Multi-Segmental Spondylosis: An Overview of Presentations at the Fifth International Conference on Lumbar Fusion and Stabilization

J. Kostuik[1]

The papers presented to the Fifth International Conference on Lumbar Fusion and Stabilization in this session on multi-segmented spondylosis were essentially divided into two groups. These include the treatment of multi-segmental instability and the treatment of degenerative lumbar scoliosis and kyphosis.

The paper presented by Professor Walter Dick of Basel, Switzerland, on patient selection for stabilization of multi-segmental stenosis, approaches the problem primarily from a psychosocial point of view. The authors acknowledge that a long lumbar spine fusion is followed inevitably by some degree of functional impairment and residual pain. They emphasize the importance of subjective assessment by the patient. The importance of correlating this with the patient's aims and place in society is also emphasized. What is good for patient A may not necessarily be the same for patient B. The authors define criteria for a successful outcome as no expectation of returning to heavy manual labor. Compensation and other third-party insurance problems should be resolved prior to surgery. In fact, they state no one should be expected to return to work who has to undergo multi-segmental instrumentation. The restoration of a reasonable goal in independence in activities of daily living should be the aim of treatment. Age is not a contraindication, and surgery should be performed only when non-operative modalities of treatment have failed to achieve a suitable aim. They further state osteoporosis is not a contraindication to fusion. As well, the operative team must be fully familiar in dealing with complex problems of multi-segmental instability, particularly in the elderly.

We would not agree with the point of view that returning to work is impossible following multi-segmental stabilization. In our own experience, we

[1]Department of Orthopaedic Surgery, Johns Hopkins Outpatient Center, Fifth Floor, Rm 5231, 601 North Caroline Street, Baltimore, MD 21287-0882, USA

have encountered, in separate series, up to 40% of such people being able to return to their full-time occupation.

It is unfortunate that, although the criteria, nine in number, are given by the authors, no rating system is applied.

Unfortunately, the numbers treated are small and variable and there is only a short-term follow-up. The authors do not give us any results in terms of outcome, except to state that the self-rating by the patient was excellent to good in 19 of 22 patients. This in itself is excellent, but I think the criteria are not adequately defined. The author notes screw loosening in five patients. In our experience, this may mean pseudoarthrosis.

Unfortunately, the paper suffers from being philosophical rather than being factual and providing us with outcome for patients requiring stabilization for multi-segmental disease.

Drs. Steffee and Enker, et al. provide us with their vast experience dealing with multi-level degenerative disease by their techniques.

A large number, 90 patients in total, underwent operative intervention, with 48 having a minimum of 2 years follow-up. It is unfortunate the full group could not be described. Thirty-nine of these 48 patients had undergone previous surgery.

This is a good paper which describes the technique accurately.

The only difficulty with reference to the surgical technique is the fact that, in assessing the results, lordosis overall was reduced, which in my experience in multi-segmental disease can often lead to deformity, resulting in bent forward or so-called flat back syndrome. Their average lordosis preoperatively was 58 degrees and 43 degrees at follow-up. Unfortunately, they did not describe how many patients did have a flat back syndrome. The authors describe cement supplementation to enhance pedicle screw purchase in 17 of 49 patients but do not describe the technique of doing this. They state that no local complications were noted. Application of cement to the pedicle is likely to lead, in a number of cases, to neurological problems, as up to 20% of pedicles do have deficiency as a result of screw placement, which may allow bone cement to exude into the canal. This can be overcome by passing an angled curette through the pedicle into the vertebral body, evacuating part of the vertebral body, and then passing a catheter into the vertebral body by the pedicle and injecting 2–3 cc of liquid bone cement into the vertebral body, thus avoiding direct placement of the cement in the pedicle. This tip of the screw will then fix into the bone cement, which then acts as a plug.

The authors admit their procedure as described is technically difficult, particularly doing a posterior lumbar interbody fusion in someone with previous surgery, which, in my estimation, can have a high degree of morbidity in terms of root involvement and neurological complications.

In terms of lordosis, although this was within physiological limits and the authors state that Stagnera stated that, in normal volunteers, the maximal lordotic curve is 50 degrees, this has not been true in our experience and it depends how lordosis is measured.

In our experience, any decrease in lordosis, unless the patient is significantly hyperlordotic, may result in difficulties in terms of posture. The authors report a satisfactory result in 83% of primary cases and 67% of revision cases and state this is comparable to single level instability. This is a high degree of success.

This paper represents a variety of patients, including those with degenerative scoliosis, degenerative spondylolisthesis, failed back surgery, and primary surgery, and it is difficult to break down and truly analyze the success in the various subgroups. The authors describe their paper in terms of percentages, which, if broken down into the 49 patients followed for more than 2 years, would render some of these subgroups very small and would probably mean that the results were not statistically significant. Although the authors state a high degree of success, they state this can be improved by further use of discographic evaluation. In their protocol, however, they stated they did descriptive discography of the affected levels. This does not correlate.

Of the patients reported in their Table 1, it is difficult to ascertain how many actually had multi-level fusions. Generally multi-level is meant to include more than two levels.

Drs. Nakai et al. provided an interesting paper on posterior stabilization for lumbar degenerative kyphosis utilizing types of fusion in maximum extension on a Hall frame. The problem as described seems to be unique to people of Japanese origin. Thirteen patients were reviewed, ranging in age from 39 to 71 years, with an average age of 60 years. The majority were female. All patients were described as being osteoporotic, yet it is unusual to find any significant degree of osteoporosis in the younger age groups described here. It is unfortunate that bone density measures were not made.

In all cases, the kyphosis was flexible, which therefore made it more amenable to correction using a posterior tension band principle.

The authors do describe two types of kyphosis, that in the lower lumbar spine and that in the upper lumbar spine.

The number of segments fused was variable, ranging from five to one segment, and the total number of patients was only 13. It is my feeling that, in the lower lumbar type, a more extensive fusion may have been of greater value, as it is my feeling that not enough lordosis was restored. As a result, the level above the fusion may be at risk of developing compression fracture, which is known to occur in between 11 and 20% of people with osteoporosis proximal to a fusion, unless a patient is fully rebalanced. This did happen in one case described in this paper. Regardless, this paper is of interest, particularly as we deal with an aging population with increasing osteoporosis. The authors should be encouraged to develop greater numbers, to incorporate bone density, and to subdivide their groups into number of levels of fusion, and outcome in terms of societal function, related both to the upper and lower lumbar kyphosis-type problems.

Professor Takemitsu, et al., have described the operative treatment for lumbar degenerative kyphosis using a variety of techniques. This is also an interesting paper and again describes a problem peculiar to the Japanese population, to a large degree. The authors describe three methods, including a posterior approach involving multi-level shortening, osteotomy and fusion with instrumentation associated with decompressive laminectomy, an anterior approach, and a combined approach. Again, the number of cases was small, with three, two, and three being reported for the various techniques described above. Unfortunately, the degree of flexibility of the kyphosis was not described preoperatively. The best results were obtained with the combined anterior and posterior approach. The authors state that the patient should be less than 65 years of age. We feel surgery should not be denied on the basis of age if the patient is otherwise healthy and the appropriate surgical team is available. The authors noted that decompression was important to perform if there were neurological symptoms as well as painful deformity present.

In the treatment of kyphotic deformity, posterior tension band, unless the curve is flexible, will often fall.

In these older age groups, it would be surprising if the majority were flexible. Anterior interbody fusion without either anterior instrumentation or supporting second-stage posterior tension band will fail, since many of the grafts will collapse into the osteoporotic bone, or may themselves collapse. As a result, the combined procedures had the best results, which is not surprising.

The final two papers in this section dealt with degenerative lumbar scoliosis. This is a problem increasing in magnitude as our population lives to a greater age, and it is particularly associated with a high degree of neurological symptoms in approximately two-thirds of cases, secondary to associated spinal stenosis.

Both these papers, by Dr. Toyama of Keio University, Japan, and Dr. Moon et al., of the Catholic University Medical College of Seoul, Korea, provide excellent descriptions of the problems of degenerative lumbar scoliosis.

Dr. Toyama describes lateral translation.

Although there is some degree of lateral translation, most of the changes, in my feeling, are essentially rotational in nature in degenerative scoliosis, although there is no doubt there is more translation in degenerative scoliosis than would occur in adult idiopathic scoliosis.

Dr. Toyama is to be congratulated for having used the rating system and for having classified degenerative lumbar scoliosis into three types. These consist mainly of wedging of the disk at the L4 level with some changes at the L3 level, i.e., mild scoliosis; type two, with increased rotation and multiple level degenerative disease; and type three, of a more generalized and severe nature. This author has defined instability on the basis of changes from the supine to standing position, which is admirable.

Dr. Toyama has described a number of surgical techniques for his 23 patients, including decompression in only six patients, decompression and fusion in three patients, type two decompression in six patients, plus decompression and fusion in seven, and anterior fusion in one. There were no cases of type three patients included, which is unusual. It is my feeling that type two is simply an extension of type one, and type three probably represents the other two types as a result of progressive degeneration. The authors noted that, with curved magnitude over 25 degrees, the curve progressed with posterior decompression, and we would agree with this. Indeed this an important point. It is unfortunate in this excellent paper that the differentiation into the various subgroups of decompression plus decompression with fusion for types one and two was not analyzed more closely. Nor were indications given regarding why decompression only was done and why fusion was not incorporated in all or no cases. A variety of techniques using Luque instrumentation, as well as Cortrel-Dubousset (CD) instrumentation, were used, and obviously CD instrumentation showed significant improvement. The statistics for improvement, as defined by recovery rate using the scoring scale provided, would indicate no great differences between the various groups. Again, however, the numbers were somewhat small for the various subgroups and therefore do not have statistical validity.

If symptomatology is related to one root, then we feel single root decompression is warranted; however, if multiple roots require decompression, then stabilization of the entire curve that is flexible should be incorporated. If the curve is rigid, then limited stabilization may be of value.

With reference to the article by Drs. Moon and Lee, et al. on degenerative lumbar scoliosis, this is an excellent article. In general, review of the topic is well handled. Again, the number of patients is small, consisting only of 31 people. Unfortunately, only 11 patients were treated surgically for a minimum follow-up of 1 year. The authors have subdivided the patients, based on the severity of degenerative changes radiologically, into four groups, which renders the subgroups, again, extremely small and does not allow for comparison with other published material. Their criteria for operative intervention appeared to be uncontrollable radicular pain in 11 of the 31 patients presented. Five of the 11 underwent associated fusion with instrumentation in conjunction with decompression. Similarly to other authors, these authors noted increasing severity of radiological changes combined with increasing severity of deformity. The authors, in discussion of the results of their operative procedures, did not define the criteria by which success would be achieved, but it was noted that all patients had excellent to good results. This is extremely high for this complex type of problem. I note the number of levels fixed internally averaged two segments. The authors do not describe lumbar lordosis, either pre- or postoperatively, and considering most of these people have an associated kyphosis secondary to loss of disk height, one would be concerned about this fact. This article is essentially an excellent review of the literature, but provides little insight into what to do with these patients, how many levels to decompress, how many levels to fuse, or the influence of instrumentation on lordosis, which I find most essential information in order to provide adequate functional outcome.

Professor Tsuji, et al. discuss expansive laminoplasty for lumbar spinal stenosis. This is a procedure which is gaining show but steady popularity as a means of preserving stabilization in patients requiring decompression for lumbar spinal stenosis. Professor Tsuji is well known for his techniques of laminoplasty in the lumbar spine. Unfortunately, he has only treated 30 cases over 10 years, with adequate follow-up in 15 cases. The value of laminoplasty, in my estimation, is in decreasing scar epidurally, as well as providing a greater surface area for arthrodesis. There is no doubt that pedicle screw fixation could be added to this to increase stability. As the authors rightly point out, there are technical limitations to the procedure, as nerve root decompression on the hinge side is technically difficult. They recommend the nerve root on the hinged side be dealt with through decompressive laminectomy before laminar rotation. We are in agreement that this is a useful technique provided by Dr. Tsuji; it is one which we have been employing with increasing frequency over the years.

This series of articles presents a study of multi-segmental degenerative disease treated by multiple level arthrodesis, as well as problems related to lumbar degenerative kyphosis, problems commonly encountored in the Japanese population. Two papers on degenerative lumbar scoliosis, an increasing problem in our aging society, were also presented. These provided some insight into the surgical management, as well as the natural history of these problems. Unfortunately, an objective discussion of results was not provided in these two papers and the surgical care in all series was relatively small.

2.9 Patient Selection for Stabilization of Multisegmental Spondylosis

Walter Dick, Heinz Widmer, and Vincent J. Leone[1]

Introduction

Multilevel degenerative lumbar spine disease is one of the most difficult problems in lumbar spine surgery. We all know of patients with poor outcomes after surgery performed in an attempt to relieve pain. Too often we discover that the wrong intervention has been performed. We also recognize the functional and long-term disadvantages of multisegmental lumbar fusions [1], especially when they include the lumbosacral junction or induce a flatback [2].

Many attempts have been made to reduce the failure rate by better patient selection for operative treatment [3]. Extensive psychological assessment [4] and sophisticated imaging techniques, such as MRI with enhancement [5], CT-discography [6], thermography [7], as well as probatory external fixations [8–10], have shown with experience that in spite of their statistical value they are not fully reliable for each individual patient. In the end, decision-making for each patient relies on the clinical judgment and subjective impression of the surgeon.

Materials and Methods

We have tried to improve our operative results by deriving a clinical hypothesis from a different perspective: we acknowledge that a long lumbar spine fusion is followed inevitably by a certain amount of functional impairment, scarring, and residual pain. These potentially negative surgical sequelae may be viewed differently by a patient with severe spondyloarthropathy. The patient will rate his own health as good if the difference between his disability and pain before and after surgery is substantial. Secondly, the self-rating will be good if the expectations of the patient, his family, his employer, and his insurance carrier

[1] Orthopaedic Department, University of Basel, Felix Platter Spital, CH-4012 Basel, Switzerland

are met after surgery. Only realistic expectations can be fulfilled. It is true that these expectations may be clearly outlined by the surgeon, but they may also be misperceived. The subjective well-being of the patient is the only post-surgical rating that matters.

The importance of the patient's expectations can be seen in the following example. Patient A, a 40-year-old construction worker with degenerative spondyloarthropathy, is unable to work for 9 months due to leg and back pain. While at rest, he continues to have pain, but he can get along with occasional nonsteroid anti-inflammatory drugs (NSAID) and alternating between walking, sitting, and bedrest. Patient B, a 70-year-old woman also with the same disease but a much lower functional level, can walk 50 m and needs help to stand up and to dress herself in the morning. If we assume the same residual functional impairment and pain after a long lumbar fusion for both individuals, patient A will have a bad result. His improvement will not be dramatic because of a preoperative lower pain level while at rest. He will not be able to return to heavy construction work. Thus the expectation from either the patient, his family, his community, his employer or insurance carrier, or a combination of all of the above will not be met after surgery. Patient B, rather, will rate her postsurgical result as excellent since she will be able to go shopping by herself and dress herself (Fig. 1). For Patient B we are restoring an independent level of functioning in her community. This is further illustrated in Fig. 2.

The above cases point to the necessity of meeting the following criteria for a successful outcome in lumbar fusions of three or more levels:

1. Neither the patient, his family, his employer, nor his insurance carrier should expect the patient to return to heavy manual labor. This is out of the question due to the patient's age or degree of disability. Compensation and other insurance cases should be completely resolved prior to surgery. No one should expect to return to work.
2. Independence in activities of daily living is significantly impaired. Its restoration is a reasonable goal and should be the aim of treatment.
3. The patient is over 50 years of age. There is no upper age limit; the only restrictions are cardiovascular or other general health problems of the

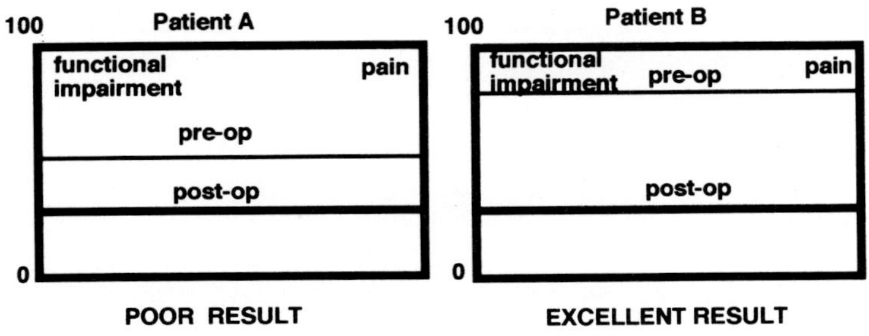

Fig. 1. The same outcome is viewed differently by patients with identical residual pain and functional impairment after multisegmental lumbar spine fusion

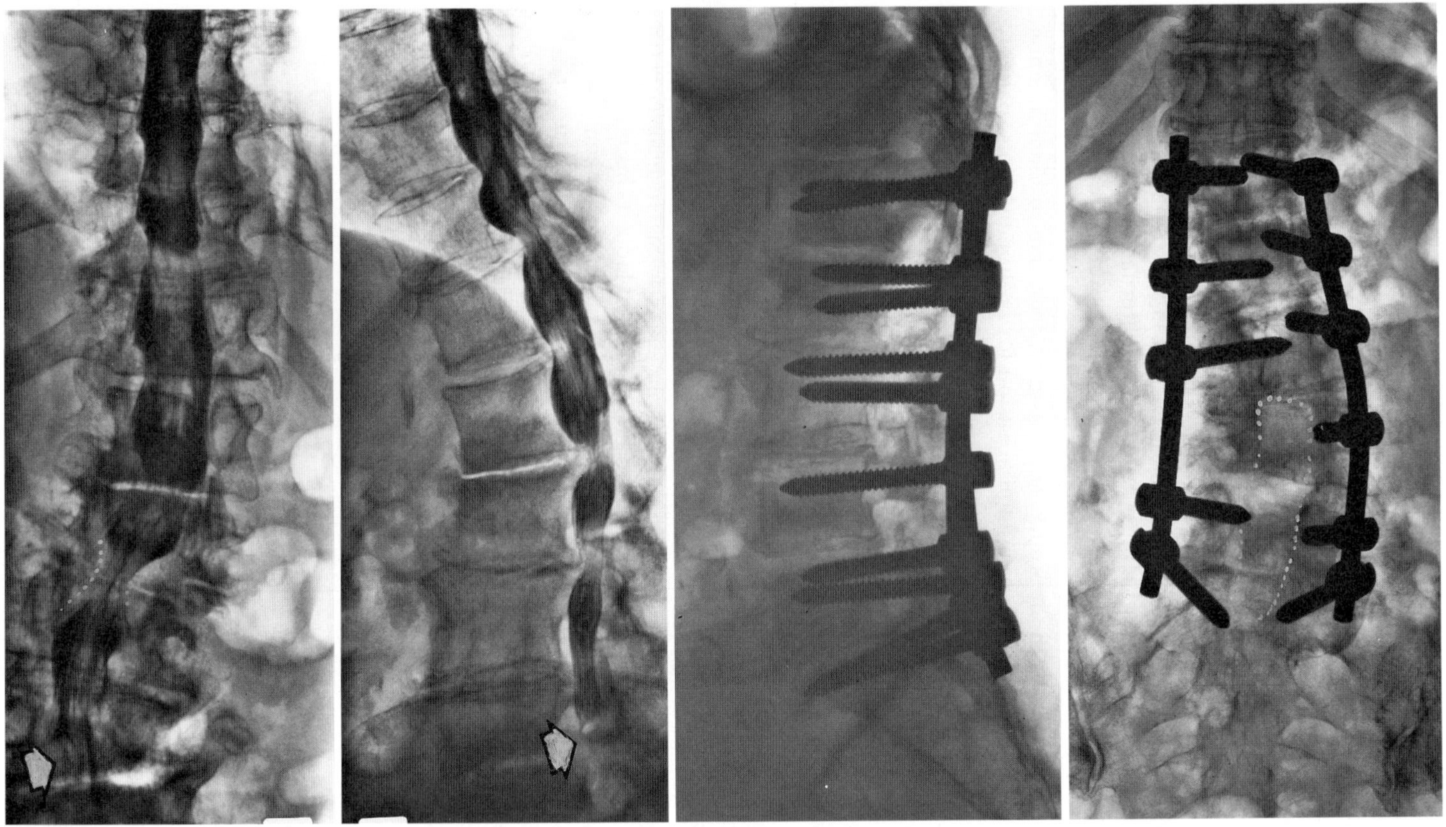

Fig. 2. A 73-year-old female with severe claudication and disabling constant pain. The patient was able to walk 10 meters with the aid of two persons, displayed trunk disequilibrium, and was narcotic dependent. At 1 year postoperative after pedicle instrumentation from L1 to S1 with laminectomy at L4–5 and flavectomy at L2–3, the patient was able to walk 2–3 km per day independently and took only nonsteroid anti-inflammatory drugs for pain. Self rating: excellent

patient. Early postoperative ambulation is always possible with adequate instrumentation, and this prevents postoperative complications by reducing bed confinement.

4. The patient suffers disabling constant pain and/or severe spinal claudication while at complete rest. Surgery should be performed when conservative treatment such as elastic braces, kinesitherapy, and weight control have been ineffective.
5. A surgically treatable finding is present and is the source of the disability and pain. This may be one or a combination of the following:
   a. Trunk imbalance
   b. Degenerative scoliosis, often with rotatory offset
   c. Spinal stenosis
   d. Kyphosis
   e. Multilevel instability
   f. Root entrapment in narrowed foramina
6. The predominance of leg or back pain is not as important as in a middle-aged patient with a herniated nucleus pulposis since the operative treatment addresses the causes of both problems.
7. Deformity, instability, and disk collapse are too severe for ligamentoplasties to ameliorate. Rigid stabilization is the only means of correction.
8. Osteoporosis (except for extreme cases), age, or previous surgery are not contraindications to long lumbar fusions. However, hip arthrodesis and cerebral palsy are contraindications to this operation.
9. The surgeon must be familiar with posterior lumbar instrumentation, which allows for three dimensional correction and solid immediate fixation. For these reasons we feel that pedicle-based instrumentation is mandatory.

Relying on these nine criteria is helpful when deciding whether or not to proceed with multisegmental operative treatment. A decision to operate may be made solely on careful evaluation of the patient's history, indepth clinical and functional examination, and plain radiographs. Bending films and MRI studies may be helpful preoperatively to determine the vertebral levels to be included in the lumbar fusion. As all degenerative changes may lead to spinal stenosis, additional decompressive measures may need to be included in a large percentage of patients. Myelography remains the single most predictive roentgenographic examination. It should be performed under axial load, distraction, flexion, and extension. Myelography aids in deciding whether reduction and distraction is sufficient in a given segment or whether canal decompression is necessary.

Results

From our outpatient clinic population 22 consecutive patients met the criteria outlined above and had lumbar instrumentation and fusion of three or more segments. They were followed prospectively for 1.5 years (range 6–36 months). There were 15 females and 7 males. The mean age was 63 years; ranging from 49 to 83 years. Four patients had Fixateur Interne instrumentation [11]; 18 had Spinefix instrumentation. Spinefix is a CD-like system currently under multicenter clinical investigation. In 14 cases, instrumentation was extended to the sacrum. In 14 cases, additional canal decompression was also performed. Five motion segments were instrumented in 6 patients, four segments in 9 patients, and three segments in 7 patients. The mean hospital stay was 26 days, ranging from 13 to 46 days. One patient died 4 months postoperatively due to myocardial infarction. All others are residing independently at home without the need for assistance in their daily living activities. All take regular local walks and have at least tripled their walking distance. Most have reached at least 2 km per day. All patients but one report pain relief as either significant or complete; the remaining patient reports moderate pain relief. Overall, the self-rating was excellent or good in 19 patients, fair in 2 and poor in none. All state that they have no regrets and would consent again to their operation.

The following complications were encountered. There was one loosening of the screw-rod connection, necessitating re-instrumentation 9 months postoperatively. There were two screw fatigue fractures, one at the level of S1 1 year after surgery, and the other at the level of L5 2 years after surgery. Both were not realized by the patients and did not interfere with their favorable outcomes. There were roentgenographic signs of screw loosening in 5 of 14 sacral instrumentations with no related pain problems. One patient had asymptomatic osteoporotic spontaneous vertebral compression fractures above the instrumented levels at 1 year's follow-up. There were no neurologic or vascular complications, and no infections.

Conclusion

In conclusion, there exists a well defined group of patients with severe disability and multilevel lumbar spondylosis which deserve operative treatment. The larger the disability, the better is the indication for surgery and a favorable subjective outcome. The improvement in the quality of life far outweighs the residual pain as well as the sequelae of long fusion surgery. It is very rare that these patients complain of postoperative stiffness. On the contrary, many of them report better mobility secondary to pain relief as they can now use the rest of their locomotive system more effectively and may find themselves able to pick up items from the floor. To date, loosening of the sacral screws did not affect the favorable outcomes encountered in this group of patients.

This group of patients is often considered surgically untreatable by general practitioners and the lay public alike and therefore are not generally referred to spine surgeons. They merit our attention.

References

1. Balderston RK, Winter RB, Moe JH (1986) Fusion to the sacrum for non-paralytic scoliosis in the adult. Spine 11:824–829
2. LaGrone MO, Bradford DS, Moe JH, Lonstein JE, Winter RB, Ogilvie JW (1988) Treatment of symptomatic flatback after spinal fusion. J Bone Joint Surg [Am] 70:569–580
3. Bigos SJ, Battié MC, Spengler DM, Fischer LD, Fordyce WE, Hansson TH, Nachemson AL, Wortley MD (1991) A prospective study of work perceptions and psychosocial factors affecting the report of back injury. Spine 16:1–6
4. Hazard RG, Fenwick JW, Kalisch SM, Redmond J, Reeves V, Reid S, Frymoyer JW (1989) Functional restoration with behavioral support. A 1-year prospective study of patients with chronic low back pain. Spine 14:157–161
5. Brant-Zawadzki M, Norman E (1982) Magnetic resonance imaging of the central nervous system. Raven, New York
6. Millette PC, Raymond J, Fontaine S (1990) Comparison of high-resolution CT with diskography in the evaluation of lumbar disk herniations. Spine 15:525–533
7. Hoffman RM, Kent DL, Deyo RA (1991) Diagnostic accuracy and clinical utility of thermography for lumbar radiculopathy: A meta-analysis. Spine 16:623–628
8. Esses ST, Botsford DG, Kostuik YP (1989) The role of external skeletal fixation in the assessment of low back disorders. Spine 14:594–601
9. Magerl F (1982) External skeletal fixation of the lower thoracic and lumbar spine. In: Uhthoff HK (ed) Current concepts of external fixation of fractures. Springer, Berlin, pp 353–366
10. Olerud S, Sjöström L, Karlstrom G, Hamberg M (1986) Spontaneous effect of increased stability of the lower lumbar spine in cases of severe chronic back pain: The answer of an external transpedicular fixation test. Clin Orthop 203:67–74
11. Dick W (1987) The "Fixateur interne" as a versatile implant for spine surgery. Spine 12:882–900

2.10 A Clinical Study of Degenerative Lumbar Scoliosis

Myung-Sang Moon, Kyu-Sung Lee, Chong-In Lim, Young-Bum Kim, and Heon-Sang Lee[1]

Introduction

There have been several epidemiologic studies showing that scoliosis is most common in the elderly over 50 years of age [1,2]. Vanderpool et al. reported that scoliotic curves in the elderly were due to osteoporosis or osteomalacia [3], but Robin found no direct correlation between the presence or progression of scoliosis and osteoporosis [2].

Although the etiology of elderly scoliosis is controversial, there is one form of adult onset lumbar curve secondary to severe degenerative disk disease with no evidence of previous scoliosis. Kostuik reviewed the thoracolumbar and lumbar curves of adult scoliosis [4]. He reported that the incidence of low back pain was 59%, which is approximately the same as that in the general population, and there was a high correlation between pain and degenerative changes in the apex of the curve or lumbosacral junction. Jackson et al. assessed back pain associated with adult idiopathic scoliosis and indicated that pain increases with age, is more frequent with compensatory lumbosacral fractional curves, and comes mainly from the concavity of the curves [5].

Even though it is not known whether the source of pain in adult scoliosis is diskogenic, mechanical or from degenerative facet arthritis, patients with degenerative lumbar curves frequently develop signs of compression of the neural canal caused by height loss in the disk space, facet hypertrophy, marginal osteophytes, and lateral translation of the body. In addition, patients usually have radicular pain and neurological claudication with advanced degenerative stenotic symptoms involving multiple levels of the lumbar spine [2,6–9]. Curves may progress in adulthood due to several factors, one of which is possibly disk degeneration. Robin reported that the increase in scoliotic curves in elderly patients ranged from 3° to 18°, with average of 7°, over a 10-year follow up period, but there was no direct relationship between scoliosis and degenerative changes [2].

[1] Department of Orthopaedic Surgery, Catholic University Medical College, 505 Ban-Po-Dong, Seo-Cho-Ku, Seoul, Korea

Epstein et al. described radiographic and clinical findings of degenerative lumbar scoliosis and effective relief of compressive neuropathy by surgical decompression [7]. However, there is no consensus concerning the site and length of decompression and the need for additional procedures such as fusion or deformity correction for the degenerative lumbar scoliosis. Benner and Ehni reviewed 14 cases of degenerative lumbar scoliosis in which decompression has provided good relief of the radicular symptoms, but they recommended that the procedure be augmented with spinal instrumentation and fusion where there are instances of increased postoperative instability [6]. Bradford recommended decompression and fusion for the stenotic symptoms of lumbar curvature in adult scoliosis because decompression alone increases instability and postoperative instability usually leads to recurrence of radicular pain from pedicular kinking and nerve root entrapment [10].

The purpose of this study is to clarify more precisely the clinical symptoms and extent of surgery required. We determined the locations of neural compression in degenerative lumbar scoliosis and assessed the curve progression related with the severity of degenerative changes. In addition, we analyzed the results of surgical intervention with degenerative lumbar curves and evaluated the need for additional fusion and instrumentation in combination with the decompressive procedure.

Materials and Methods

We reviewed 31 symptomatic elderly idiopathic scoliosis patients with degenerative lumbar curves that were referred over a period of 5 years. There were 23 females (75%) and 8 males (26.5%) ranging in age from 51 to 75 years with a mean of 63 years. Criteria for inclusion in this study were that the patient (1) was over 50 years of age, (2) had no associated congenital or developmental spinal anomalies, (3) had no compression fractures in the osteoporotic spine, and (4) had not undergone prior surgery. Patients were excluded if they had a history of scoliosis while they were young or if radiographic findings showed lateral vertebral wedging and alterations of the lamina suggesting that the patient had undiagnosed idiopathic scoliosis at a young age.

Clinical syndromes in 31 patients were reviewed based on history, physical examination, and radiographic findings including plain film and CT myelograms. The type, side, and location of the pain, and the site of neural compression were assessed from the patient history and neurological findings.

Posteroanterior and lateral radiographs of all patients were examined for the analysis of the direction, apex, and number of involved segments of the lumbar curve. The degree of scoliosis, kyphosis, and lordosis were measured by Cobb's method. Degenerative changes in the lumbar spine were evaluated and also graded on a scale of 1–4 modified from Jackson's criteria [11] (Table 1). To determine the location of neural compression, we analyzed the predominant site of radiographic changes in the degenerative process including disk space

Table 1. Grades of degenerative changes in the lumbar curve (modified from Jackson's criteria [11]).

Grade 1	Only mild disk narrowing with evidence of degenerative changes.
Grade 2	Moderate disk degeneration, end-plate sclerosis, osteophyte-associated slipping
Grade 3	Severe disk degeneration, sclerosis, osteophytic lipping, degenerative slipping, associated vertebral wedging
Grade 4	Marked disk degeneration, sclerosis, osteophytic lipping, slipping and vertebral body wedging

narrowing, unilateral traction spurs, facet hypertrophy, and lateral, anterior and posterior translation of vertebral bodies within the curve, as well as CT myelographic findings of stenosis of the neural canal and foramen. In addition, to investigate the course of progression of degenerative curves, curve progression was observed and the relationship between the degree of scoliosis and severity of degenerative changes, and the degree of scoliosis and the patients' age were analyzed statistically.

Among the 31 patients, 11 surgically treated patients were followed up for at least 1 year using a questionaire according to Gill's criteria. The levels and the number of segments included in surgical decompression were analyzed and the surgical result for each patient was reviewed to determine the preferable area and extent of surgery. According to the types of operation, the surgical results were compared between patients that underwent decompression only and patients that underwent decompression and additional fusion with instrumentation.

Results

Pain and Neurological Symptoms

All patients had low back pain of variable severity: 27 patients (87%) had back pain associated radicular pain or intermittent claudication and 4 patients (13%) had back pain only. In terms of location of the pain, 24 patients (77%) had radicular pain in the lower extremities: 14 had pain in the leg corresponding to the convex side of the primary curve (concave side of the compensatory curve), 4 had pain in the leg corresponding to the concave side of the primary curve, and 8 had pain on both sides. There were symptoms of neurogenic claudication in 13 patients (42%), and 12 patients (39%) had motor or sensory deficits. Of all patients, only 3 showed positive results in the Laseque test (Table 2).

Curve Features

All of the curves involved lumbar segments, except two curves extending to the lower thoracic spine, and none had compensatory thoracic curves. We recorded c-shaped primary lumbar curves over the sacrum in 18 patients (58%), and

Table 2. Clinical symptoms.

Clinical features	No. of patients (%)	Total
Low back pain		
Low back pain only	4 (13)	
Associated neuropathy	27 (87)	31 (100)
Radiating pain		
Convex side	12 (50)	
Concave side	4 (17)	
Both sides	8 (33)	24 (77)
Claudication	13	13 (42)
Motor and/or sensory		
Lower compensatory curve	7 (70)	
At the apex	3 (30)	10 (32)
Laseque test positive	3 (10)	3 (10)

Table 3. Curve features.

Curve pattern	No. of patients (%)
Shape of curve	
C-shape	18 (58)
S-shape	13 (42)
Direction of curve	
Right Side	17 (55)
Left Side	14 (45)
Apex of curve	
L2	5 (16)
L3	20 (65)
L4	6 (19)
Number of segments involved	
5	1 (3)
4	5 (16)
3	9 (26)
2	16 (55)
Mean: 2.8 segments	
Range: 2–5 segments	
Degree of curve	
11–20°	22 (70)
21–30°	8 (26)
31–40°	1 (4)
Mean: 16.4°	
Range: 10–32°	

short compensatory s-shaped lumbosacral half curves involving the segments above the 4th lumbar vertebra in 13 patients (42%). The curves were right-sided in 17 patients (55%) and left-sided in 14 patients (45%). The apex of the curve was located at the 2nd lumbar vertebra in 5 patients (16%), at the 3rd lumbar vertebra in 20 patients (65%), and at the 4th lumbar vertebra in 6 patients (19%). The number of segments involved ranged from 2 to 5 with an

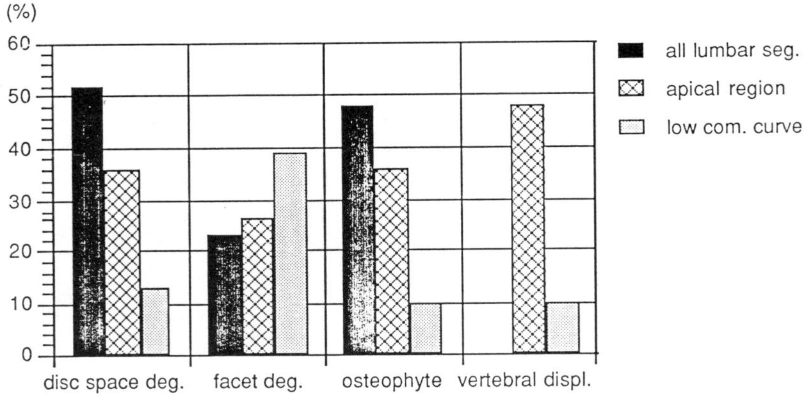

Fig. 1. Degenerative changes seen in plain radiographs. *Hatched area*, apical region; *dotted area*, lower compensatory curve; *solid area*, apical all lumbar segments

average 2.8 segments. The mean degree of curvature was 16.4°, ranging from 11° to 32°, and all curves were less than 40° (Table 3).

Degenerative Changes of Curvature

All 31 patients showed mild to severe degenerative arthritic changes in the lumbar curve. The severity of the degenerative changes were subdivided into 4 grades with grade 4 being the most severe: 7 patients (22%) were ranked grade 1; 13 patients (42%), grade 2; 9 patients (29%), grade 3; and 2 patients (6%), grade 4. Degenerative changes including unilateral height loss of disk space, formation of osteophytes, and facet hypertrophy were predominantly located over the concave side of the primary curve or compensatory curve. Height loss of disk space, seen in 16 patients (52%), and osteophyte formation, seen in 15 patients (48%), were commonly demonstrated over the lumbar segments, as seen in 15 patients (48%), but were more prominent at the apex, as seen in 11 patients (36%). However, facet hypertrophy was most common at the lower end of the primary curve or lower compensatory curve, as seen in 12 patients (39%). Lateral translations of vertebral bodies combined with or without forward or posterior displacement were commonly found at the apical region, as seen in 15 patients (48%), and infrequently at the lower end of curve, as seen in 3 patients (10%) (Fig. 1).

Fig. 2a–d. **a** X-ray of a 61-year-old male with mild left lumbar scoliosis. **b** Same patient at 66 years (5 years later) showing mild curve progression with mild degenerative changes. **c** X-ray of a 54-year-old female with mild right lumbar scoliosis. **d** Same patient at 61 years (7 years later) showing more progression of the curve than in the above case, with more advanced degenerative changes

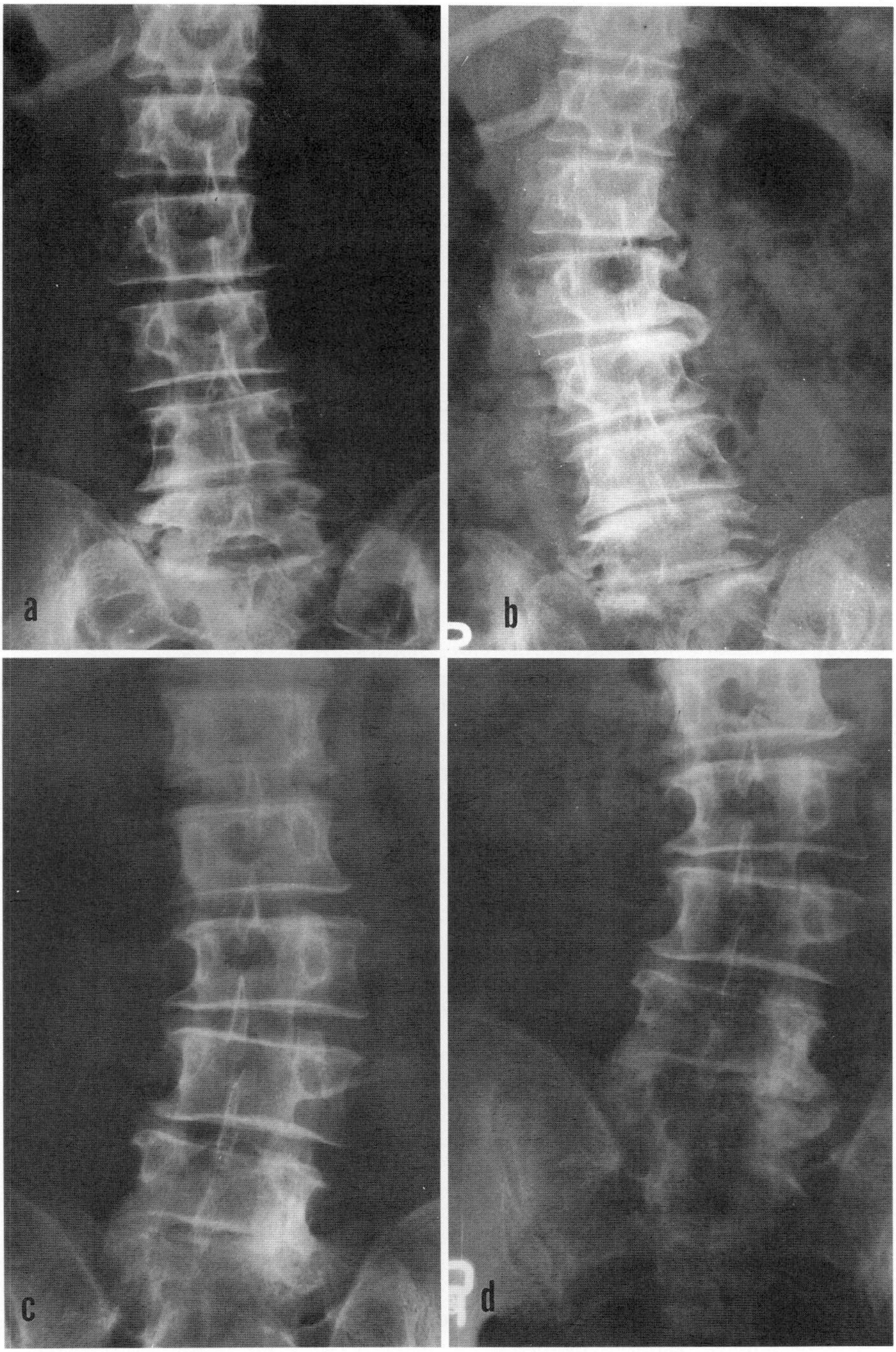
a
b
c
d

CT Myelographic Findings

CT myelography of 13 patients disclosed multiple level compression of the lumbar spinal canal as shown by the findings in the stenotic neural canal and in foraminal defects produced by osteophytes and facet hypertrophy. In 13 patients, 1 to 4 segments, were involved, with a mean of 2.1 segments, and in 9 of these 13 patients (69%), multiple levels of intervertebral disk spaces from the apex of the curve to the lower junctional area were involved. The most commonly involved levels were L4–5, as seen in 12 patients (92%), and L3–4, as seen in 8 patients (62%).

Curve Progression

Accurate determination of the rate of curve progression was impossible because long-term follow-up for all patients was not carried out except for with three patients who showed constant curve progression over a minimum follow-up period of 5 years (Fig. 2). Patients were grouped by age according to decades and the degree of curvature in each decade was studied. The mean degree for each decade was 15° (range 11°–22°) in 13 patients in the 6th decade, 16° (range 10°–25°) in 13 patients in the 7th decade, and 20° (range 11°–32°) in 5 patients in the 8th decade. The degree of curvature increased with increasing age but the results were not statistically significant ($P > 0.05$, $r = 0.28$).

The degree of curvature in each grade of degenerative change was studied. The mean degree of curvature was 13° (range 10°–22°) in 7 grade 1 patients, 15° (range 10°–26°), in 13 grade 2 patients, 18° (range 10°–25°) in 19 grade 3 patients, and 26° (range 20°–32°) in 2 grade 4 patients. The degree of curvature increased linearly with the severity of degenerative changes and the results were statistically significant ($P < 0.01$, $r = 0.45$) (Fig. 3). However, the data of

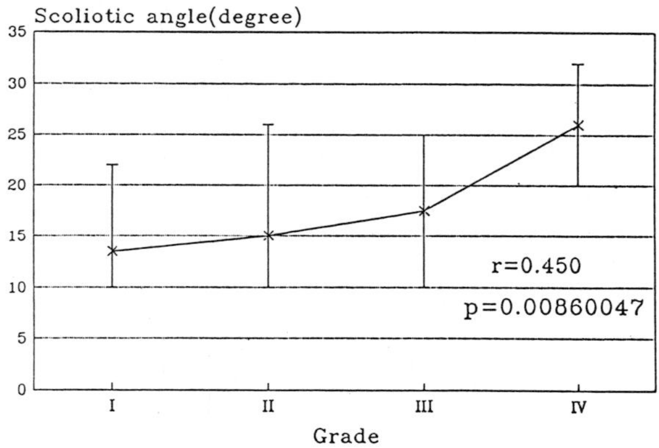

Fig. 3. Scoliotic angle versus degenerative change. The degree of curvature in degenerative lumbar scoliosis increased significantly with the grade of degenerative changes. $P = 0.00860047$; $r = 0.450$

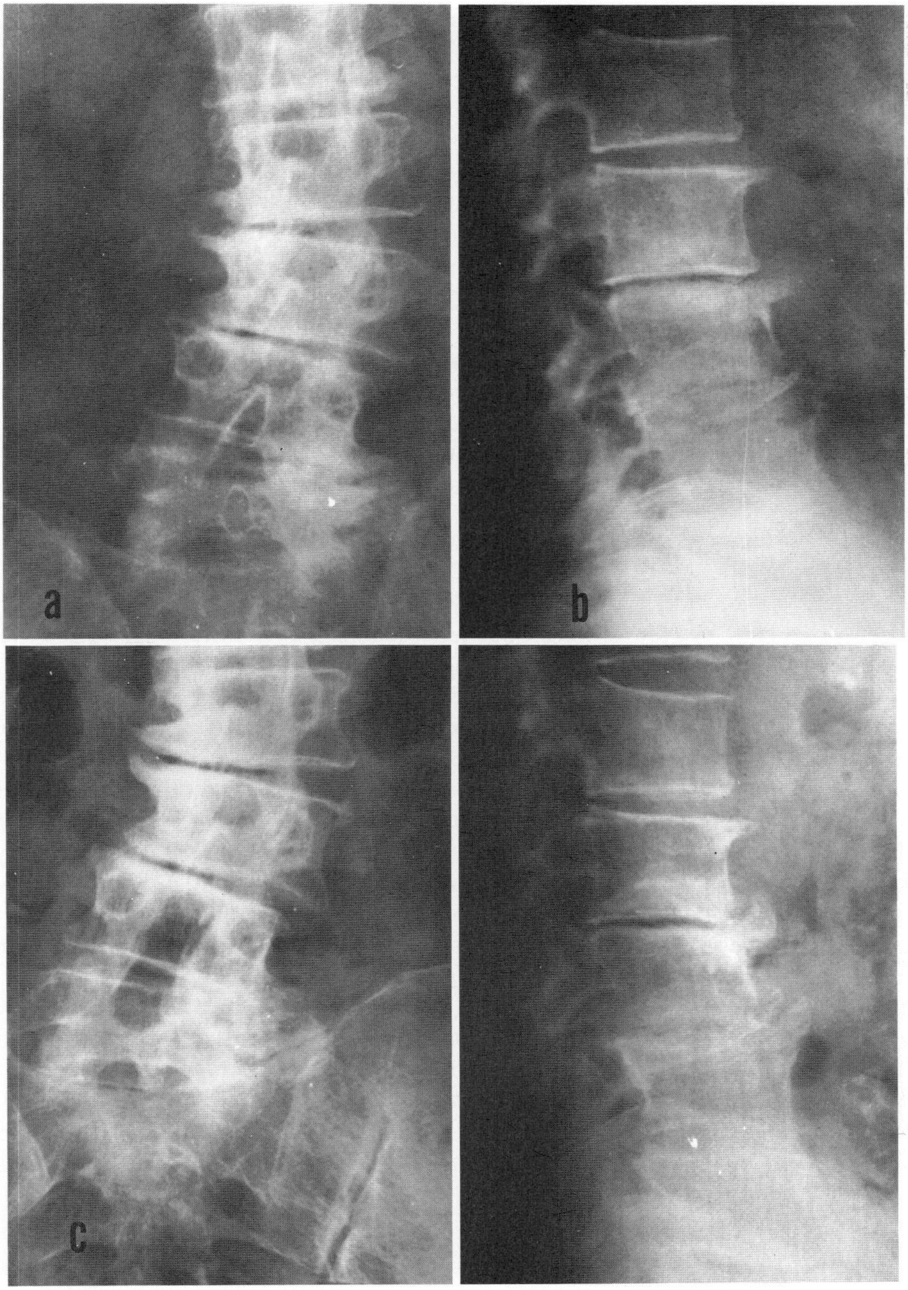

Fig. 4a–d. a,b X-rays of a 63-year-old female patient who underwent laminectomy at L3–L5. **c,d** There was no curve progression except mild retrolisthesis during the 5-year postoperative period

this series showed that the most severe curve was 32° and curve progression did not exceed 40°.

Surgical Intervention

Of 31 patients, 11 (35%) were treated surgically because of uncontrollable radicular pain and/or neurological claudication as opposed to low back pain or progression of deformity. All patients underwent posterior decompressive laminectomy (Fig. 4). The mean number of segments included in decompression was 1.9 segments (range, 1–3 segments). Decompressive laminectomy combined with posterolateral fusion and posterior instrumentation was carried out on 5 of these patients and posterior interbody fusion and instrumentation on 1 patient (Fig. 5). The implant system used in stabilization included four Cotrel-Dubousset (C–D) systems, and two modular segmental spinal instrumentation (MOSS) systems (Fig. 6). The mean number of segments included in internal fixation was 2.0 segments. The results are shown in Table 4.

Discussion

There are relatively few studies of elderly scoliosis in the literature [2,3,6–9]. Although scoliosis in the elderly seemed to be similar in some aspects to adult idiopathic scoliosis, degenerative lumbar curve has characteristic clinical manifestations and radiographic findings different from those seen in adult idiopathic scoliosis [6–9]. Degenerative lumbar scoliosis develops from disk degeneration and in patients that have not had any preexisting scoliosis or trauma. Benner and Ehni used the term degenerative lumbar scoliosis for this type of scoliosis [6]. The degenerative lumbar curve frequently has a secondary compensatory curve (42% of patients in this series) at the L4–S1 area, while compensatory thoracic curves are rarely combined.

Low back pain is the most common symptom of adult idiopathic scoliosis on presentation. The causes of pain are multiple and complex. Several authors have reported back pain in scoliosis to be mainly diskogenic in nature [12,13] and to be correlated directly with increasing age [1,14,15]. Kostuik [14] and Jackson et al. [11] noted that the incidence of pain from nerve root entrapment is quite low in adult scoliosis. In our series of 31 eldery patients with scoliosis, 87% were referred to surgeons with complaints of radicular symptoms or claudication from compressive neuropathy. CT myelography of 13 patients disclosed nerve root compression at the spinal canal or the neural foramen.

Fig. 5a–d. a,b X-rays of a 57-year-old female patient with left degenerative lumbar curve. There was severe sclerosis and forward slipping of L4 on L5. **c,d** Posterior lumbar interbody fusion was carried out

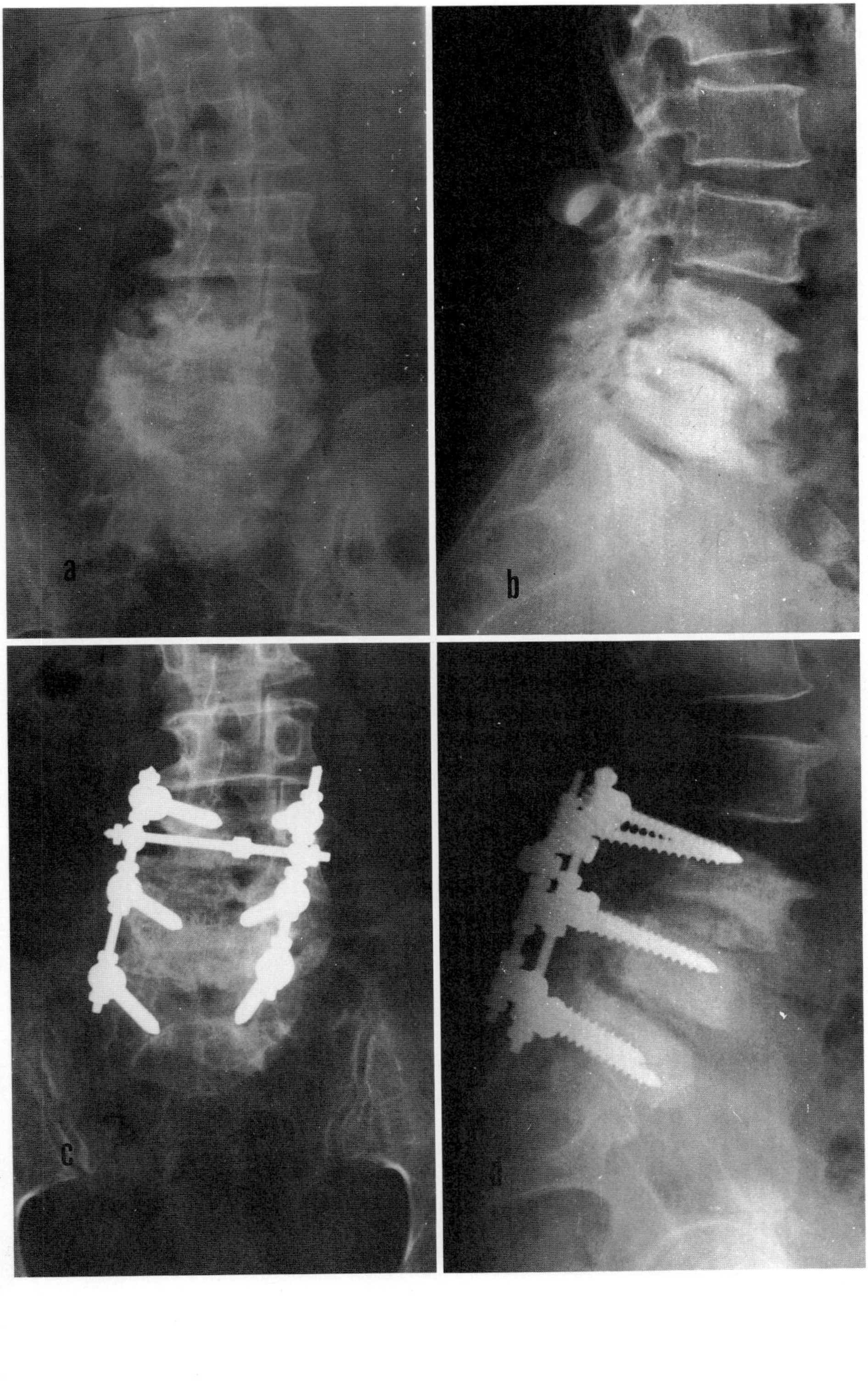
a
b
c

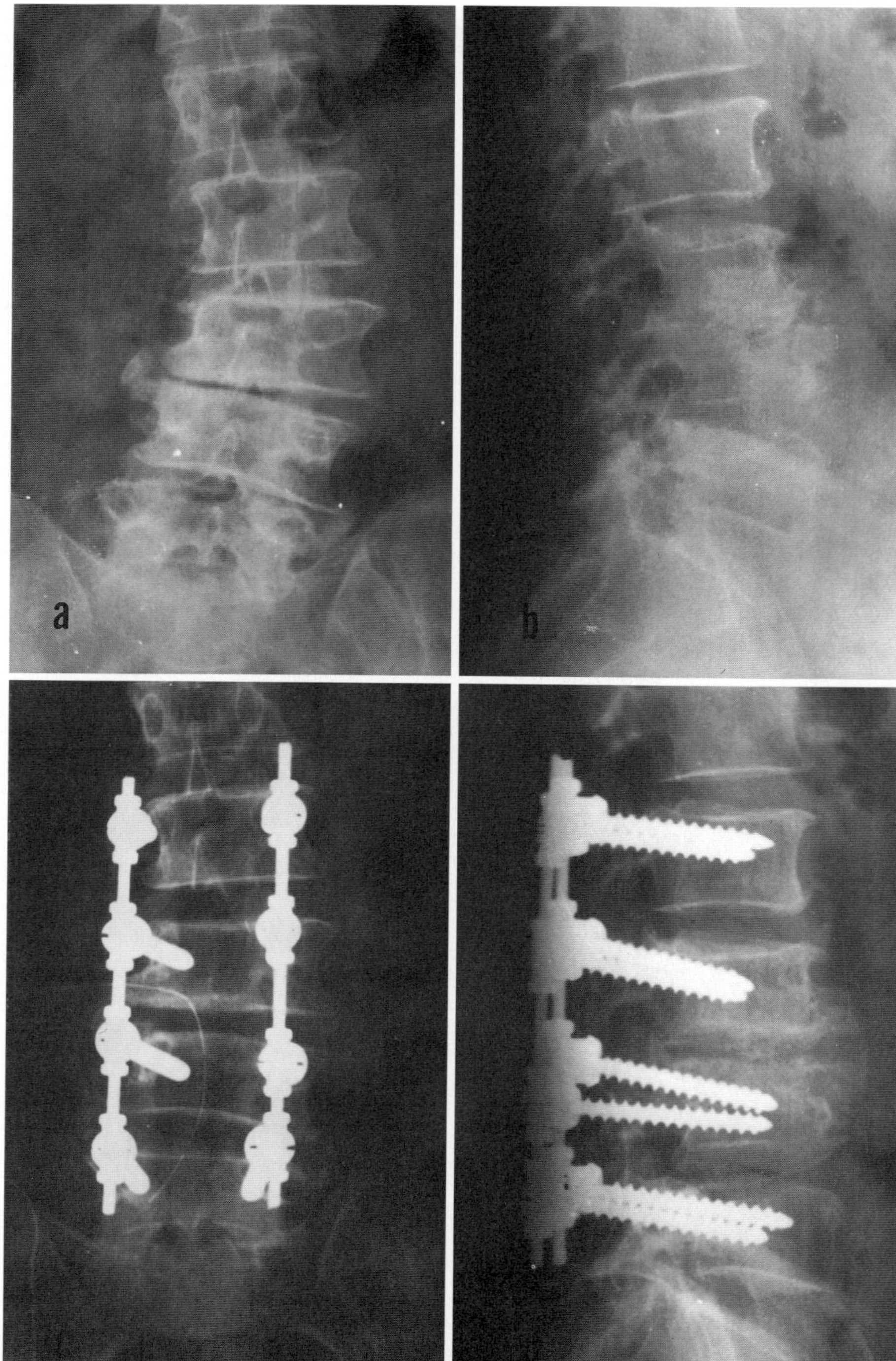
a
b

Surgical decompression over multiple lumbar segments was carried out in 11 patients. These findings illustrate that there is a significantly higher incidence of nerve root compression in degenerative lumbar scoliosis in the elderly than that in adult scoliosis in the middle aged. Furthermore, disabling stenotic symptoms rather than low back pain or curve progression are major surgical indications in this deformity.

Sites of clinical complaint in the back change according to whether the disease is in the early or late degenerative stage. Several studies have suggested that back pain is localized at the concavity of the curve and radiating pain arises from the concavity of the primary curve or lower compensatory curve [5,7,8,11,16]. All of our patients treated surgically also had radiating pain and neurological deficit predominantly in the leg corresponding to the concave side of the lower compensatory curve (convex side of the primary curve) or the primary curve.

In assessing the origin of radicular or stenotic symptoms in degenerative lumbar curves, metrizamide myelography combined with CT scanning should be carried out to ensure the pathology of the canal distal to the block [10,14]. The finding of stenosis in the neural canal and neural foramen in CT myelograms was most common at L4–5, as seen in 92% of patients, and next at L3–4. These levels are sites commonly involved with usual degenerative lumbar spinal stenosis.

Whether disk degeneration in scolosis in the elderly is a resultant anatomical fact or a cause of curve progression is as yet undetermined. Risser [17] and Wiltse [18] suggested that degeneration and thinning of the intervertebral disks at points of great stress was a common cause of increasing scoliotic deformity in adults. Degenerative changes affecting the lumbar curve were variable. Unilateral height loss in intervertebral disks and osteophyte formation on the concave side were found all over the lumbar segment of the major curve, but more markedly at the apex of the curve. In the other hand, facet hypertrophy was more common on the concave side of the lower junctional area of the primary curve or compensatory curve. Lateral translation was found in more severe degenerative curves and involved multiple segments around the apex, and was often combined with forward displacement or retrolisthesis. However, 58% of patients had vertebral body translations which demonstrated the possibility of instability with this type of lumbar curve.

It has been reported that scoliotic curves in the elderly population progressed, although the actual incidence and rate of progression have not been determined [2,9,19]. The relationship between age and degree of curvature and between degenerative changes and degree of curvature were analyzed in this study. There was no direct relationship between age and degree of curvature,

Fig. 6a–d. a,b X-rays of a 54-year-old male patients with left degenerative lumbar curve. **c,d** The curve was corrected with mild distraction using a MOSS system and pedicular screw fixation

Table 4. Results in 11 patients treated surgically.

Case No.	Age/Sex	Curve length	Curve shape	Curve side	Curve (°)	Back pain	Radicular symptom	Neurological sign	C-T mvelogram	Decompression level	Fusion + instrumentation	Prognosis
1	55/F	L1–4	S	Lt	22	Yes	Lt	L4–S1 lt	L3–L5	L3–L5	–	E
2	66/F	L2–4	C	Lt	19	Yes	Lt	L5 lt	L3–S1	L4–L5	L4–L5	E
3	54/M	L2–4	S	Lt	15	Yes	Rt	L4–S1 lt	L2–L5	L2–L5	L2–L5	E
4	74/M	L2–4	C	Lt	14	Yes	Rt	–	L2–L5	L2–L5	–	G
5	64/F	L2–4	C	Lt	18	Yes	Both	L5–S1 both	L4–L5	L4–L5	–	G
6	65/M	L2–5	S	Lt	15	Yes	Lt	L4–S1 both	L5–S1	L4–S1	L4–S1	G
7	53/M	L2–5	C	Lt	12	Yes	Lt	L5–S1 lt	L4–L5	L4–L5	–	G
8	62/F	L3–5	C	Lt	13	Yes	Both	–	L5–S1	L5–S1	–	E
9	58/F	L1–4	C	Lt	21	Yes	Rt	–	L3–L5	L3–L5	L3–L5	G
10	66/F	L2–5	C	Lt	14	Yes	Rt	L2–S1 rt	L2–S1	L4–S1	L4–S1	E
11	57/F	L2–5	S	Lt	20	Yes	Both	L5–S1 lt	L4–S1	L4–S1	L4–S1	E

Rt, right; Lt, left; E, excellent; G, good

whereas there was a linear relationship between the severity of degenerative changes and increase in curvature. This result showed that degenerative changes of the intervertebral disk can cause scoliotic deformity and progression of curvature without any other factors, and degenerative curvature does not continue to progress spontaneously according to increasing age. Progression of the degenerative changes produce osteophyte formation from the vertebral margin on the concave side, and this appears to prevent rapid progression of the curve, but it also causes stenotic neuropathy of the neural foramen and spinal canal.

Epstein et al. has reported effective relief of radicular pain and recovery of function in 4 elderly patients with lumbar scoliosis following only surgical decompression of the lateral recess of the spinal canal [7]. In our series, decompression surgery alone was satisfactory in patients that had a lesion involving one level, but fusion with instrumentation was added in one case that had forward slipping on that level. Kostuik recommended curve correction with instrumentation because many patients with spinal stenosis or root pain who underwent only posterior decompression had significant collapse or curve progression [14,15]. He indicated that curves with a short c shape over the sacrum and sharp and angulated compensatory curves have poor prognosis, and rebalancing the short compensatory curve rather than the primany curve was recommended. Bradford recommended a combined approach consisting of anterior interbody fusion followed by posterior decompression with instrumentation in significant lumbar curvature over 40° associated with radicular stenotic pain [10]. But for minor degrees, he recommended posterior decompression and instrumentation with a transpedicular implant. In degenerative lumbar curves in our series, a greater number of preoperative patients were seen with instability from translation, and further risk of instability was expected from wide decompression over multiple levels. To prevent collapse of the curve, we prefered stabilization with instrumentation rather than curve correction by which compression of other nerve roots might occur. In addition, fusion and transpedicular screw fixation were carried out with moderate distraction on patients with lesions involving multiple levels.

References

1. Kostuik JP, Bentivoglio J (1981) The incidence of low back pain in adult scoliosis. Spine 6:268–273
2. Robin GC, Span Y, Steinberg R, Makin M, Menczel J (1982) Scoliosis in the elderly. A follow up study. Spine 7:355–359
3. Vanderpool DW, James JIP, Wynne Davis R (1969) Scoliosis in the elderly. J Bone Joint Surg [Am] 51:446–455
4. Kostuik JP (1980) Recent advances in the treatment of painful adult scoliosis. Clin Orthop 147:238–252
5. Jackson RP, Simmons EH, Stripinis D (1983) Incidence and severity of back pain in adult idiopathic scoliosis. Spine 8:749–756

6. Benner B, Ehni G (1979) Degenerative lumbar scoliosis. Spine 4:548–552
7. Epstein JA, Epstein BS, Lavine LS (1974) Surgical treatment of nerve root compression caused by scoliosis of the lumbar spine. J Neurosurg 41:449-454
8. Epstein JA, Epstein BS, Jones MD (1979) Symptomatic lumbar scoliosis with degenerative changes in the elderly. Spine 4:542–547
9. Grubb SA, Lipscomb HJ, Coonrod RW (1988) Degenerative adult onset scoliosis. Spine 13:241–245
10. Bradford DS (1988) Adult scoliosis: Current concepts of treatment. Clin Orthop 229:71–87
11. Jackson RP, Simmons EH, Stripinis D (1989) Coronal and sagittal plane spinal deformities correlating with back pain and pulmonary function in adult idiopathic scoliosis. Spine 14:1391–1397
12. Sponseller PD, Cohen MS, Nachemson AL, Hall JE, Whol MEB (1987) Results of surgical treatment of adults with idiopathic scoliosis. J Bone Joint Surg [Am] 69:667–675
13. Swank S, Lonstein JE, Moe JH, Winter RB, Bradford DS (1981) Surgical treatment of adult scoliosis. J Bone Joint Surg 63:268–287
14. Kostuik JP (1990) Adult scoliosis. In: Weinstein JN, Wiesel SW (eds) The Lumbar Spine. Saunders, Philadelphia, pp 882–915
15. Kostuik JP, Isreal J, Hall JE (1973) Scoliosis surgery in adults. Clin Orthop 93:225–234
16. Simmons EH, Jackson RP (1979) The management of nerve root entrapment syndromes associated with the collapsing scoliosis of idiopathic lumbar and thoracolumbar curves. Spine 4:533–541
17. Risser JC (1964) Scoliosis past and present. J Bone Joint Surg [Am] 46:166–199
18. Wiltse LL (1971) The effect of common anomalies of the lumbar spine upon disk degeneration and low back pain. Orthop Clin North [Am] 2:569–582
19. Collins DK, Ponseti IV (1969) Long-term follow-up of patients with idiopathic scoliosis not treated surgically. J Bone Joint Surg [Am] 51:425–445

2.11 Surgical Management of Degenerative Lumbar Scoliosis

Yoshiaki Toyama[1]

Introduction

Among the spinal deformities in the aged, degenerative lumbar scoliosis (DLS) has been attracting attention together with degenerative lumbar kyphosis, and there has been active discussion on the pathogenesis and treatment of DLS in recent years. The purpose of this study was to investigate the surgical management of symptomatic DLS in the light of how symptoms develop, and we have placed emphasis on the indications for correction and spinal fusion. We also discuss the selection of posterior instrumentation surgery, including the problems arising from it.

Materials and Methods

DLS was defined as scoliotic deformity with a curve magnitude of a Cobb angle of at least 10° based on intervertebral disk degeneration in the lumbar spine. DLS has the following characteristic findings on radiographs: severe degenerative changes of the lumbar spine, such as the formation of osteophytes; wedge-shaped disks and narrow disk heights; lateral translation of vertebrae; vertebral rotation; and a short curve in the lumbar spine. Residual deformity caused by clear idiopathic scoliosis was excluded from this study. Patients with symptomatic DLS accompanied by caudal and nerve root compressions, such as intermittent claudication, sciatica, or numbness, were selected as subjects of the present investigation. The total number of patients was 23, 12 men and 11 women. Their age at the time of surgery ranged from 48 to 82 years, with an average of 64 years.

The patients were examined by functional X-ray, myelography, CT myelography, and radiculography, and the results were compared to clinical symp-

[1]Department of Orthopaedic Surgery, School of Medicine, Keio University, 35 Shinanomachi, Shinjuku-ku, Tokyo, 160 Japan

toms and operative findings. The following six items were examined in the X-rays of standing patients: Cobb angle, vertebral rotation, wedging of the intervertebral disk, lateral translation of vertebrae, degeneration of the facet joint, and osteophyte formation. When the presence of nerve root involvement in DLS was suspected, comprehensive evaluation of clinical findings, myelography, CT myelography, electromyography, and selective nerve root blocks were necessary to diagnose these conditions with certainty.

Clinical evaluation of the operative results was done according to a score rating system designed by the Japanese Orthopaedic Association (JOA) [1]. This scale has a total of 29 points, but this study used only 15 of these points and excluded restrictions in activities of daily living that account for 14 points. Severity of low back pain and sciatica was rated as follows: 9 to 0 points, subjective symptoms (low back pain, sciatica, and gait disturbance); 6 to 0 points, clinical signs (SLR test, sensory, and motor disturbance); and 0 to −6 points, urinary bladder function.

DLS was classified into three types on the basis of the radiographic findings. Type I consists mainly of wedging of the intervertebral disk at L4–L5 and lateral translation at L3–L4, with a slight curve of scoliosis recognized at the upper lumbar spine. Type II is a scoliotic deformity associated with vertebral rotation and lateral translation based on multiple disk degeneration in the middle lumbar spine (Fig. 1). Type III includes all other deformities. The 23 patients included 9 with Type I and 14 with Type II DLS, but there were no cases of Type III DLS in this study.

Instability associated with DLS was defined as the following angular or translational changes from the supine position to the standing position on radiographs:

1. A change in curve magnitude of scoliosis of more than 5°
2. A change in lateral translation of vertebrae of more than 3 mm
3. A change in disk wedging of more than 3°

The surgical methods used for the 23 patients with symptomatic DLS were as follows: (a) in Type I, fenestration was carried out in 6 and laminectomy and posterolateral fusion (PLF) in 3 cases; and (b) in Type II, posterior decompression without fusion was carried out in 6, posterior decompression and correction plus spinal fusion with instrumentation in 7, and anterior spinal body fusion (ASF) in 1 case.

The patients operated on with instrumentation were all women with Type II DLS, and the curve magnitude on standing was a Cobb angle of 26° on average. The posterior instrumentation used was Luque in 3 cases and Cotrel-Dubousset (C-D) using the multisegmental pedicular screw fixation in 4 cases. The follow-up period ranged from 6 months to 8 years with an average of 3 years.

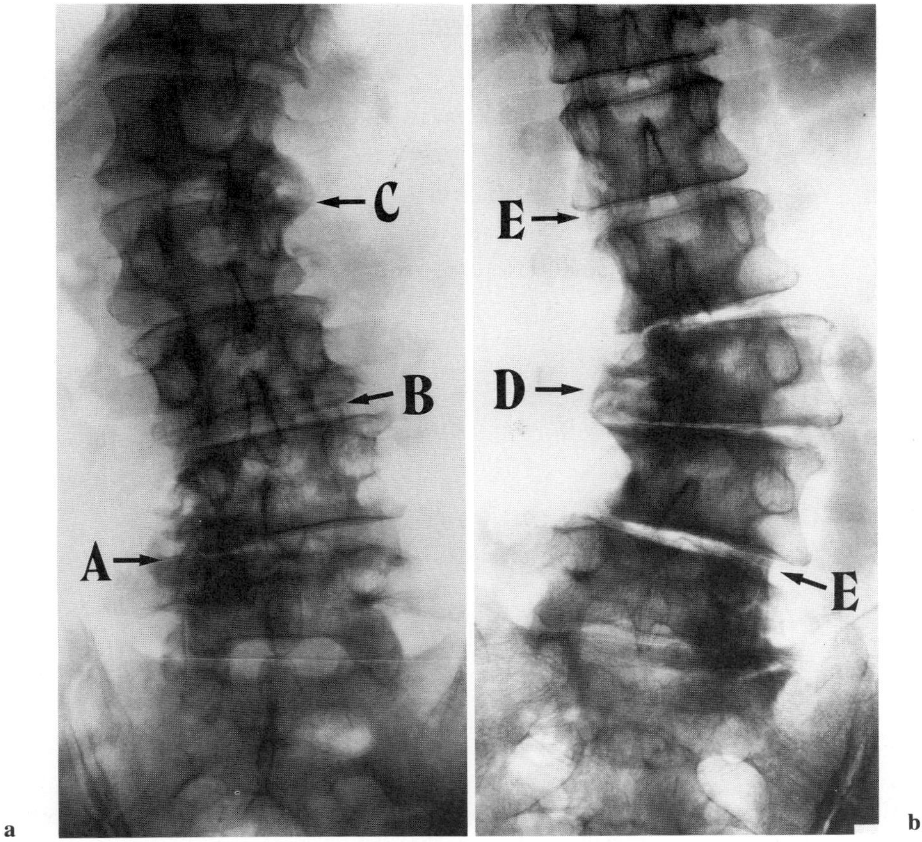

Fig. 1a,b. Morphological classification of DLS based on the radiographic findings. **a** Type I consists mainly of L4/L5 disk wedging (*A*) and L3/L4 lateral translation (*B*) with mild scoliosis (*C*) in the upper lumbar spine. **b** Type II is a scoliotic deformity associated with vertebral rotation (*D*) and lateral translation (*E*) based on multiple disk degeneration in the middle lumbar spine

Results

Radiographic Findings and Clinical Symptoms

The most characteristic findings of DLS on the radiographs were wedging of the intervertebral disk, lateral translation of vertebrae, and vertebral rotation. The curve magnitude was 18° in Type I, 25° in Type II, and an average of 22° in all cases of DLS. The rotation of the apical vertebra was evaluated using the system described by Nash and Moe (zero to Grade VI) [2]. Vertebral rotation was greater in Type II, and 11 cases in Type II were Grade II rotation according to this method. There were no cases of severe Grade III rotation or more, and no differences in lateral translation between the two types. Trans-

Table 1. Radiographic findings and clinical symptoms of DLS.

No. of cases (*n*)	Type I 9	Type II 14	Total 23
Curve pattern			
Right convex	7	8	15
Left convex	2	6	8
Curve magnitude (Cobb angle)			
Average	18°	25°	22°
Range	10–29°	12–42°	10–42°
Vertebral rotation (Moe and Nash method)			
Grade I	6	3	9
Grade II	3	11	14
Lateral translation			
1–5 mm	4	6	10
6–10 mm	6	13	19
Over 11 mm	1	3	4
Leg pain			
Right	5	4	9
Left	2	3	5
Both	2	7	9
Nerve compression			
Cauda equina	2	8	10
Nerve root	7	6	13
Intermittent claudication (for 100 m or less)	3	7	10
Sensory disturbance	5	13	18
Motor disturbance	6	10	16
Low back pain	8	11	19

lation of 6–10 mm was recognized in 6 disk spaces in Type I and 13 disk spaces in Type II. Analysis of our clinical cases showed no problem in cases with 10% or 5–6 mm lateral translation, but if translation went beyond 20% or 10 mm, the spinal canal was clearly constricted and stenotic. Although no clear correlation was seen between the curve pattern and neurologic disturbance, nerve root compression tended to appear more frequently in Type I and caudal lesions in Type II (Table 1). Especially in Type I, neurologic disturbance showed a higher incidence in L5 nerve root compression on the concave side of disk wedging at L4–L5, and cauda equina compression was often recognized at the level of vertebral rotation or lateral translation in Type II (Fig. 2). Low back pain occurred in 19 cases (83%) and there was an obvious correlation between the curve pattern and site of low back pain. However, more than 80% of patients with low back pain showed onset or worsening on standing.

Results by Operative Methods

Concerning the progress of postoperative scoliotic deformity treated by posterior decompression without fusion, there were few problems in DLS cases with a preoperative curve magnitude of about 20°. However, if the curve

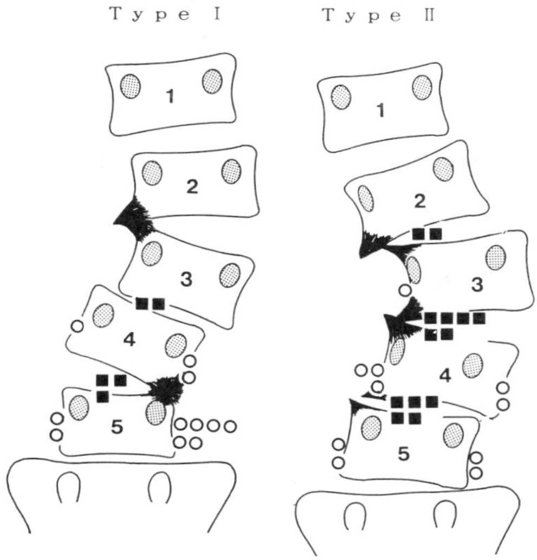

Fig. 2. Site and location of the cauda equina and nerve root compression associated with DLS in the lumbar spine. *Solid square*, caudal lesion (Type I, $n = 2$; Type II, $n = 8$); *open circle*, root lesion (Type I, $n = 7$; Type II, $n = 6$)

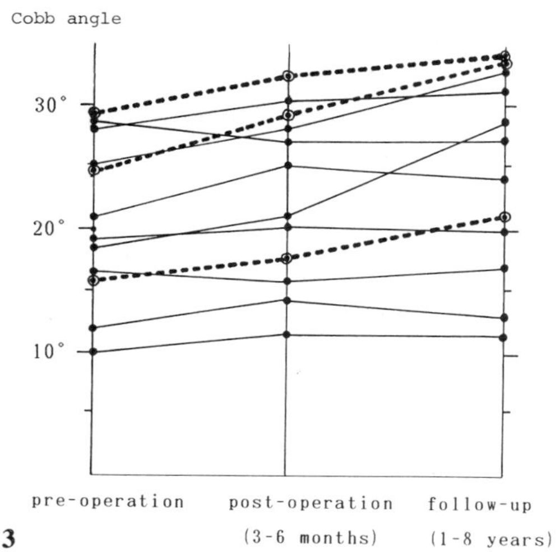

3

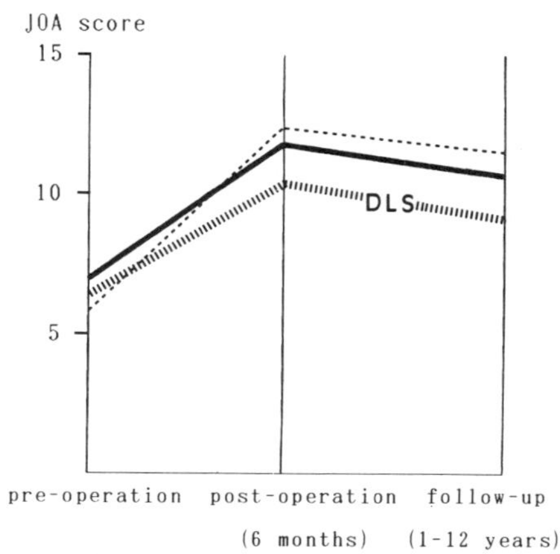

4

Fig. 3. Curve progression after posterior decompression without fusion for DLS ($n = 12$). *Dotted line*, laminectomy ($n = 3$); *solid line*, fenestration ($n = 9$)

Fig. 4. Postoperative results of lumbar spinal stenosis in the elderly. *Striated line*, DLS ($n = 15$; recovery rate = 46%); *solid line*, degenerative spondylolisthesis ($n = 36$; recovery rate = 62%); *dotted line*, central and lateral stenosis in degenerative type of acquired stenosis ($n = 37$; recovery rate = 68%)

magnitude was over 25°, the curve progressed with posterior decompression. Deformity progressed in all three patients treated with laminectomy, indicating that laminectomy should not be used in such cases (Fig. 3).

Seven cases of posterior instrumentation surgery are summarized in Table 2. Because of the fragility of bone caused by osteoporosis in aged patients and the possibility of developing postoperative neurological complications, it is essential not to overcorrect the deformity. The correction rate was 20% by the Luque method and 54% by the C-D method. Bone union was achieved in 6 cases, but one case operated on by the Luque method required a salvage operation due to non-union at the lumbosacral region (Table 2).

Although we chose the most adequate operative method for each individual case, the recovery rate was 46% on average in all cases of DLS: 56% in fenestration, 21% in laminectomy, 45% in laminectomy and PLF, 41% in posterior decompression and correction plus spinal fusion with instrumentation, and 68% in ASF. The recovery rate in DLS was clearly lower than that in other diseases, such as 62% in degenerative spondylolisthesis and 68% in the degenerative type of acquired stenosis ($P < 0.05$) (Fig. 4).

Discussion

Reports on this disease started with that of Müller [3] in 1931 who referred to lateral translation of vertebrae associated with lumbar scoliosis as "Drehgleiten." In 1969, Vanderpool and Wynne-Davis [4] reported on lumbar scoliosis in patients over the age of 50 years old under the title "Scoliosis in the Elderly." In 1974, Epstein et al. [5] reported on the surgical treatment of root compression associated with lumbar scoliosis. Since then, many clinical and radiological studies have been performed, mainly on clinical cases [6–9]. However, many of the cases in such reports included degenerative scoliosis and residual deformity following idiopathic scoliosis. Benner and Ehni [10] reported on DLS first in 1979 using the same criteria as those used in the present study. Mild scoliosis is generally seen at high frequencies in the elderly, but clinically, most of these cases are asymptomatic or show only mild low back pain. However, some cases are associated with persistent low back pain or sciatica, and clarification of the pathogenesis and mechanism of neurologic disturbance is necessary for the surgical management of DLS.

Pathomechanism of Neurological Symptoms

As a result of the investigation of clinical symptoms, myelography, radiculography, CT myelography, and the study of operative findings, the mechanism by which neurologic disturbance develops was found to be as follows: the most frequent condition observed that led to the development of symptoms in DLS was nerve root compression accompanied by narrowing of the lateral recess mainly due to degeneration of the facet joints and disk protrusion at the

Table 2. Summary of seven cases operated on with posterior instrumentation surgery.

Case	Age (years)	Sex	DLS type	Neurologic disturbance	Instrumentation	Cobb angle pre → postoperation (correction rate)	JOA score (15 points) pre → postoperation (recovery rate)
1	69	F	II	Nerve root	Luque[a]	17° → 13° (24%)	9 → 10 (17%)
2	66	F	II	Cauda equina	Luque	18° → 15° (17%)	9 → 11 (33%)
3	48	F	II	Cauda equina	Luque	23° → 17° (26%)	0 → 7 (47%)
4	70	F	II	Cauda equina	C-D	28° → 13° (54%)	2 → 8 (46%)
5	63	F	II	Cauda equina	C-D	33° → 18° (45%)	5 → 11 (60%)
6	59	F	II	Combined	C-D	42° → 15° (64%)	9 → 13 (67%)
7	71	F	II	Nerve root	C-D	26° → 16° (38%)	9 → 10 (17%)

[a] Non-union

C-D, Cotrel-Dubousset instrumentation

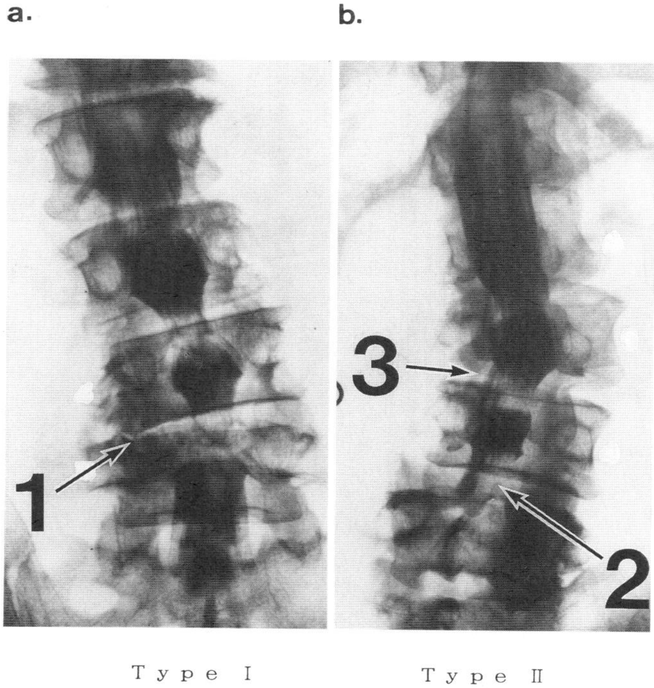

Fig. 5a,b. Nerve root and cauda equina compression associated with Type I (**a**) and Type II (**b**) DLS developed from wedging of the intervertebral disk (*1*), lateral translation of vertebrae (*2*), and vertebral rotation (*3*)

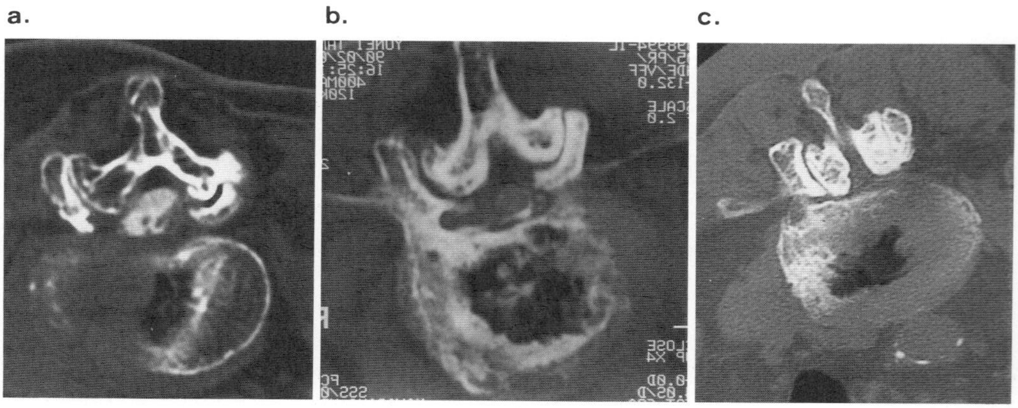

Fig. 6. Grading of lumbar spinal stenosis caused by DLS with vertebral rotation on CT myelogram. **a** Grade I. Nerve root compression should be treated by fenestration. **b** Grade II. Nerve root compression is greater than cauda equina compression and this should be treated by wide fenestration. **c** Grade III. Severe caudal lesions should be treated by wide laminectomy and spinal fusion

concave side of *disk wedging*. This often occurs at the level of L4–L5 in DLS Type I.

Reporting on *lateral translation* of vertebrae, Simmons and Jackson [11] noted that neurologic disturbance is caused by pedicular kinking of the translated vertebrae and traction of the nerve root at the inferior vertebrae. However, there has been no detailed report that includes changes in the dural sac. From analysis of our clinical cases, the spinal canal of DLS with lateral translation of over 10 mm or 20% was clearly constricted and stenotic (Fig. 5).

The neurologic disturbance accompanying *vertebral rotation* develops from subluxation of the facet joint. From analysis of the CT myelograms, I divided the severity of spinal canal stenosis into three grades, from Grade I with nerve root compression to Grade III with severe cauda equina compression (Fig. 6). The articular processes are rotated by coupling motion, and subluxation occurs in the facet joint on the frontal surface. As a result, nerve roots and cauda equina on the concave side are subjected to compression by the lower articular

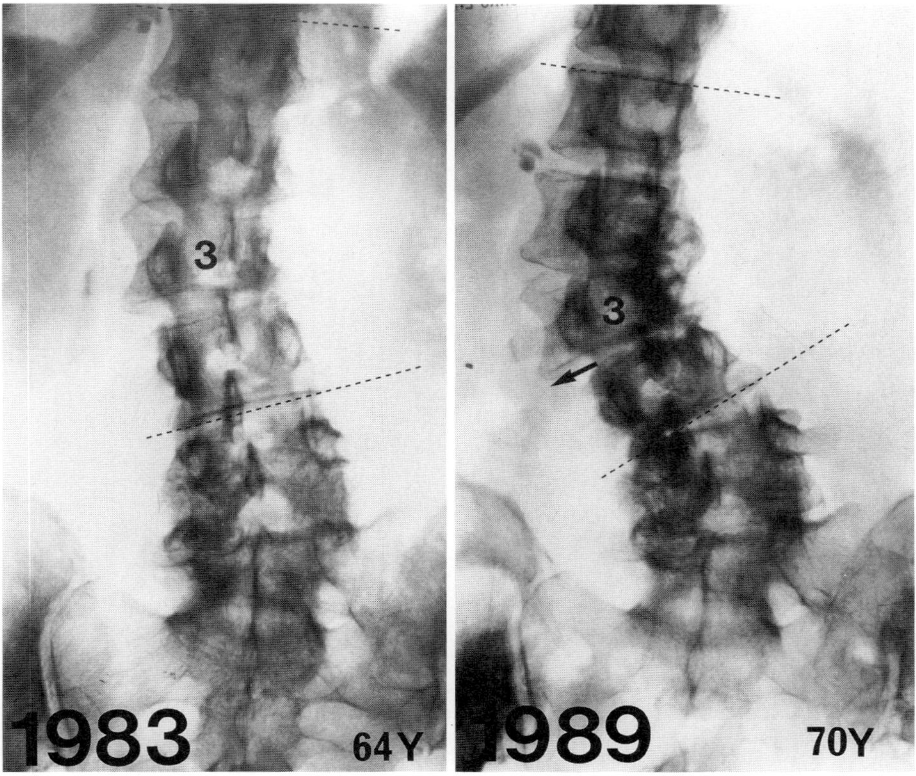

Fig. 7. A 64-year-old woman with progressing deformity. In the last 6 years, curve magnitude has increased from 20° to 41° and lateral translation from 4 mm to 12 mm at L3/L4

processes of the upper vertebrae. This compression is further worsened by hypertrophy of the facet joint on the concave side.

Choice of Operative Procedures

To sum up the main points on surgical management of DLS, fenestration is indicated for patients with a single nerve root compression and a stable spine when the curve magnitude is under 20°, and also this procedure is applicable to patients with Grades I or II on our grading of lumbar spinal stenosis. No spinal

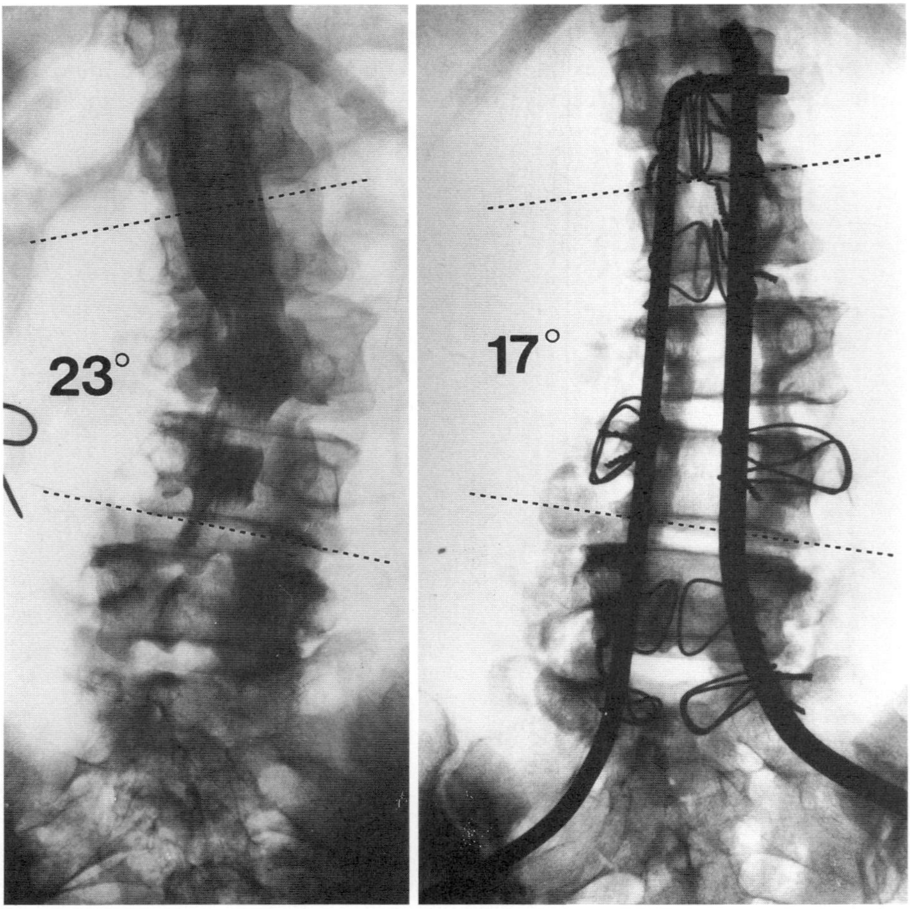

a b

Fig. 8. A 48-year-old woman (case 3 in Table 2) with DLS Type II and a 0 point preoperative JOA score. Cauda equina compression at the level of L3/L4 vertebral rotation and L4/L5 lateral translation was diagnosed (**a**). Laminectomy with correction and fusion using Luque's method were performed (**b**). Correction rate = 26%; recovery rate = 47%

fusion is required in these patients. On the other hand, correction and spinal fusion are required in DLS patients with an unstable spine and progressing scoliosis with a curve magnitude of over 25° or with lateral translation of over 10 mm (Fig. 7). Wide laminectomy including the facet joints and spinal fusion with instrumentation are indicated for patients with a multisegmental focus or severe spinal stenosis, such as Grade III on a CT myelogram.

The Luque method is seldom indicated for various reasons, including the extensive fusion area required, the inability to fix the wide decompressed lumbar spine, and the difficulty of rigid fixation in the lumbosacral region (Fig. 8). I am presently using the C-D method with multisegmental pedicular screws

a 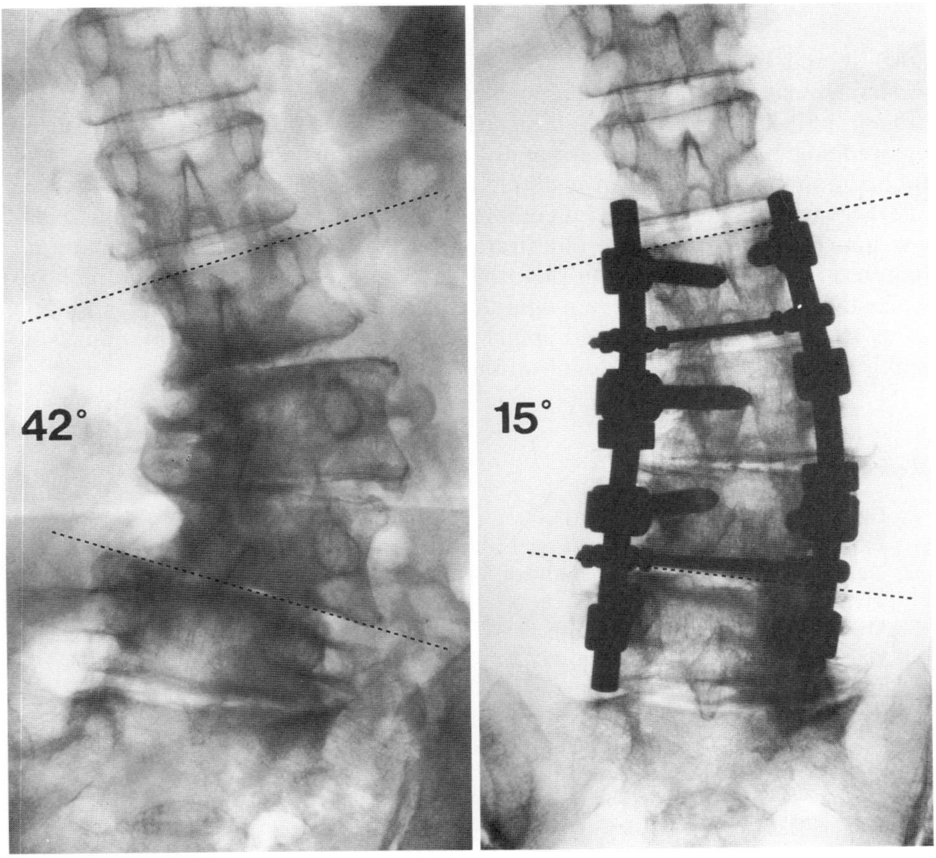 b

Fig. 9. A 59-year-old woman (case 6 in Table 2) with DLS Type II and a 9 point preoperative JOA score. Cauda equina and nerve root compression (Grade II on CT myelogram) at the level of L3/L4 vertebral rotation were diagnosed (**a**). Wide fenestration with correction and fusion using C/D instrumentation with multisegmental pedicular screw were performed (**b**). Correction rate = 64%; recovery rate = 67%

[12] because it is applicable to three-dimensional deformities, rigid and short segmental fixation is possible, and it is capable of fixing the wide decompressed lumbar spine (Fig. 9) [13]. With this method, control of the systemic condition before and after operation is important since the patient is usually aged. Loosening of screws or fracture of the pedicle as a result of osteoporosis may occur, and adequate, moderate correction with short segmental fixation and reliable bone grafting are important. In addition, we should not overestimate the strength of instrumental fixation, and rigid bracing should be used if necessary.

Conclusions

DLS should be recognized as a new category among the various types of lumbar spinal stenosis. We classified DLS into three types on the basis of radiographic findings. Neurologic disturbances associated with DLS were caused by wedging of the intervertebral disk, lateral translation of vertebrae, and subluxation of the facet joint resulting from vertebral rotation. The stable type of DLS with a single nerve root compression in which the curve magnitude was less than 20° should indicate fenestration. No spinal fusion and correction are required in these patients. On the other hand, in cases of progressive scoliosis or unstable DLS with a curve magnitude of over 25° or with lateral translation of over 10 mm, correction and spinal fusion with C-D instrumentation using multisegmental pedicular screw fixation were effective.

References

1. Inoue S, Watanabe T, Goto S, et al. (1988) Degenerative spondylolisthesis – Pathophysiology and results of anterior interbody fusion. Clin Orthop 227:90–98
2. Nash C, Moe J (1969) A study of vertebral rotation. J Bone Joint Surg [Am] 51:223–229
3. Müller W (1931) Spontane seitliche Wirbelkorperverschiebungen (Das Drehgleiten von Lendenwirbeln bei Skoliosen der altern Leute). Z Orthop Chir 55:351–364
4. Vanderpool DW, Wynne-Davies R (1969) Scoliosis in the elderly. J Bone Joint Surg [Am] 51:446–455
5. Epstein JA, Epstein BS, Lavine LS (1974) Surgical treatment of nerve root compression caused by scoliosis of the lumbar spine. J Neurosurg 41:449–454
6. Grubb SA, Lipscomb HJ, Coonrad RW (1988) Degenerative adult onset scoliosis. Spine 13:241–245
7. Toyama Y, Hirabayashi K, Wakano K (1987) Pathogenesis and surgical treatment of lumbar canal stenosis in elderly patients (in Japanese). Bessatsu Seikei-Geka 12:142–149
8. Toyama Y, Hirabayashi K, Wakano K (1987) Pathogenesis and operative methods for lumbar canal stenosis associated with degenerative scoliosis (in Japanese). Cent Jpn J Orthop Traumat 30:54–56

9. Toyama Y, Nakamura T, Yorimitsu E (1990) Clinical studies on the pathogenesis of degenerative lumbar scoliosis with caudal and nerve root compression (in Japanese). Clin Orthop Surg 25:407–416
10. Benner B, Ehni G (1979) Degenerative lumbar scoliosis. Spine 4:548–552
11. Simmons EH, Jackson RP (1979) The management of nerve root entrapment syndromes associated with the collapsing scoliosis of idiopathic lumbar and thoracolumbar curves. Spine 4:533–541
12. Simmons EH, Capicotto WN (1988) Posterior transpedicular Zielke instrumentation of the lumbar spine. Clin Orthop 236:180–191
13. Toyama Y, Nakamura M, Nakazawa H, Yorimitsu E (1991) Indication of posterior instrumentation surgery for degenerative lumbar scoliosis (in Japanese). Bessatsu Seikei-Geka 20:84–88

2.12 Treatment of Multilevel Anterior and Retrolisthesis of the Lumbosacral Spine

Paul Enker, Arthur D. Steffee, Louis Keppler, Robert S. Biscup, and Scot D. Miller[1]

Introduction

Instability of the adult lumbosacral spine, commonly due to degenerative spondylolisthesis and post-laminectomy instability, affects single levels more frequently than multiple levels [1–6]. Treatment options applied to single-level instability have been applied to multiple-level instability, with the cornerstone of treatment being decompression. Notwithstanding the consensus on the need for decompression, the extent necessary is controversial, as are the indications for concurrent fusion, deformity correction, and the use of instrumentation [1,4,5,7–24].

The purpose of this paper is to present a retrospective review of a large series of patients with multilevel instability, treated by single-stage posterior decompression, segmental pedicle fixation [25], deformity correction, and interbody and intertransverse fusion.

Materials and Methods

Between July 1983 and December 1990, 90 patients underwent operative treatment with 48 having a minimum 2-year follow-up. There were 34 females and 14 males with an average age of 60 years (range: 38–88 years) and an average follow-up of 3.5 years (range 2–7 years). Of the 48 patients, 9 underwent primary surgery and 39 underwent revision surgery. Prior surgeries included single or multilevel decompressive laminectomy (27/39), diskectomy (7/39), posterolateral fusion (4/39), and laminectomy and fusion (1/39).

Clinical evaluation included determination of pain severity using a ten-point analog pain scale. Results of analog pain scores were classified as follows:

[1] Division of Orthopaedics, Cleveland Spine and Arthritis Center, 2709 Franklin Boulevard, Cleveland, OH 44113, USA

excellent (9–10), good (7–8.9), fair (5–6.9), and poor (4.9 or less). Excellent and good were rated as satisfactory, and fair and poor as unsatisfactory.

All patients underwent roentgenographic assessment with standing anteroposterior and lateral views, myelography and follow-up CAT scan, and provocative and descriptive diskography of the affected levels. The following measurements were made: Cobb angle, percent slip, percent slip correction, and lumbar lordosis. Postoperative roentgenographs were evaluated for fusion.

Surgical Procedure

All patients underwent somatosensory evoked potential assessment preoperatively and monitoring intraoperatively. Operative findings, use of cement and complications were recorded.

The surgical technique consisted of decompression over the required levels by complete removal of the laminae, partial to complete facetectomy bilaterally, and in revision cases, complete scar removal around the dural sac and exiting and descending nerve roots. Bipolar coagulation was used to control the epidural vessels. Pedicle screws (VSP System, AcroMed Corp., Cleveland) were inserted at all the required levels and their positions verified by control radiography. In cases where osteopenic vertebra precluded sound pedicle purchase, the pedicles and posterior vertebral bodies were prepared using a curved Penfield dissector to compact the cancellous bone in these regions. Cement was then injected through one pedicle until it was visible exiting the contralateral pedicle. The pedicle screws were then reinserted and the cement allowed to cure.

Starting at the most inferior level, diskectomy was carried out. Disk space distraction was accomplished in 1-mm increments using Collis interspace shapers (V. Mueller, Niles, IL), disk spreaders, and a lamina spreader to separate the pedicle screws, with the endpoint of distraction being the inability of the next size shaper or spreader to be rotated to its maximum vertical height. The shapers or spreaders were left in place and 3- or 5-mm washers were applied to the inferior and superior sets of screws. Working plates contoured to the appropriate degree of lordosis were then applied to the pedicle screws and secured by tightening tapered nuts. Control radiographs were taken to assure appropriate positioning of the screws, lumbar lordosis and slip correction. The disk shapers and spreaders were then removed leaving the disk space distracted to its maximum height achieved through ligamentotaxis. The intervertebral foramona were decompressed by removing posterolateral annulus and marginal osteophytes anterior and inferior to the exiting nerve roots.

A posterior lumbar interbody fusion (PLIF) was performed using a broach set (ADS PLIF Broach System, AcroMed Corp., Cleveland) to prepare rectangular troughs bilaterally either 11 , 13, or 15 mm in height and width. Length of the allograft block was adjusted to the depth of the disk space so as to allow the graft to be countersunk 3–5 mm. Control radiographs were then taken to assess the position of the grafts, percent correction of the olisthesis, position of the screws, and lumbar lordosis. The superior set of tapered nuts were then loosened resulting in visible compression of the PLIF grafts by recoil of the distracted vertebral bodies. The tapered nuts were then retightened.

The next superior level was addressed in an identical fashion. The modification required consisted of applying 3- or 5-mm washers to the next set of pedicle screws in order to elevate the next set of working plates posterior to the inferior set of working plates. The disk space was distracted in the same manner and the tapered nuts on the pedicle screws now overlapped by two plates were then tightened. The tapered nuts on the pedicle screws at the superior end of the second set of working plates were then tightened and PLIF carried out in the same manner.

Additional levels were addressed by stacking successive sets of working plates one on top of the other. After completion of the required levels and starting on one side, the multiple working plates were removed and the intertransverse bed prepared using a high speed burr. The intertransverse graft consisted of morcellized autograft from bone removed during the decompression and allograft. A single contoured plate was then applied. These steps were then repeated on the contralateral side. Foraminal patency was then verified by the ability to pass a 6-mm foraminal probe, and additional decompression of the foramina carried out until this was possible. A percutaneous epidural catheter was then inserted and gelfoam applied over the exposed PLIF blocks and dura. One or two deep drains were placed and closure was carried out.

Results

Seventy-two percent of patients presented with back and radicular symptoms, either unilateral (35%) or bilateral (37%), 22% with back pain only, and 6% with leg pain only. Eighteen percent had objective neurological findings.

Somatosensory evoked potentials were abnormal in all patients including those with back pain only. In patients with unilateral leg symptoms, 75% demonstrated bilateral abnormalities on somatosensory evoked potential testing while 100% of patients with bilateral leg symptoms demonstrated abnormalities on somatosensory evoked potential testing. There were no cases of single-root abnormalities.

Table 1. Instability patterns classified by direction.

Unidirectional listhesis (n = 29 of 48 patients)		Bidirectional listhesis (n = 19 of 48 patients)	
2-level anterior	20	1-level anterior and 1-level retro	6
3-level anterior	4	1-level anterior and 2-level retro	6
2-level retro	3	1-level anterior and 1-level lateral	2
3-level retro	2	2-level anterior and 1-level retro	4
		2-level anterior and 2-level retro	1

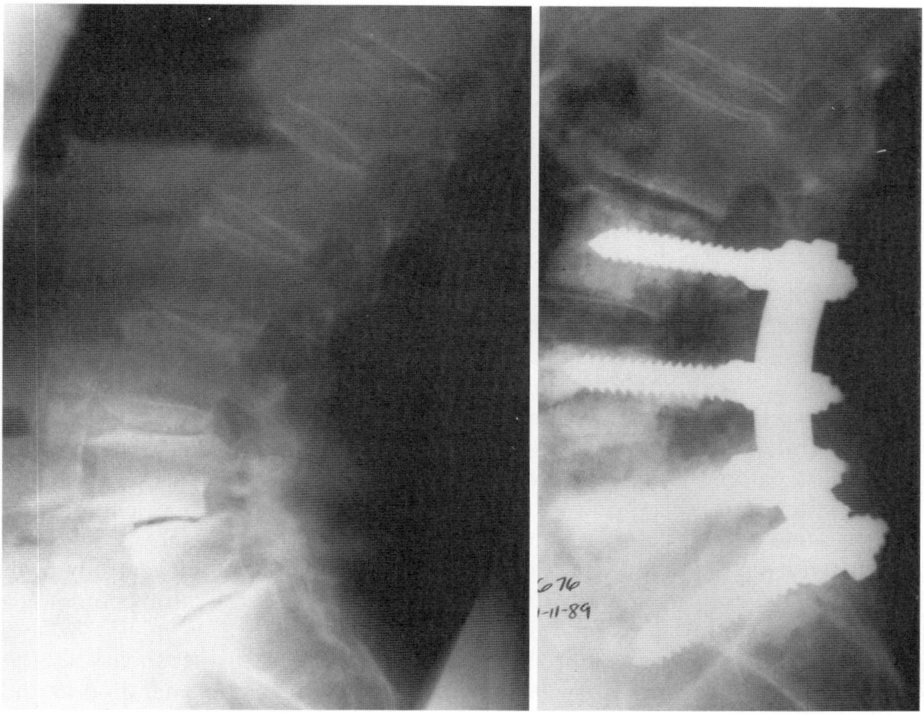

a b

Fig. 1a,b. a Lateral radiograph of a 72-year-old women who had undergone prior L4–5, and L5–S1 decompressive laminectomy, displaying spondylolisthesis at L3–4, L4–5 and L5–S1. **b** Lateral view at 2-year follow-up demonstrating complete reduction of the olisthesis at the L3–4, L4–5, L5–S1 levels with cement supplementation of pedicle screw fixation

Instability patterns were divided into unidirectional and bidirectional groups (Table 1).

The average percent slip and percent slip correction for the anterior listhesis levels was 22% (8%–42%) and 71% (54%–100%) respectively, and for the retrolisthetic levels 23% (9%–71%) and 75% (26%–100%). While in the early part of the series deformity correction was incomplete, in the latter part, with refinement in the surgical technique, the percent slip correction was 100% at all levels in all patients (Fig. 1).

Degenerative scoliosis, present in 6 of 48 patients, averaged 12° (5–15°) preoperatively and 4° (2–8°) postoperatively.

Lumbar lordosis averaged 58° preoperatively and 43° at follow-up.

Intraforaminal stenosis secondary to bulging posterolateral annulus and posterior osteophytes was found in 48 of 48 patients, both primary and revision cases. In the primary surgery group, there was also lateral recess stenosis in 9 of 9 patients secondary to facet joint overgrowth, compromising the foramen in an anteroposterior direction. The descending nerve root was compressed in the anteroposterior direction, while the exiting nerve root was compressed in both the anteroposterior and superoinferior direction. In the revision surgery group, the subgroup with midline decompression only, demonstrated residual lateral recess and intraforaminal stenosis, while 29 of 39 patients with partial or total facetectomy, demonstrated residual intraforaminal stenosis in the floor of the foramen secondary to posterolateral annulus with or without osteophyte.

The interbody (100% allograft) fusion rate was 91% and the intertransverse (50%–70% allograft) fusion rate was 67%.

Cement supplementation was used to enhance pedicle screw purchase in 17 of 49 patients. No local complications were noted. At review all 434 screws were contained within the pedicle, while 5 screws were fractured.

There were no systemic complications. Local complications consisted of dural lacerations in 12 patients, all revision cases. Despite primary repair in all patients, 2 patients required secondary repair and had uneventful outcomes. There were 2 superficial and 2 deep wound infections requiring incision and drainage and wound debridement. Instrumentation was not removed in either patient with deep wound infection. They went on to heal uneventfully with wound healing by secondary intention following long-term intravenous antibiotic therapy and serial wound debridement.

Revision surgery was required in 5 patients for bursitis secondary to the plates, and in 7 patients for pseudarthrosis or fusion for degeneration at the next mobile segment adjacent to the instrumented segments.

Satisfactory results were obtained in 83% of the primary group and 67% of the revision group.

Discussion and Conclusion

The patient population in this series shares the same demographic characteristics as reported in series on the treatment of single-level degenerative spondylolisthesis [1–5,9,12,15]. The majority of patients with multilevel degenerative spondylolisthesis had undergone prior surgery, which is in contrast to a minority of patients in other reported series [8,9,22]. We feel this reflects the referral nature of this practice. Back and leg pain, either unilateral or bilateral, was the most common clinical presentation and is consistent with previous series of single-level instability [8,9].

Physical examination revealed neurologic deficits in a minority of patients despite radicular symptoms in the majority, a discrepancy noted previously [2,3]. Somatosensory evoked potentials were abnormal in all patients in this series, demonstrating a discrepancy between the clinical examination and neurophysiologic testing, also reported previously [3]. Neurophysiologic testing is, therefore, more sensitive than clinical examination in assessing nerve-root compromise and should be part of the evaluation process.

The 4 : 1 ratio of revision to primary cases in this series implicates isolated decompressive laminectomy, with or without diskectomy, as a principal etiologic factor in multilevel instability.

Decompression with partial or total facetectomy in single-level degenerative spondylolisthesis has been shown to lead to increased listhesis [2,8,12,15,18,20, 26–30]. Controversy exists regarding the affect of post-decompression olisthesis on clinical outcome [9,12,18,19,26,30,31].

In this series all revision patients had been referred because of increased symptoms post-decompression with documented progression of olisthesis. As such, we agree with those authors who feel there is a correlation between post-decompression listhesis and symptoms [9,12,18,19,26,30,31].

While the causal relationship between the extent of facet removal and instability has been established, the priority must be adequate exposure of the canal and foramen bilaterally in order to perform sufficient decompression of the neural structures.

Arthritic enlargement of the facet joints at the level of the olisthesis is responsible for lateral recess stenosis compromising the descending nerve root, and intraforaminal stenosis compromising the exiting nerve root in the foramen. This has prompted the recommendation for facetectomy [3,5,8,20,23,32,33].

Patients in the revision group who had prior facetectomy all demonstrated residual stenosis in the intraforaminal zone related to vertical compression against the inferior surface of the pedicle by posterolateral protruding annulus with or without associated posterolateral osteophytes. This lesion was not addressed at the time of their initial surgery. This lesion was found in the primary patients in addition to stenosis in the central and lateral recess zones. These findings are in contrast to Reynold's and Wiltse's [19] who felt that the exiting nerve root at the level of an olisthesis is not impinged because it occupies the upper half of the neural canal. The significance of this lesion is emphasized by Burton et al. [34] who concluded that this was the most common cause of failed back surgery syndrome. The findings in this series support his conclusion.

The persistence of this site of compression in the revision group who had already had part or all of their facets removed emphasizes the failure of facetectomy, partial or complete, to decompress this lesion.

This form of intraforaminal stenosis in single-level degenerative spondylolisthesis has been described, and removal of the posterolateral corner of the vertebral body and the inferior portion of the pedicle has been advocated as a direct method of decompression [2,11,32,34]. Indirect decompression of the intraforaminal zone by using instrumentation to distract the affected disk space has been reported as an alternate method [14,21,22,24].

The technique used in this series provides for distraction of the disk space resulting in restoration of disk height, enlargement of the foramen, and variable relief of anteroposterior intraforaminal compression due to facet osteoarthritis and subluxation. Distraction optimizes visualization of intraforaminal pathology. Decompression inferior and anterior to the exiting nerve root, difficult to achieve in the nondistracted state, is facilitated by the increased room to position appropriate instruments to remove posterolateral osteophytes which will not subside with distraction alone. Disk space distraction has the benefit of correcting olisthesis by using tension of the collapsed annulus as the end point (i.e., ligamentotaxis). By repeating the technique one motion segment at a time, multilevel deformity is corrected, one segment at a time, irrespective of whether the translation is anterior, posterior, or lateral.

The average percent listhesis in our series was similar to that in other series [1,2,15,20].

While in the early part of this series, corrections were incomplete, in the latter part, with refinement in the technique, complete correction was achieved at all levels in all patients. By comparison, reported series using other instrumentation techniques [14,16,22] have all described residual olisthesis with incomplete correction and distraction-induced local kyphosis [14,22].

By distracting anterior to the center of rotation of the motion segment, local kyphosis is minimized. Appropriate lordosis is assured by securing plates that have been contoured to the appropriate degree of lordosis. In this series, lordosis was restored to more normal values and associated degenerative scoliosis was reduced or completely corrected. Stagnara et al. [35] reported that in a study of normal volunteers the maximum lordotic curve is 50°. In this series, patients presented with an average hyperlordosis and were all corrected to values of less than 50°.

In this series, all patients underwent fusion to minimize the incidence of post-decompression instability and to maintain the achieved correction. Posterolateral fusion has been reported to improve clinical results [12,15] despite concerns of a suboptimal biomechanical environment [11,13].

Segmental pedicle fixation has been reported to enhance posterolateral fusion rates [22,24]. In addition, this series demonstrates that, in conjunction with disk space distraction, deformity correction in the x-, y-, and z-axes is possible.

Unsupported disk space distraction, by increasing the bending moment on the posterior column, may lead to pseudarthrosis and instrumentation failure. Posterior lumbar interbody fusion addresses these concerns by virtue of being load sharing. The high PLIF fusion rate demonstrated in this series offsets posterolateral pseudarthrosis. Notwithstanding these advantages, this is a demanding technique, and if faced with a suboptimal environment, an alternative is staged anterior interbody fusion.

We feel that degeneration in adjacent levels is minimized by optimized spinal balance achieved through restoration of spinal alignment. Longer follow-up will be needed to assess this point.

Dural laceration was the most common intraoperative complication. Despite 2 patients requiring secondary repair, as a group there were no patients with long-term morbidity, a finding consistent with previous reports on incidental durotomy repaired primarily [36].

Satisfactory results were obtained in 83% of primary and 67% of revision cases which is comparable to reported results of single-level instability [8,14,

15]. We feel that results can be improved further by diskographic evaluation to assess adjacent levels for degeneration. This may reduce the number of patients with poor results secondary to unrecognized coexisting disk degeneration adjacent to the anticipated fusion levels.

Acknowledgments. The authors thank Ed Lashomb for preparing the manuscript.

References

1. Alexander E Jr, Kelly DL Jr, Davis CH Jr, McWhorter JM, Brown W (1985) Intact arch spondylolisthesis. A review of 50 cases and description of surgical treatment. J Neurosurg 63:840–844
2. Cauchoix J, Benoist M, Chassaing V (1976) Degenerative spondylolisthesis. Clin Orthop 115:122–129
3. Epstein NE, Epstein JA, Carras R, Lavine LS (1983) Degenerative spondylolisthesis with an intact neural arch: A review of 60 cases with an analysis of clinical findings and the development of surgical management. Neurosurgery 13:555–561
4. Fitzgerald JAW, Newman PH (1976) Degenerative spondylolisthesis. J Bone Joint Surg [Br] 58:184–192
5. Newman PH (1976) Surgical treatment for spondylolisthesis in the adult. Clin Orthop 117:106–111
6. Rosenberg NJ (1975) Degenerative spondylolisthesis. Predisposing factors. J Bone Joint Surg [Am] 57:467–474
7. Bradford DS (1986) Instrumentation of the lumbar spine. An overview. Clin Orthop 203:209–218
8. Brown MD, Lockwood JM (1983) Degenerative spondylolisthesis. Instr Course Lect 32:162–169
9. Dall BE, Rowe DE (1985) Degenerative spondylolisthesis. Its surgical management. Spine 10:668–672
10. Epstein JA, Epstein BS, Lavine LS, Carras R, Rosenthal AD (1976) Degenerative lumbar spondylolisthesis with an intact neural arch (pseudospondylolisthesis). J Neurosurg 44:139–147
11. Farfan HF, Kirkaldy-Willis WH (1981) The present status of spinal fusion in the treatment of lumbar intervertebral joint disorders. Clin Orthop 158:198–214
12. Feffer HL, Wiesel SW, Cuckler JM, Rothman RH (1985) Degenerative spondylolisthesis. To fuse or not to fuse. Spine 10:287–289
13. Frymoyer JW, Selby DK (1985) Segmental instability. Rationale for treatment. Spine 10:280–286
14. Hanley EN (1986) Decompression and distraction-derotation arthrodesis for degenerative spondylolisthesis. Spine 11:269–276
15. Herron LD, Trippi AC (1989) L4–5 degenerative spondylolisthesis. The results of treatment by decompressive laminectomy without fusion. Spine 14:534–538
16. Kaneda K, Kazama H, Satoh S, Fujiya M (1986) Follow-up study of medial facetectomies and posterolateral fusion with instrumentation in unstable degenerative spondylolisthesis. Clin Orthop 203:159–167

17. Lettin AWF (1967) Diagnosis and treatment of lumbar instability. J Bone Joint Surg [Br] 49:520–529
18. Lombardi JS, Wiltse LL, Reynolds J, Widell EH, Spencer C III (1985) Treatment of degenerative spondylolisthesis. Spine 10:821–827
19. Reynolds JB, Wiltse LL (1979) Surgical treatment of degenerative spondylolisthesis. An abstract. Spine 4:148–149
20. Rosenberg NJ (1976) Degenerative spondylolisthesis. Surgical treatment. Clin Orthop 117:112–120
21. Selby DK (1983) When to operate and what to operate upon. Orthop Clin North Am 14:577–588
22. Simmons EH, Capicotto WN (1988) Posterior transpedicular Zielke instrumentation of the lumbar spine. Clin Orthop 236:180–191
23. Soren A, Waugh TR (1985) Spondylolisthesis and related disorders. A correlative study of 105 patients. Clin Orthop 193:171–177
24. Zielke K, Strempel AV (1986) Posterior lateral distraction spondylodesis using the twofold sacral bar. Clin Orthop 203:151–158
25. Steffee AD, Biscup RS, Sitkowski DJ (1986) Segmental spine plates with pedicle screw fixation. A new internal fixation device for disorders of the lumbar and thoracolumbar spine. Clin Orthop 203:45–53
26. Johnsson KE, Willner S, Johnsson K (1986) Postoperative instability after decompression for lumbar spinal stenosis. Spine 11:107–110
27. Johnsson KE, Redlund-Johnell I, Udén A, Willner S (1989) Preoperative and postoperative instability in lumbar spinal stenosis. Spine 14:591–593
28. Lee C (1983) Lumbar spinal instability (olisthesis) after extensive posterior spinal decompression. Spine 8:429–433
29. Shenkin HA, Hash CJ (1979) Spondylolisthesis after multiple bilateral laminectomies and facetectomies for lumbar spondylosis. Follow-up review. J Neurosurg 50:45–47
30. Sienkiewicz PJ, Flatley TJ (1987) Postopertive spondylolisthesis. Clin Orthop 221: 172–180
31. Wiltse LL, Kirkaldy-Willis WH, Mclvor GWD (1976) The treatment of spinal stenosis. Clin Orthop 115:83–91
32. Kirkaldy-Willis WH, Wedge JH, Young-Hing K, Reilly J (1978) Pathology and pathogenesis of lumbar spondylosis and stenosis. Spine 3:319–328
33. McIvor GWD, Kirkaldy-Willis WH (1976) Pathological and myelographic changes in the major types of lumbar spinal stenosis. Clin Orthop 115:72–76
34. Burton CV, Kirkaldy-Willis WH, Yong-Hing K, Heithoff KB (1981) Causes of failure of surgery on the lumbar spine. Clin Orthop 157:191–199
35. Stagnara P, De Mauroy JC, Dran G, Gonon GP, Costanzo G, Dimnet J, Pasquet A (1982) Reciprocal angulation of vertebral bodies in a sagittal plane: Approach to references for the evaluation of kyphosis and lordosis. Spine 7:335–342
36. Jones AAM, Stambough JL, Balderston RA, Rothman RH, Booth RE (1989) Long term results of lumbar spine surgery complicated by unintended incidental durotomy. Spine 14:443–446

2.13 Posterior Stabilization for Lumbar Degenerative Kyphosis: In Situ Fusion in Maximum Extension on Hall's Frame

Osamu Nakai, Isakichi Yamaura, Yoshiro Kurosa, Hiromichi Komori, Atsushi Ookawa, Hiroshi Sakai, and Masahiro Abe[1]

Introduction

The most common form of spinal deformity in Japan, especially in rural areas, was coined lumbar degenerative kyphosis (LDK) by Takemistu et al. [1], from among the various types of kyphosis that have been recognized and investigated [2]. LDK had not been delineated regarding pathology and treatment, simply because this spinal deformity has historically been viewed as a result of the inevitable aging process. The pathology of this disease thus remains unknown and treatment remains undetermined. On the other hand, the everyday disabilities of patients with LDK are much more severe than those who are healthy can imagine; even essential daily activities such as standing and walking are seriously affected by LDK. The solution of this problem is therefore a natural target of study for Japanese spinal surgeons.

In this study, a surgical procedure for LDK was developed to satisfy the following conditions: (1) minimum risk of neurological involvement, (2) minimum invasiveness because of the patients' advanced ages, (3) reduced effects on the patients' inability to stoop or bend after operation, and (4) reduced reliance on the correction force of the spinal instrumentation system due to simultaneous existence of osteoporosis. The method employed was posterior stabilization in a position of maximum lumbar extension using Cotrel-Dubousset (C-D) instrumentation. No attempt at further correction during the operation was made.

[1]Department of Orthopaedic Surgery, Kudanzaka Hospital, 2-1-39 Kudan-Minami, Chiyoda-ku, Tokyo, 102 Japan

Subjects and Methods

Clinical Subjects

We reviewed 13 patients who had been treated with this method for LDK. The patients ranged in ages from 39 to 71 years (average of 60 years), and 2 patients were male and 11, female. Follow-up periods ranged from 10 months to 45 months (average of 27 months).

Clinical Symptoms

All patients complained of difficulty in walking and standing, due to their trunks leaning forward. They complained of their inability to hold things in front of them; they had to support themselves with their elbows in order to wash dishes. Difficulty in climbing slopes was also frequently mentioned. The cosmetic aspect of their stooped posture was a problem, especially for middle-aged women. These patients said that they were surprised when they saw themselves in a shop window, and they corrected their posture as a result.

Low back pain was a symptom in the early stages of this disease, but only 5 of 13 patients complained of low back pain just before the operation. Radicular symptoms were presented in seven cases. Cases in which lumbar kyphosis was caused mainly by radicular pain were excluded from this study.

Radiographic Findings

Operative cases were classified radiographically into three types: (1) lower lumbar, in which kyphosis existed below the level of L3, and the upper lumbar or thoracic spine was lordotic; (2) upper lumbar, in which thoracic kyphosis extended downward, and included the upper lumbar spine although lordosis remained at the level of L4–L5 or L5–S1; and (3) mixed, in which L4–L5 exhibited instability and became kyphotic during lumbar flexion, although a neutral X-ray was classified into the upper lumbar type.

There were eight cases of lower-lumbar-type LDK, three cases of upper-lumbar-type LDK, and two cases of mixed-type LDK. In all cases, the kyphotic curve was flexible and could be corrected in the lumbar extension position.

Myelography

Myelography was performed in all cases in order to detect a predisposition for problems resulting from hyperextension. Central stenosis was found in seven cases. In two cases, foraminal constriction was suspected and confirmed by a selective nerve root block.

Operative Method

Under general anesthesia, patients were kept prone on a Hall frame with the lumbar spine hyperextended. Posterior stabilization using C-D instrumentation was performed in situ, with no attempts at further correction during operation. Below the L3 level, posterolateral fusion and facet fusion were combined, and above the L2 level, only facet fusion was used with autogenous iliac bone grafting. Circular wiring of spinous processes was applied for augmentation at the end of the fused areas in cases of multisegmental fusion.

Decompression was performed at levels in which spinal stenosis existed or might occur postoperatively. Wide fenestration at one level was performed in seven cases, unilateral unroofing of the intervertebral foramen at one level was performed in one case, and total laminectomy and bilateral unroofing of the intervertebral foramen at two levels were performed in one case.

In most cases, the fusion area was determined to coincide with the kyphotic area. This is because many older sufferers of this kyphotic condition continue to work in farming, and must still spend long hours in a stooped position for planting and so on. For these patients, the fusion was made as short as possible. On the contrary, in patients who were not involved in farming work, whole lumbar fusion was chosen. In lower-lumbar-type LDK, the fusion area coincided with the kyphotic area in seven patients and the whole lumbar was fused in one. In upper-lumbar-type LDK, the unstable segments of the upper lumbar spine were fused in one, and the whole lumbar was fused in two patients in which the curve was rigid. In mixed-type LDK, the fusion area was limited to only the unstable L4–L5 segment (Table 1).

The numbers of segments fused were five in one patient, four in three patients, three in one patient, two in three patients and one in five patients.

The operations ranged from 175 min to 420 min for an average of 258 min. Blood loss ranged from 145 ml to 1780 ml, for an average of 634 ml, and four patients required blood transfusions.

Postoperative management consisted of bed rest for 3–8 weeks and application of rigid orthosis for 4–6 months.

Table 1. Fusion area in each LDK type and results.

LDK type	Fusion area		Results	
Lower lumbar	Kyphotic site only	7	Good 4	Poor 3
	Whole lumbar	1[a]	Good	
Upper lumbar	Unstable segments only	1[b]	Good	
	Whole lumbar	2	Fair	Poor
Mixed	Unstable L4–L5 only	2[c]	Good 2	

[a] Case 1, [b] Case 2, [c] Case 3

Results

Clinical Symptoms

Eight patients exhibited subjective improvement in both walking and standing, and also improvement in appearance. These were rated as good results. One patient exhibited subjective improvement in walking and standing, but no improvement in appearance. This case was rated as fair. The remaining four patients showed improvement neither subjectively nor objectively. These were rated as poor. These four patients included three with lower-lumbar-type LDK in the advanced stage, and one with the upper-lumbar-type LDK in which the curve was rigid (Table 1).

Complications

There were no complications. However, a 68-year-old woman sustained a compression fracture at the L1 level 3 months after the L4–L5 fusion operation. She recovered with no residual symptoms and was rated good, although she exhibited an increase in kyphosis at the L1 level.

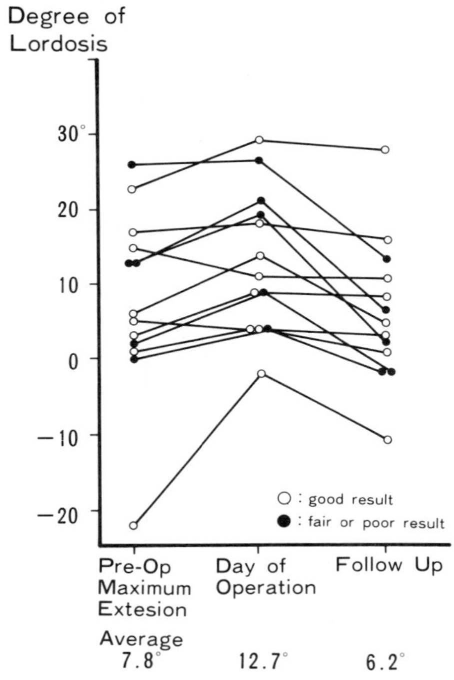

Fig. 1. Fluctuation of the degree of lordosis in the fusion area. The degree of lordosis immediately after operation exceeded preoperative anticipated degrees in the majority of cases. Loss of correction was observed 2–4 months after operation. Patients in which loss of correction was high were unsatisfied with the results

Bony Union

Complete union was obtained in twelve patients. Psuedarthrosis was found in one patient who had had arthrodesis from the L3 level to the sacrum. Loosening of the sacral screws caused a failure of union at the L5–S1 level and a poor clinical result.

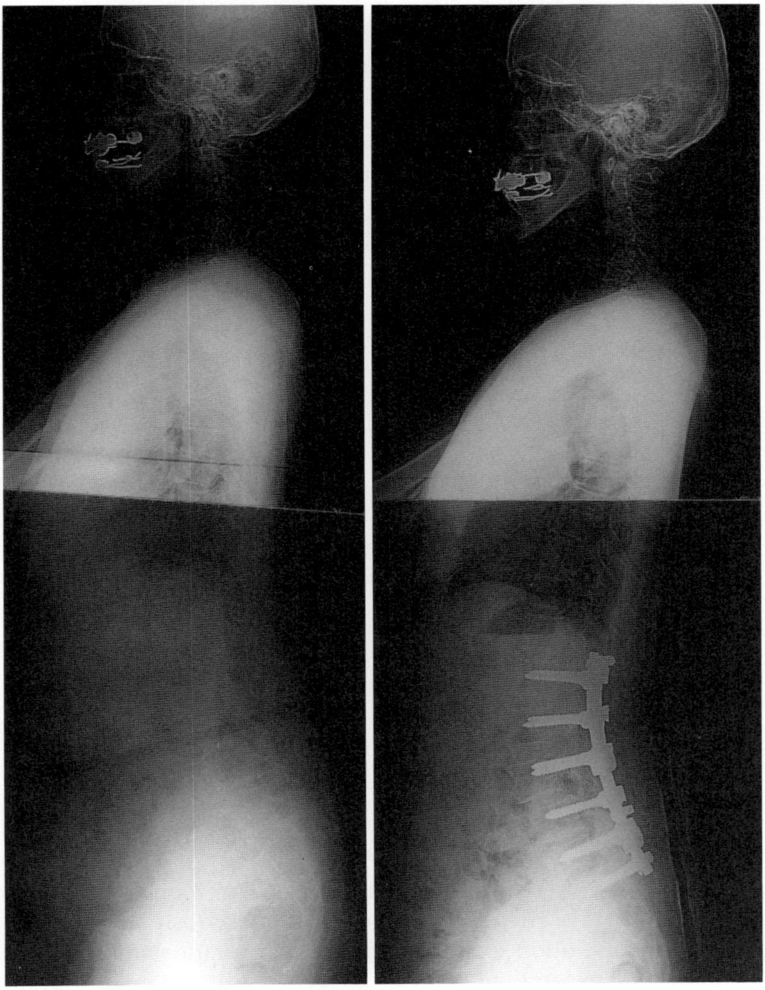

a b

Fig. 2a–e. Case 1: a 55-year-old woman with lower-lumbar-type kyphosis. Preoperative (**a**) and postoperative (**b**) X-rays, and preoperative (**c**) and postoperative (**d**) appearance are shown. The patient had no complaints about limited lumbar flexion (**e**)

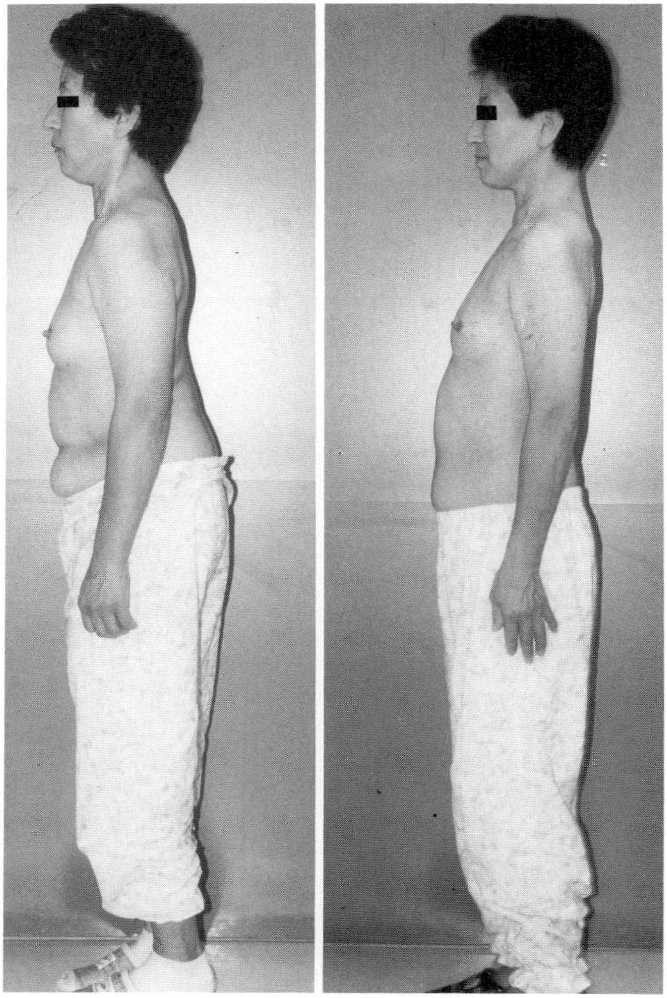

c d

Fig. 2. (*continued*)

Loss of Correction

In nine patients, loss of correction was observed 2–4 months after operation, ranging from 3° to 17°. However, the degree of lordosis in the fusion area immediately after operation exceeded preoperative anticipated degrees in the majority (10 of 13 patients). Therefore, at the time of follow-up, preoperative anticipated lordosis was obtained in eight patients, when the error was considered to be within ±3°. Seven of these eight patients showed good clinical results (Fig. 1).

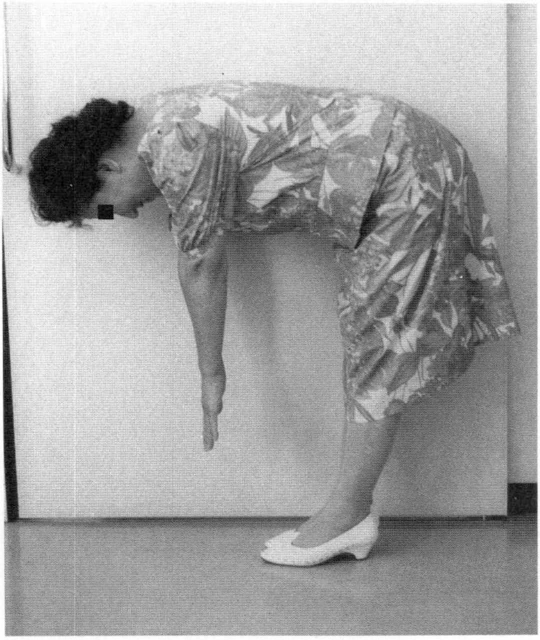

e

Fig. 2. (*continued*)

Loss of correction occurred mainly at the most distal segment of multisegmental fusion, due to the pedicle screws being loosened or bent. Bone union was obtained in the position of loss of correction in all but one patient.

Case Report

Case 1: A 55-year-old woman with lower-lumbar-type LDK. Kyphosis existed from the L3 to the S1 level, although the thoracic and upper lumbar curve was lordotic. In a standing position, she compensated by bending her knees and hyperextending her hips. While walking, she gradually leaned further forward and periodically had to stop to try and straighten herself, otherwise she could not continue to walk. The fusion area was chosen to be from the L1 to S1 levels, including the lordotic upper lumbar level. This was because she had changed from farming work to a job as an office clerk, and so she did not require the bending posture during daily activities. The degree of lordosis between the L1 and S1 level was 23° at the preoperative maximum extension, 29° on the day of operation (supine), and 28° at 20 months after the operation when complete union was obtained.

The result was satisfactory both subjectively and objectively. She had no complaints about limited lumbar flexion or stiffness (Fig. 2).

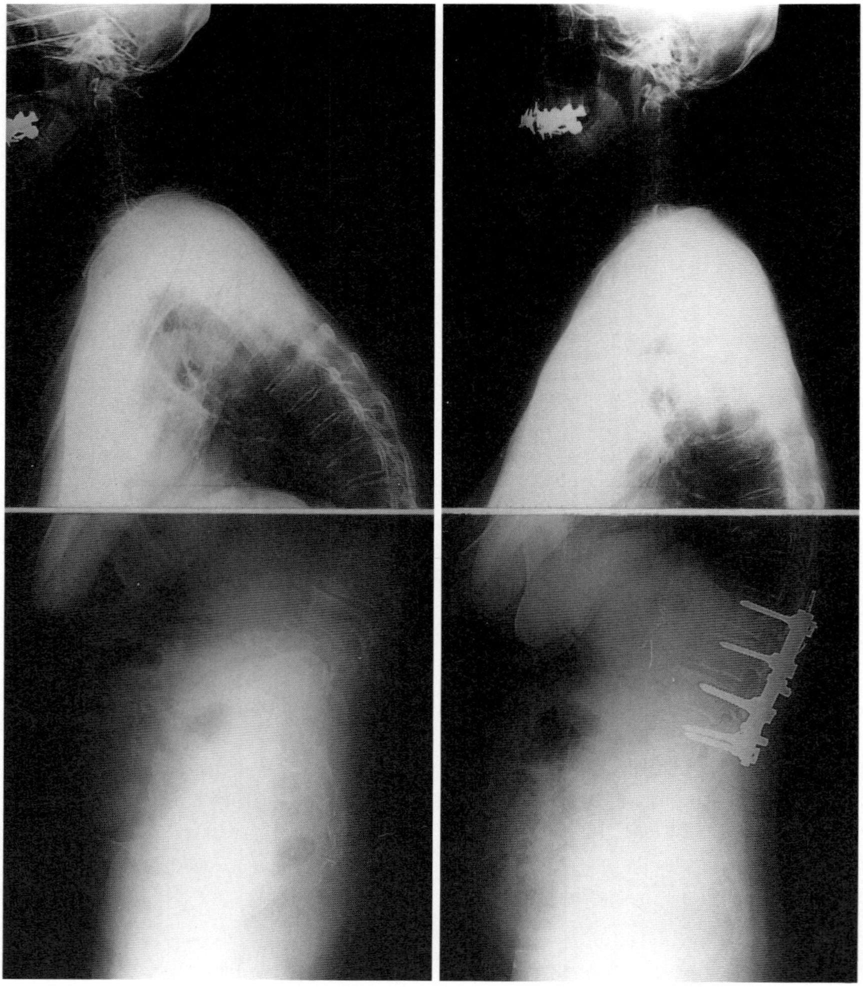

a b

Fig. 3a–f. Case 2: a 68-year-old woman with upper-lumbar-type kyphosis. Preoperative (**a**) and postoperative (**b**) lateral X-rays in a standing position, along with the preoperative appearance (**c**) are shown. She could not carry heavy things in front of her (**d**). Her appearance was remarkably improved and her symptoms were relieved (**e**,**f**)

Case 2: A 68-year-old woman with upper-lumbar-type LDK. Thoracic kyphosis extended to the L4 level and both segments at the L2–L3 and L3–L4 levels showed marked instability. She complained of difficulty when walking and standing, and of the inability to carry things in front of her. Posterior stabilization from L1 to L4 in the position of maximum lumbar extension using C-D

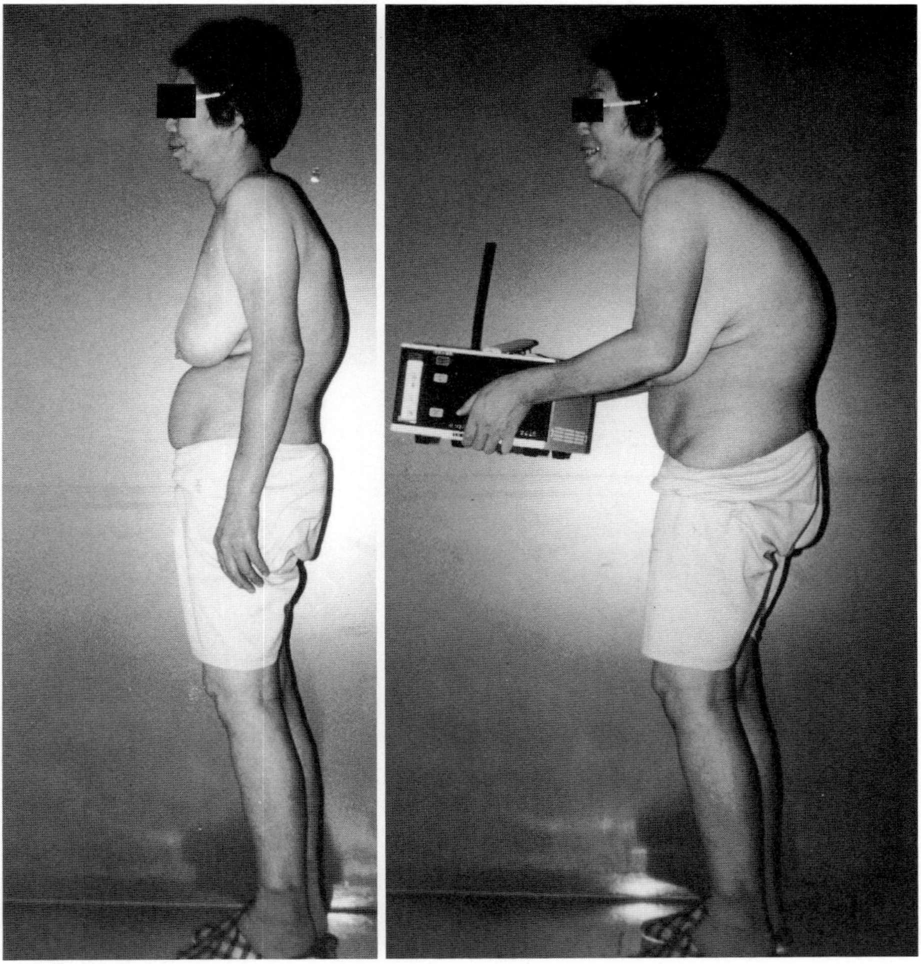

c d

Fig. 3. (*continued*)

instrumentation was performed, supplemented by interspinous wiring between T12 and L1.

The degree of lordosis in the fusion area which was from the T12 to L4 levels was −22° at preoperative maximum extension, −2° on the day of the operation (supine), and −11° at 12 months after the operation when complete union was obtained. Her appearance was remarkably improved and her disturbance when walking and standing was relieved. She could carry heavy things in front of her and was satisfied with the results (Fig. 3).

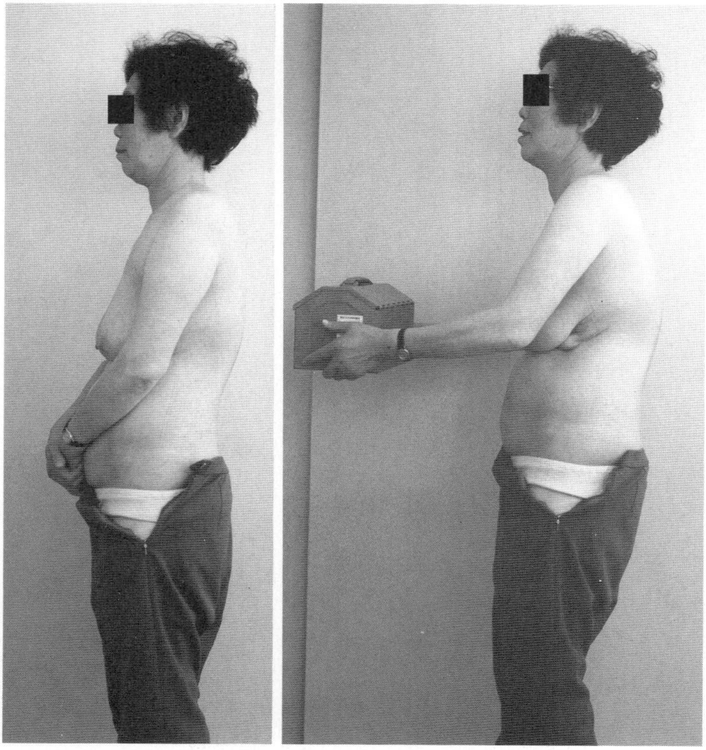

e f

Fig. 3. (*continued*)

Case 3: A 56-year-old woman with mixed-type LDK. Thoracic kyphosis extended downward to the L4 level, and lordosis remained only at the L4–L5 and L5–S1 levels in a neutral standing position. However, the L4–L5 segment exhibited marked instability and it was becoming kyphotic in the lumbar flexion position. Her symptoms were the same as seen in other patients.

The fusion area was determined to limit only the unstable L4–L5 segment because she desired to continue farming and required a bending posture in her postoperative life. Her appearance did not improve very much, but subjective symptoms were markedly improved after the operation. She returned to her farm work, and continues that work now, 2 years after the operation (Fig. 4).

Discussion

The etiology of LDK remains unknown [3]. We speculate that the etiology of the upper lumbar type is different from that of the lower lumbar type because there are some different characteristics for each type: onset is earlier in the

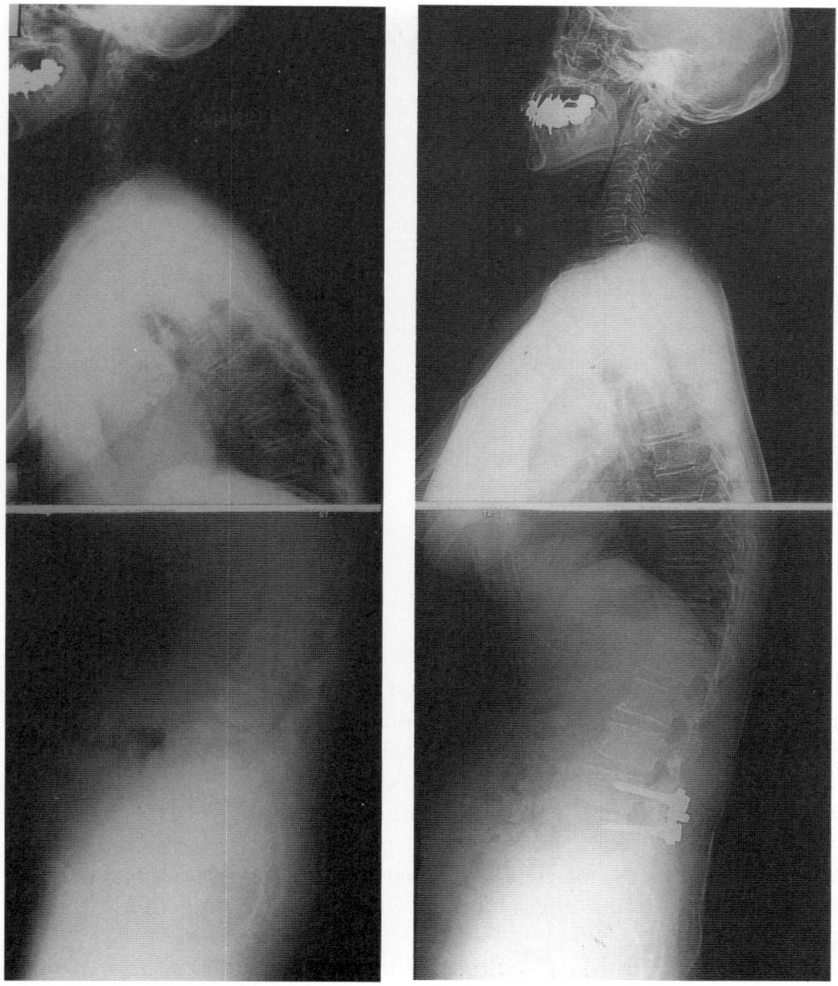
a b

Fig. 4a–d. Case 3: a 56-year-old woman with mixed-type LDK. Thoracic kyphosis extended downward to the L4 level in a neutral standing position (**a**). L4-L5 showed marked instability, and became kyphotic in lumbar flexion (**c,d**). Her symptoms were relieved with only L4-L5 fusion, although her appearance did not improve very much (**b**)

lower lumbar type than in the upper lumbar type; thoracic curve is lordotic in the former, although kyphotic in the latter; and disk degeneration is more prominent in the former than in the latter. Whole thoracolumbar kyphosis including even the sacrum is the final stage of both types.

In the lower lumbar type, kyphotic deformity usually starts at the L4–L5 level, and is caused by disk degeneration. Kyphosis extends downward to the

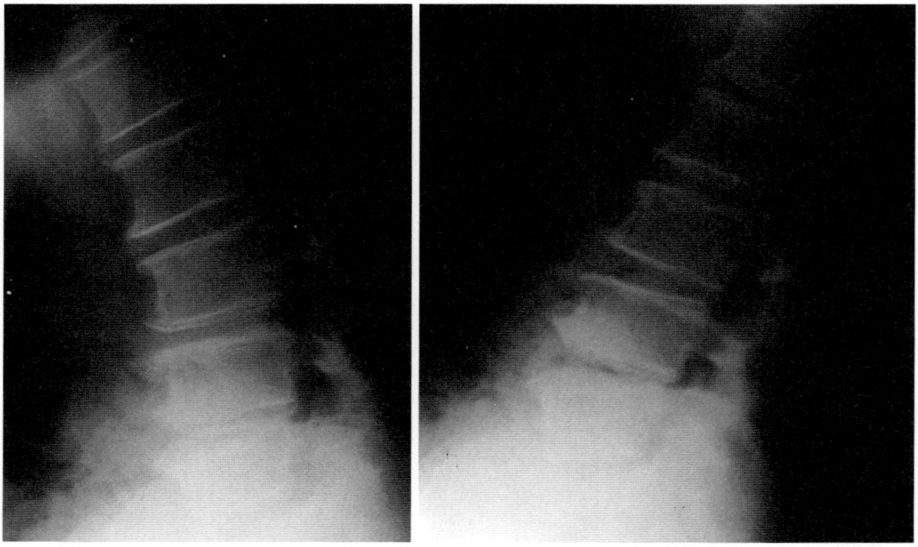

c d

Fig. 4. (*continued*)

L5–S1 level and upward to the L3–L4 level. Anterior slipping is usually combined at the L3–4 level. In the beginning, kyphosis is corrected by lumbar extension; however, kyphosis becomes rigid later.

The stage of disease can be determined using the following two lines obtained by measurement in lateral X-ray films: line F from the center of the vertebral body of L1 to the superior anterior iliac spine, and line B from the same point to the spinous process of S1. The length of line F represents that of the abdominal muscles, and the length of line B represents that of the back muscles (Fig. 5).

The length of line F is always longer than that of line B in normal subjects. However, in lower-lumbar-type LDK patients, F becomes shorter than B on lumbar flexion in the beginning. Later, F becomes shorter than B also in the neutral position, and finally F becomes shorter than B even on lumbar extension. We call these three stages early, intermediate, and late, respectively.

Eight patients of the lower lumbar type in this series were classified as follows: four patients were in the early stage, two were in the intermediate stage, and two were in the late stage. The four patients in the early stage were successfully treated by fusion of the kyphotic site in the extension position. However, similar treament of three of the patients in the intermediate or late stages was unsuccessful. This was because correction of kyphosis in the lower lumbar levels was canceled out by the postoperative appearance of kyphosis in the upper lumbar levels (Fig. 6). Therefore, in the intermediate stages, fusion

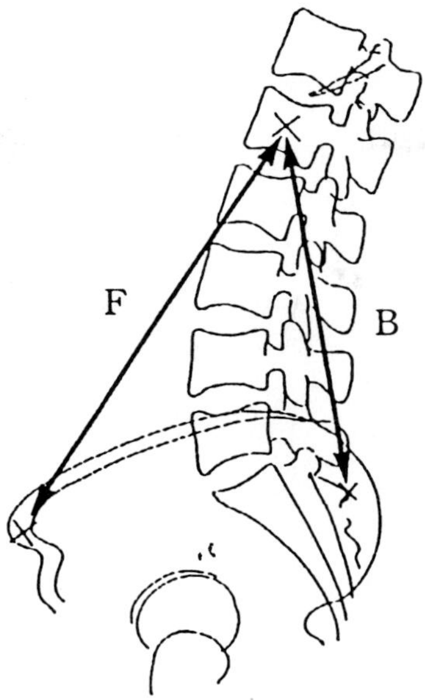

Fig. 5. Measurement of a lateral X-ray for determination of the stages of disease in lower-lumbar-type kyphosis. The stages of disease in lower-lumbar-type kyphosis can be determined by comparing the length of line *F*, representing the abdominal muscles, and line *B*, representing the back muscles

should cover the entire lumbar spines in the extension position as in case 1, so that line F is longer than B after operation.

In the late stages, even in the extension position, alignment with F longer than B cannot be obtained, and therefore there is no indication for this operative method. More radical methods, such as anterior and posterior release and corrective stabilization for rigid kyphotic sites, are necessary [4–6].

One case in the late stage who had a fusion at only the kyphotic site was rated poor and is shown in Fig. 6. She was 68 years old, presenting with symptoms of a compromised right L4 root and also typical symptoms of lumbar kyphosis. Decompression surgery combined with fusion from L1 to S1 in a maximum extension position was recommended. However, she refused long lumbar fusion because she desired to continue working in farming. Therefore, only the kyphotic site fusion in maximum extension was associated with decompression surgery at the L3–L4 level. Her anterior thigh pain on the right disappeared completely after the operation, but the symptoms of lumbar kyphosis remained unchanged.

Upper-lumbar-type LDK does not start from degeneration of a certain disk, but progresses gradually by thoracic kyphosis extension. Usually disks are relatively well preserved. Lower lumbar spines become hyperlordotic and

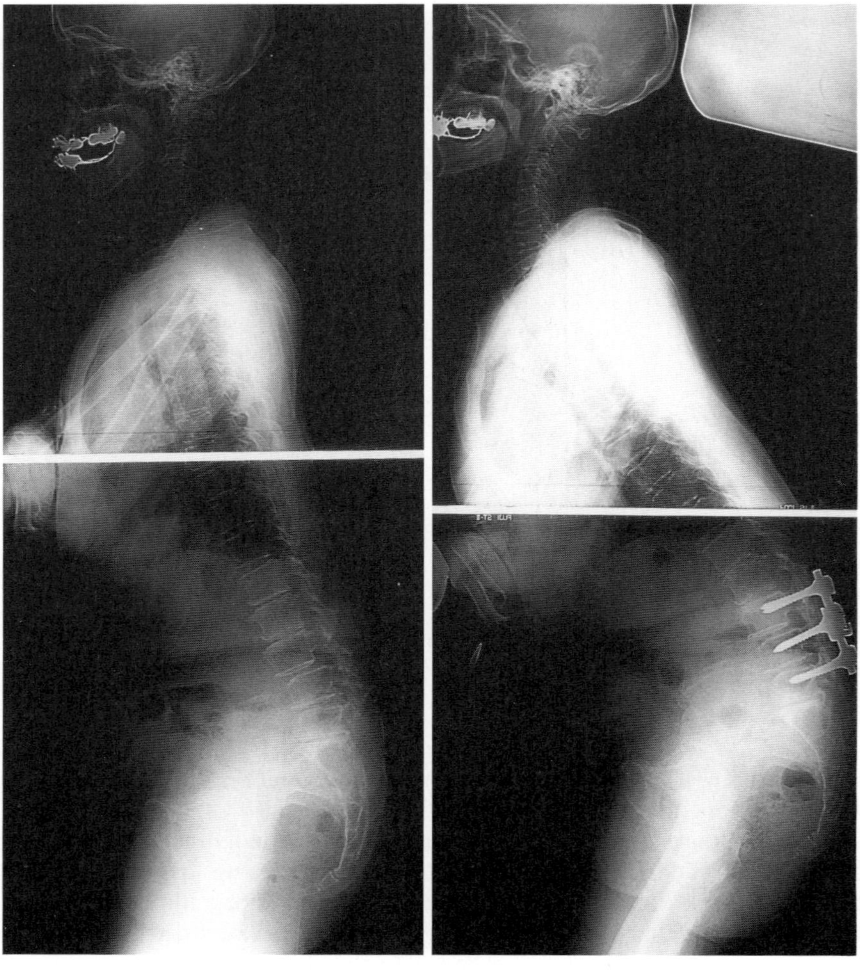

a b

Fig. 6a,b. Patients in the intermediate or late stage of lower-lumbar-type kyphosis were unsuccessfully treated by fusion at only the kyphotic site. This was because correction of kyphosis in the lower lumbar levels was canceled out by postoperative appearance of kyphosis in the upper lumbar levels

compensate. If there are not any unstable segments, the patient's disability is not as great as his appearance suggests. However, if any unstable segments exist in kyphosis or compensatory lordosis, such as at the L4–L5 level, disability becomes greater. Stabilization of the unstable segments in the extension position is an effective treatment in this case.

In upper-lumbar-type LDK with no unstable segments, determination of the fusion area is difficult [7,8]. If the curve is rigid, this operative method is not indicated. If extension produces over 30° correction, stabilization from the mid or lower thoracic spine to the lower lumbar spine in this method is indicated.

Combined osteoporosis is also an important factor for operative indication. Advanced osteoporosis is a contraindication for this method. If two or more compressive fractures of the vertebral body at the thoracolumbar level are found, this operation is not recommended, since postoperative bed rest causes disuse bone atrophy in the spine and causes a risk of multiple compression fracture resulting in deterioration of kyphosis. Early ambulation was pursued in this study. Nevertheless, one patient suffered from a compression fracture during the postoperative rehabilitation program. It is unknown how C-D instrumentation influences progression of senile osteoporosis over long periods. In order to evaluate this, longer follow-up will be necessary.

References

1. Takemitsu Y, Harada Y, Iwahara T, Miyamoto M, Miyatake Y (1988) Lumbar degenerative kyphosis: Clinical, radiological, and epidemiological studies. Spine 13: 1317–1326
2. Kostuik JP (1991) Adult kyphosis. In: Frymoyer JW (ed) The adult spine: Principle and practice. Raven, New York, pp 1369–1403
3. Milne JS, Willamson J (1983) A longitudinal study of kyphosis in older people. Age Ageing 12:225–233
4. Thomasen E (1985) Vertebral osteotomy for correction of kyphosis in ankylosing spondylitis. Clin Orthop 194:142–152
5. Kostuik JP, Maurais GR, Richardson WJ, Okajima Y (1988) Combined single stage anterior and posterior osteotomy for correction of iatrogenic lumbar kyphosis. Spine 13:257–266
6. Kokubun S, Sakurai M, Suzuki T, Masuda K, Ishii Y, Tani M (1990) One-stage anterior and posterior correction of lumbar degenerative kyphosis (in Japanese). East Jpn J Clin Orthop 2:80–82
7. Bernhardt M, Bridwell KH (1989) Segmental analysis of the sagittal plane alignment of the normal thoracic and lumbar spines and thoracolumbar junction. Spine 14: 717–721
8. Stagnara P, De Mauroy JC, Dran G, Gonon GP, Costanzo G, Dimnet J, Pasquet A (1982) Reciprocal angulation of vertebral bodies in a saggital plane: Approach to references for the evaluation of kyphosis and lordosis. Spine 7:335–342

2.14 Operative Treatment of Lumbar Degenerative Kyphosis

Yoshiharu Takemitsu, Yuji Atsuta, Yuki Kamo, Toshihito Iwahara, Osamu Sugawara, Yoshio Harada, and Yasumasa Miyatake[1]

Introduction

Lumbar degenerative kyphosis (LDK) is a clinical entity in which abnormal kyphosis, including flat back, occurs in the lumbar region due to degenerative changes of the spine and supporting structures [1]. Clinical features include a kyphotic change of the lumbar spine and trunk stooping increases while walking, and in the upright posture labor is disturbed by pain and dullness in the lumbar region which disrupt daily activities. Patients cannot lift their trunk up from the prone position. Vertebral wedging and multiple disk space narrowing are commonly seen in the LDK lumbar spine. Also a characteristic atrophy of the lumbar extensors has been noted. This deformity is frequently seen among farmers who have worked in a trunk flexion position for many years. Therefore this kind of working posture is supposed to be intimately related with the development of an LDK posture, possibly through its affect on the lumbar extensors.

Most LDK patients are treated conservatively by passive lumbar extension, exercise, and braces. However, with this treatment, correction is difficult to achieve and maintain in progressive cases. A rarely reported operative treatment has been done in a few cases [2] (see Chap. 2.13). With the increasing number of aged people, this kind of surgery might increase in the future. Our indications include (1) ambulatory disability with the stooped posture in patients who stand for long periods at work, (2) patients who are still active and under 65 years of age, and (3) severe low back pain that makes work difficult. However, patients who have osteoporosis with a round back are to be excluded. Local factors such as the range of lumbar motion, extent of lumbar muscle weakness, and extent of spondylosis combined with lumbar canal stenosis do not limit indications for operative treatment. The aim of the operation is to correct the kyphotic deformity and to cure low back pain by obtaining stab-

[1] Department of Orthopaedic Surgery, Asahikawa Medical College, Nishikagura 4-5, Asahikawa, Hokkaido, 078 Japan

ility. If lumbar canal stenosis is also present, we advocate simultaneous decompression.

Since 1979 we have operated on eight cases, seven of which were successful. Although there has been only a small number of cases, we have encountered many interesting problems which we will report here, as well as a discussion of the operative method and results achieved.

Materials and Methods

Three methods were used in this study:

1. *Posterior approach*. Multilevel shortening osteotomy and fusion using instrumentation following decompression laminectomy was performed in three cases. The posterior approach was used for patients who simply wanted to cure low back pain by obtaining solid fusion in maximally corrected spinal curvature, following adequate decompression for lumbar stenosis symptoms if they existed.
2. *Anterior approach*. Multilevel intervertebral release and fusion was carried out in two cases, in which lumbar kyphosis was not corrected by extension exercise for at least 1 week and an anterior release was needed for correction of kyphosis.
3. *Combined procedure*. Multilevel anterior and posterior correction and fusion using instrumentation was done in three cases. This surgery was used for patients with indications for sufficient correction of lumbar kyphosis to adequate lordosis, thereby, obtaining a good upright posture, supported by combined instrumentation and fusion, as well as posterior decompression for lumbar canal stenosis.

Results

The results from operated cases are shown in Table 1. The average age at operation was 58.6 years, ranging from 48 to 67 years. The average lumbar kyphosis angle measured while standing was 19.3°, ranging from 5° to 30°. At 1 year after surgery this had been improved to an average of 10.4° lordosis, ranging from 30° lordosis to 9° kyphosis. Lumbar lordosis was achieved with good results in six patients. In one of the other two patients, a 57-year-old female (case 4), significant correction was not obtained by simple posterior fusion, although the patient could walk with her trunk straight upright for long distances with good stability. In case 1, a 66-year-old female, only anterior fusion of L4–S was performed, but there was recurrence of lumbar kyphosis and progression of disease 3 years after surgery. A possible reason for such failure is that the fusion was too short due to intraoperative complications and that both extensor muscle atrophy and vertebral osteoporosis progressed after surgery.

Table 1. Results of eight operated cases of lumbar degenerative kyphosis.

Case no./init.	Age/sex	Initial diagnosis	Year	Before operation (°)	Method	After operation (°)	Instrumentation	Correction (°)	Complication
Anterior method									
1 F.S.	66 F	LDK Osteoporosis	1980	Ky: 25 (L1–L5)	Anterior (L4–S1)	Lor: 5 (L4–L5) Ky: 25 (L1–L5) 3 years postop.	None	0	Increased kyphosis
2 I.O.	57 M	LDK post-laminectomy kyphosis	1986	Ky: 30 (L1–L4)	Anterior (L2–L4)	Lor: 3 (L2–L4)	Anterior Kaneda device (without transverse fixateur)	33	
Poterior method									
3 A.D.	67 F	LDK Idiopathic scoliosis	1985	Ky: 5 (L1–L5) Scol: 61	Posterior (L1–S)	Lor: 11 Scol: 42	Harrington Luque SSI	16	
4 T.O.	57 F	LDK	1986	Ky: 12 (T12–L5)	Posterior (L1–L5)	Ky: 9 (T12–L5)	Luque Galveston SSI	3	Wire breakage in upper end of Luque rod (reoperated)
5 H.K.	64 F	LDK LCS	1991	Ky: 16 (L2–S)	Posterior (L2–S) PLIF (L3–L5) Foraminotomy	Lor: 17	C-D pedicle screw	33	L4/L5 nerve root impingement (reoperated)
Combined method									
6 M.T.	48 M	LDK	1979	Ky: 18 (L1–L5)	Combined (L1–L5)	Lor: 30	Harrington compression hook (T12–L5)	48	
7 T.N.	52 F	LDK	1987	Ky: 14 (L1–L5)	Combined Ant: L3–L5 Post: L5–S	Lor: 21 (L1–L5)	Anterior Kaneda device Steffee VSP (one stage)	35	
8 S.A.	57 F	LDK Degenerative olisthesis (L3/4, L4/5) LCS	1989	Ky: 19 (L2–L5)	Combined Ant: L2–L5 Laminectomy Post: L5–S1	Lor: 5	Anterior Kaneda device Steffee VSP (one stage)	24	L4 nerve root impingement (reoperated)

LDK, lumbar degerative kyphosis; ant, anterior; post, posterior; Ky, kyphosis; Lor, lordosis; Scol, scoliosis; PLIF, posterior lumbar interbody fusion; LCS, lumbar canal stenosis

No infection nor pseudarthrosis occurred. Two patients developed radicular pain when they started to walk a few weeks after surgery. One patient who underwent combined correction and fusion developed left L4 radicular pain after surgery. By adding foraminotomy for this complication 6 weeks after surgery, the pain was relieved. In another patient, who had a recurrence of right L5 radicular pain, a part of the C-D rod had to be removed and decompression foraminotomy was done with good results.

Anterior Correction and Fusion

Two patients had anterior correction and fusion alone, and one achieved a successful result.

Case 2: A 57-year-old male who was operated upon using the anterior procedure. The patient had difficulty in walking for more than 10 min because of low back pain and a stooped posture. His lumbar spine showed retrolisthesis at L3–L4 and postlaminectomy kyphosis. A Kaneda device was successfully used in the anterior operation, making his kyphotic lumbar spine lordotic, performing correction and fusion at two disk levels, and resulting in 23° of correction (Fig. 1).

Posterior Fusion

Three cases were treated using posterior fusion at 4.6 levels on average, resulting in a mean correction angle of 16°. In case 4, an upper junctional kyphosis occurred 1 year postoperatively, although good correction of degenerative scoliosis, better gait posture, and pain relief were maintained by solid fusion. In case 8, the L5 nerve root was involved after operation using PLIF and C-D instrumentation, and this was successfully treated by additional foraminotomy.

Case 4: A 57-year-old female who complained of servere low back pain and a flat back posture. The X-ray showed slight kyphoscoliosis due to multiple disk narrowing and wedged vertebra. Since the lumbar spinal canal stenosis was shown by myelography and was slightly symptomatic, posterior decompression was performed at 2 levels, followed by posterolateral fusion from L1 to S1 using Luque instrumentation. One year postoperatively an L rod began protruding due to upper junctional kyphosis and therefore was removed. On reflection a better result might have been obtained if anterior fusion had been done simultaneously (Fig. 2).

Case 5: A 64-year-old female school teacher who presented with LDK combined with severe lumbar spinal canal stenosis. The chief complaint was gait disturbance due to low back pain and sciatica as well as a forward leaning posture while walking. Spinal canal stenosis at two levels was demonstrated by myelography. Decompressive laminectomy was done from L3 to L5 for lumbar

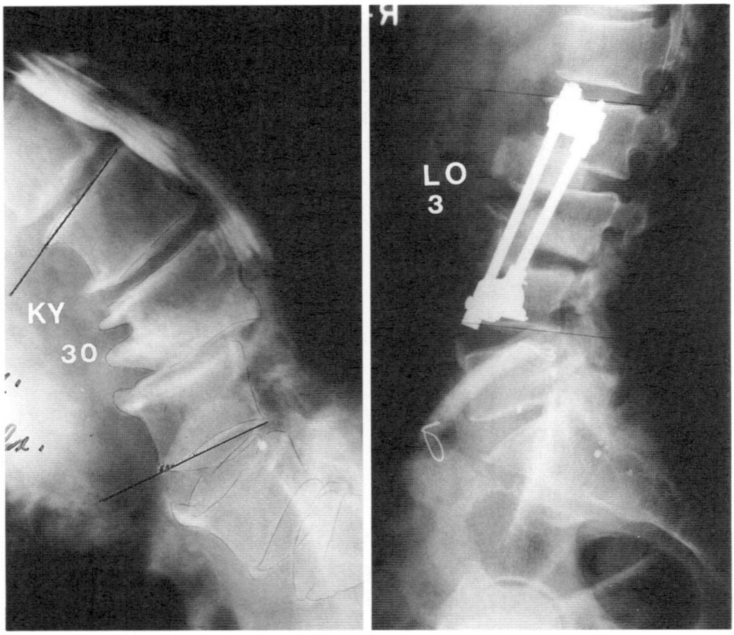

1 a b

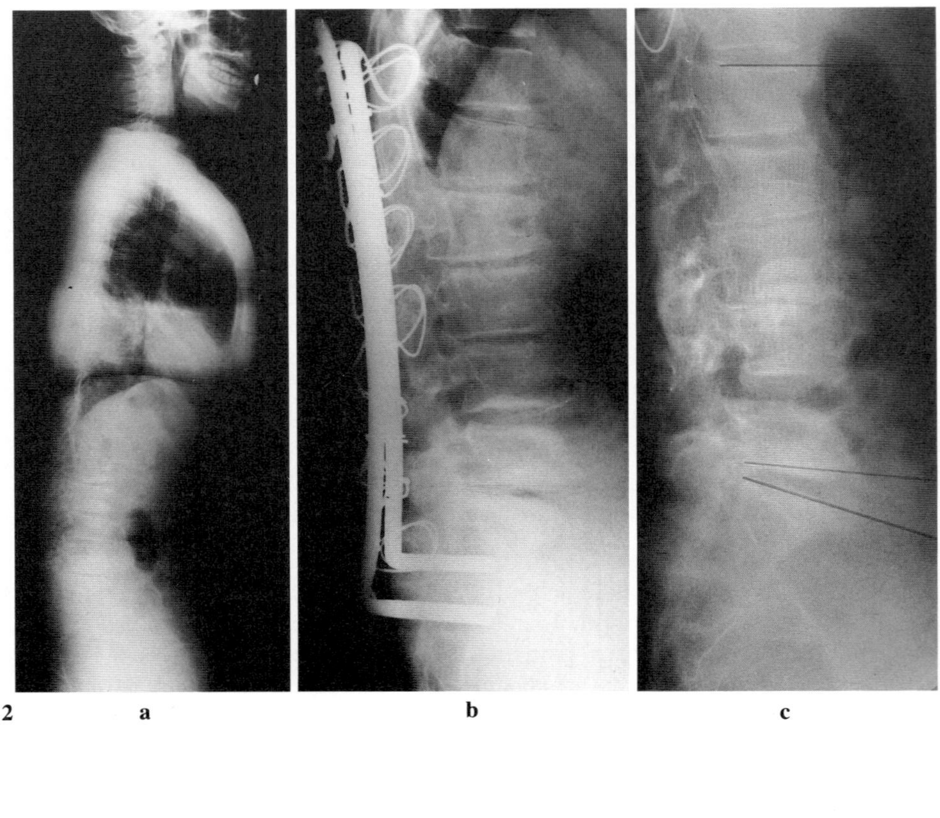

2 a b c

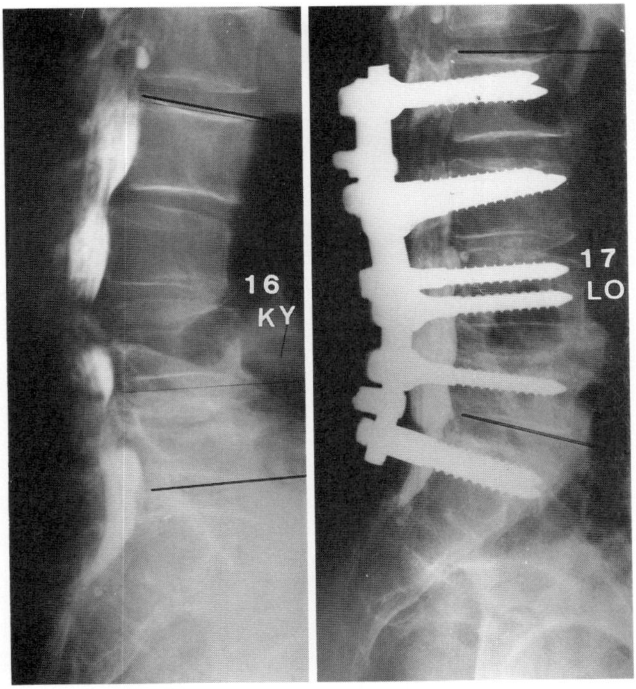

a b

Fig. 3a,b. Case 5: a 64-year-old female. **a** The patient had low back pain and lumbar canal stenosis symptoms for more than 12 months, as well as a stooped posture. Myelography showed a marked block at L3/4 and L4/5. **b** Myelography at 6 months after decompression and fusion using C-D pedicle screws and 3 months after the second foraminotomy, showing good correction with smooth myelography column. Lumbar kyphosis of 16° (*16KY*) was corrected to 17° lordosis (*17LO*)

◄———

Fig. 1a,b. Case 2: a 57-year-old male who complained of severe low back pain and stooped posture. **a** Lumbar kyphosis due to post-laminectomy instability combined with degenerative kyphosis. *ky30*, L2–L4 30°. **b** After anterior fusion at L2–L4 using an old-type Kaneda device (Mizuho Ika Kogyo, Tokyo). The patient's deformity was corrected to 3° lordosis (*LO3*) and posture was also corrected

Fig. 2a–c. Case 4: a 57-year-old female farmer. **a** The patient had low back pain and a stooped posture while walking. **b** Posterior fusion with Luque SSI instrumentation following multilevel interlaminar decompression was carried out. Lumbar kyphosis was not corrected enough by the operation, but the patient was able to walk in a stable upright posture. **c** At 1 year after removal of the instruments

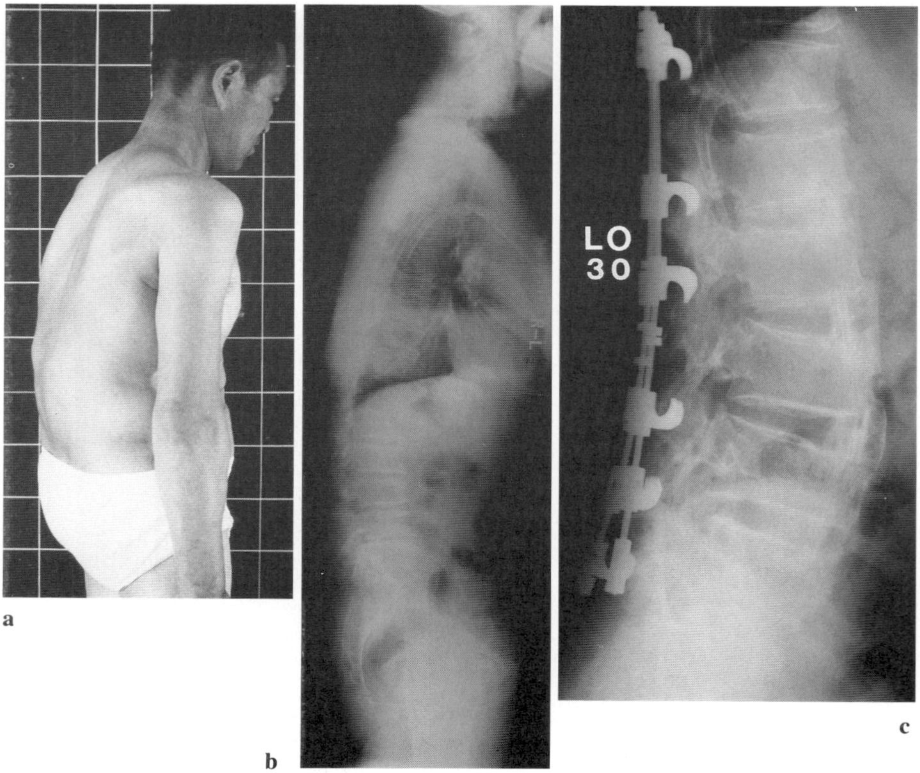

Fig. 4a–c. Case 6: a 48-year-old male. **a** The patient had low back pain for many years and found difficulty in keeping the trunk upright while standing. **b** X-ray before surgery showing 18° lumbar kyphosis due to multiple disk narrowing at L1–S. **c** At 2 years after combined anterior plus posterior fusion L1–L5 with a Harrington compression hook, done in 1979, 30° lordosis (*LO 30*) was obtained and the patient had excellent sagittal realignment

canal stenosis, followed by PLIF with osteotomy at the same levels after removal of the protruded disk. To reinforce stability we added posterolateral fusion from L2 to S1 using C-D pedicle screw fixation between the same levels. After the recurrence of moderate right radicular pain at L4 and L5 2 months after surgery, we partially removed the C-D instrument and relieved the roots. Examination of nerve-root-evoked potentials gave helpful information for detecting the root lesion during surgery (Fig. 3).

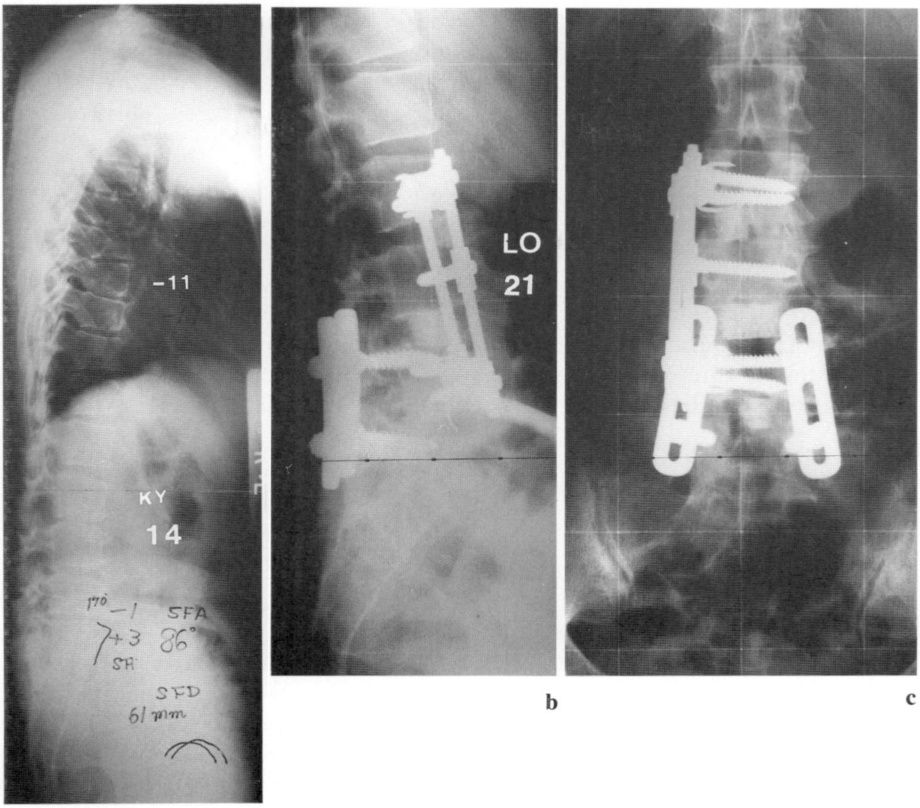

a b c

Fig. 5a–c. Case 7: a 52-year-old female with low back pain and a stooped posture. **a** Before surgery. Maximal extension in upright standing showed 14° kyphosis (*KY 14*) which was produced by marked extensor muscle atrophy and disk narrowing. **b,c** At 1 year after combined anterior and posterior fusion L2–L5 using a Kaneda device with the Steffee VSP system. Lumbar curvature improved from 14° kyphosis to 21° lordosis (*LO 21*) between L2 and L5. Excellent results were obtained. Sacralization of L5 was seen

Combined Method

In the three patients treated by the combined method, the average correction angle was 35.5°. The Harrington compression system was used for one case in 1979, and a Kaneda device plus Steffee variable screw placement (VSP) was used in the other two cases, with the best correction and solid fusion obtained by this combined procedure.

Case 6: A 48-year-old male forestry worker who complained of severe low back pain at work and an 18° kyphotic lumbar spine. Anterior ligament release, diskectomy with L2–L5 fusion plus posterior instrumentation using the Harrington compression system at L1–L5 were performed in two stages. This achieved the excellent results of 30° lordosis (Fig. 4).

Case 7: A 52-year-old female lumberer who had 14° of lumbar kyphosis in the natural standing position with marked lumbar muscle atrophy. The combined operation was done with anterior fusion at three levels, L2/3, L3/L4, and L4/L5 (L5 was fused congenitally to the sacrum), using the Kaneda device from L2 to L4, followed by posterior decompression of L4/L5 and fusion using the Steffee VSP system at L4/L5. Bioactive ceramic blocks, such as the AW glass ceramic and hydroxyapatite intervertebral spacer were used for intervertebral fusion. This resulted in 21° lumbar lordosis and excellent balanced alignment (Fig. 5).

Discussion

In Japan, especially in rural areas, many elderly women have LDK. They often complain of pain and dullness in their lower back while walking in an upright posture and for many the cosmetic aspect is also a problem. Conservative treatment such as extension functional braces and physical therapy are usually prescribed, resulting in considerable pain relief. However, the kyphosis cannot be significantly corrected and patients who have kyphosis complicated with lumbar canal stenosis are difficult to manage conservatively. We therefore began surgical treatment in 1979 on patients who are relatively young, still working, and who are determined to improve their spinal deformity and low back pain. This last indication for operation should be the most important factor for these patients. We also advocate that the patient should be less than 65 years of age. In more than 150 cases registered in our clinic we have operated upon only eight patients because we believe the operative invasion to be major even when using modern techniques. Most patients are too old and inactive to undergo such operations. In this volume Nakai et al. reports on 13 cases operated with the posterior method alone where C-D instrumentation was used, but no attempts to correct kyphosis further than that of maximal extension position shown before the operation were made (Chap 2.13). Nine patients out of 13 were treated with fusion of the lumbar spine at two segments or less. Nakai also suggested a restricted indication for the operative treatment of LDK.

In our study, low back pain and gait disturbance were significantly improved in all patients except one. Our results indicate that the most desirable method was combined fusion, which obtained 35° of correction. In patients that had lumbar canal stenosis complications, including those whose radicular pain was slight when provoked by extension of the lumbar spine, decompression foraminotomy needed to be done simultaneously based on symptoms and myelography. As shown in our series, anterior or posterior surgery alone did not result in good correction of the kyphosis. A simple anterior procedure can be chosen for cases who only have chronic low back pain with slight kyphosis. Simple posterior surgery was indicated for cases with minor kyphosis complicated with lumbar canal stenosis requiring posterior decompression at the same procedure. In cases where structural kyphosis was evident in the whole lumbar spine caused by multiple disk narrowing, an anterior ligament and disk release of all involved segments followed by intervertebral fusion with solid bone graft was preferable in those patients whose general conditions tolerated such a procedure.

Technical Considerations

We would like to emphasize some technical points of the operation:

1. In the case of structural kyphosis caused by multiple disk narrowing, an anterior release with fusion preferably of three segments and more using an instrumentation following intervertebral strut graft, with or without bioactive ceramic blocks, is recommended. This does not usually have any unfavorable effects on the spinal canal, but if necessary, posterior decompression can be done secondarily.
2. When nerve root symptoms exist or are easily produced by lumbar extension, a careful decompression procedure is required to prevent progression of postoperative root complications. Nerve root monitoring using electrodiagnostic methods such as use of extradural catheter electrodes can help prevent this.
3. Obtaining sufficient lumbar lordosis is important for maintaining good postoperative results. For this reason, the combined operation using strong instrumentation such as the Kaneda device for anterior fusion, and C-D and/or the Steffee VSP system for posterior operations have the best potential.

References

1. Takemitsu Y, Harada Y, Iwahara T, et al. (1988) Lumbar degenerative kyphosis: Clinical, radiological, and epidemiologic studies. Spine 13:1317–1326
2. Takemitsu Y, Atsuta Y, Harada Y, et al. (1990) Treatment of lumbar degenerative kyphosis. SICOT Congress, Montreal, Sept. 13–18

2.15 Non-Instrumentation Stabilization/ Decompression Procedure for Lumbar Spinal Stenosis: Significance of Expansive Laminoplasty

Haruo Tsuji, Hisao Matsui, Masahiko Kanamori, Norikazu Hirano, and Yoshiharu Katoh[1]

Introduction

In the surgical treatment of various types of spinal stenosis, adequate decompression of the nerve roots and maintenance of spinal stability are essential. When spinal instability or degenerative spinal malalignment exists, extensive laminectomy impairs the mechanical integrity of the posterior supportive structures, and acceleration of the spinal instability and symptom recurrence may occur.

The expansive laminoplasty, non-instrumentation stabilization/decompression procedure, was developed in 1982 in our department, and has been performed on 30 patients during the past 10 years. The procedure aims at obtaining sufficient expansion of the spinal canal and prevention of postoperative symptomatic instability of the lumbar spine [1–4]. Here, the technique and its significance are described based on results from 15 cases with a follow-up of 1.25–8 years.

Patients and Methods

We examined 15 patients with degenerative spinal stenosis (except one case of cauda equina tumor) by direct examination, stress radiography, and CT scanning. We diagnosed one case of developmental stenosis, four cases of degenerative stenosis accompanied by an intraspinal ossified mass, five cases of degenerative stenosis with symptomatic instability, and five cases of combined spinal stenosis with disk herniation. Of the 15 patients, 14 were male and 1 female, with an average age of 49.4 years ranging from 33 to 83 years at the time of operation. All patients underwent laminoplasty: the extent of surgery was L1–L3 in one case, L2–L5 in four cases, L3–L4 in two cases, L3–L5 in

[1] Department of Orthopaedic Surgery, Faculty of Medicine, Toyama Medical and Pharmaceutical University, Toyama City, 930–01 Japan

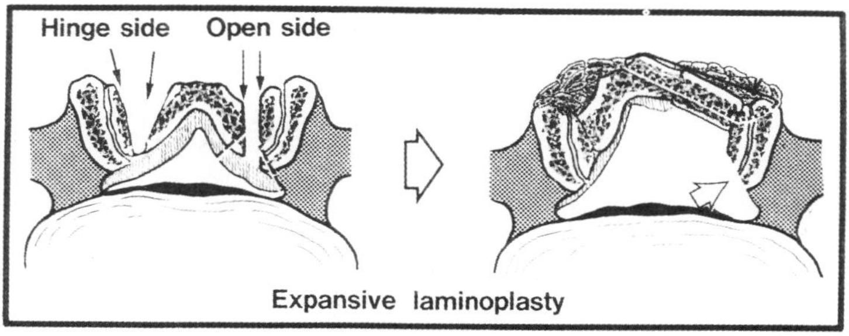

Fig. 1. Cross section of groove making and expansion of the spinal canal in expansive laminoplasty

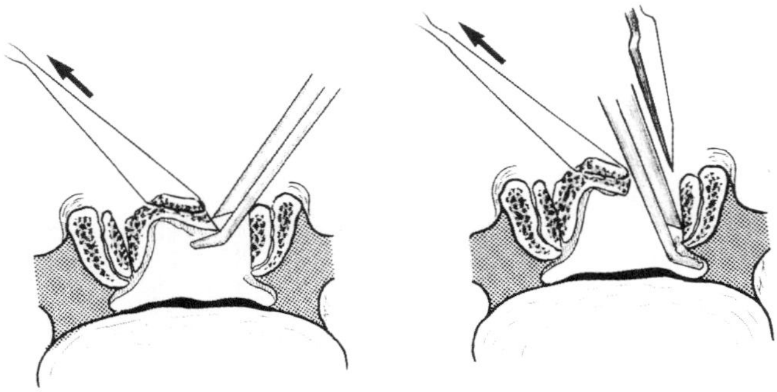

Fig. 2. Trimming of the groove edges provides lateral recess expansion and wide gaps between the laminae

seven cases, and L5 alone in one case. Mean follow up was 3.25 years ranging from 1.25 to 8 years.

Surgical Technique

After sufficient exposure of the laminae, the spinous processes are removed at the base and used as bone graft. The laminae are cut bilaterally using a high speed air drill. Those that are to be mobilized should be cut as widely as possible in the same fashion as in en bloc extensive laminectomy [2,3]. The groove on the hinged side is made wider and more conical in cross-section than the groove on the open side (Fig. 1), and tunnels for wiring are made using a special awl, pusher, and perforator [3]. A 0.3-mm braided steel wire or 0.32-mm monofilament steel wire is passed through each hole in the laminae, followed by laminar detachment at the open side and rotation through a minimum of 45°. At the open side, the edge of the groove facing the lateral recess of the spinal canal is trimmed with a Colclough rongeur and curette

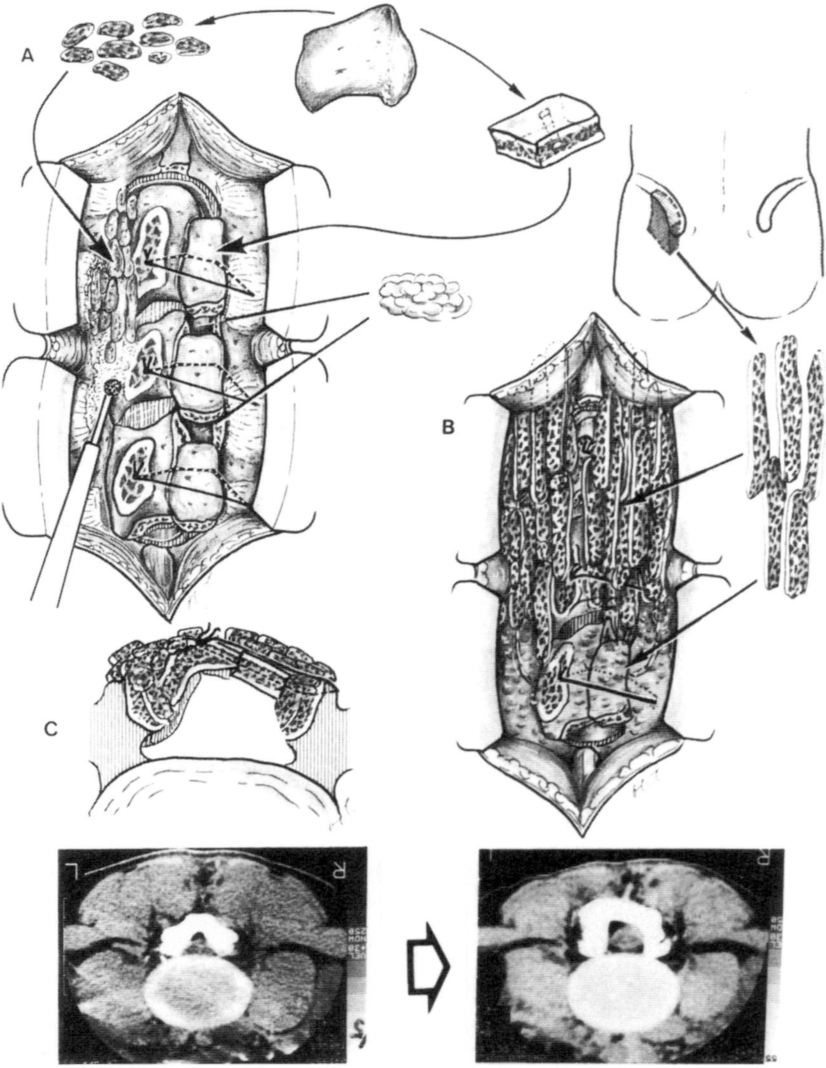

Fig. 3. Final procedure of expansive laminoplasty and the representative CT scan

(Fig. 2). If disk herniation or an intraspinal bony mass/tumor mass exists, intraspinal intervention is performed through the open gap. Unroofing of the lateral recess at the hinged side should be done before making the groove in the laminae. The wire is tied firmly after the cube bone graft from the spinous process is interposed into the open gap, followed by capsulectomy, laminar decortication using a high speed air drill and gouge, and transplantation, on both sides, of cancellous bone sticks obtained from the posterior ilium (Fig. 3).

Thus, the spinal canal is expanded in a square shape in cross-section, and posterior fusion can be achieved.

Surgical Indication

The indications for this surgery are as follows: (1) degenerative/developmental or combined stenosis in patients in whom great physical activity is required in daily life, (2) degenerative stenosis with spondylolisthesis or symptomatic instability, (3) degenerative stenosis associated with disk herniation or intra-spinal bony masses in active patients, and (4) cauda equina tumor or lumbar disk herniation with multiple disk degeneration in patients demanding strenuous work.

Aftercare Program

At 2 weeks after surgery, the patient is permitted to sit and walk while in a short body cast. The body cast is worn for 4 weeks, when it is replaced with a Williams flexion orthosis.

Results

During follow-up, no iatrogenic spinal stenosis and symptom recurrence were noted. The mean operation time was 179 min, ranging from 95 min to 210 min, and the volume of blood loss was 617 g ranging from 265 to 1,200 g.

The 15 patients remained in bed for an average of 16 days (range, 7–28 days), and were discharged at 33 days (range, 23–49 days) after surgery. The mean time spent wearing the cast was 6.5 weeks. Patients returned to their jobs or sports activities 12 weeks postoperatively. Thus the all-over results were satisfactory (Table 1).

On the CT scan, the spinal canal was found to have enlarged into a square shape (Figs. 3–5), and the expanded cross-sectional area was calculated as 2.0 cm^2 on average (range, 1.3–3.4 cm^2) before surgery, and 3.5 cm^2 (range, 2.1–6.2 cm^2) after surgery.

Table 1. Total results (1.25–8 years).

Excellent	11
Good	4[a]
Fair	0
Poor	0

[a] One case was a lumbar spinal stenosis accompanied by cervical myelopathy

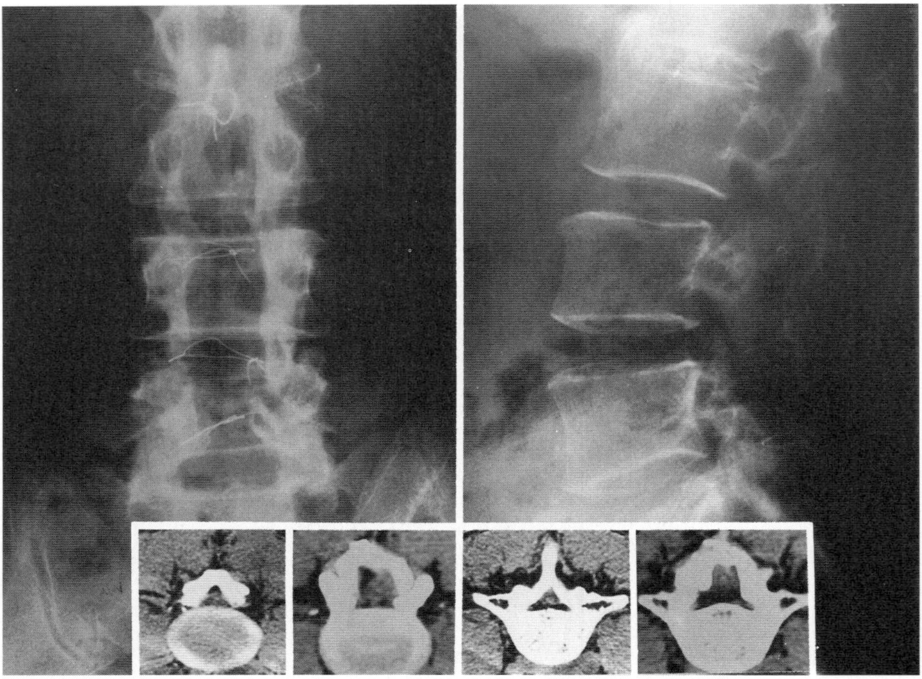

Fig. 4. A 33-year-old male, heavy manual worker with extensive spinal stenosis complained of low back and leg pains for 4 years. At 1 year before laminoplasty, he received anterior interbody fusion at L2–L3 which resulted in nonunion. Inset are shown pre- and postoperative CT scans taken 5 years after L2–L5 expansive laminoplasty. The spinal canal changed from a triangular shape to a square (*left half*, L4 level; *right half*, L5 level). Iliac bone grafting was not performed so the flexion-extension motion of the lumbar spine was reduced by about 50%

The radiological bone growth and union of the grafts became apparent after 3 or 4 months with no dislocation of floated laminae. The range of flexion-extension motion of the operated spinal areas was $19.1 \pm 7°$ (range, 6–40°) preoperatively, and $6.2 \pm 3°$ (range, 3–18°) postoperatively, and any abnormal translational movements of the vertebra were not observed.

Discussion

Decompressive laminectomy destroys the posterior supportive structure of the lumbar spine. In degenerative spine diseases, irrespective of the presence [5–8] or absence of instability, extensive laminectomy may affect spinal stability, resulting in symptom recurrence [6–8].

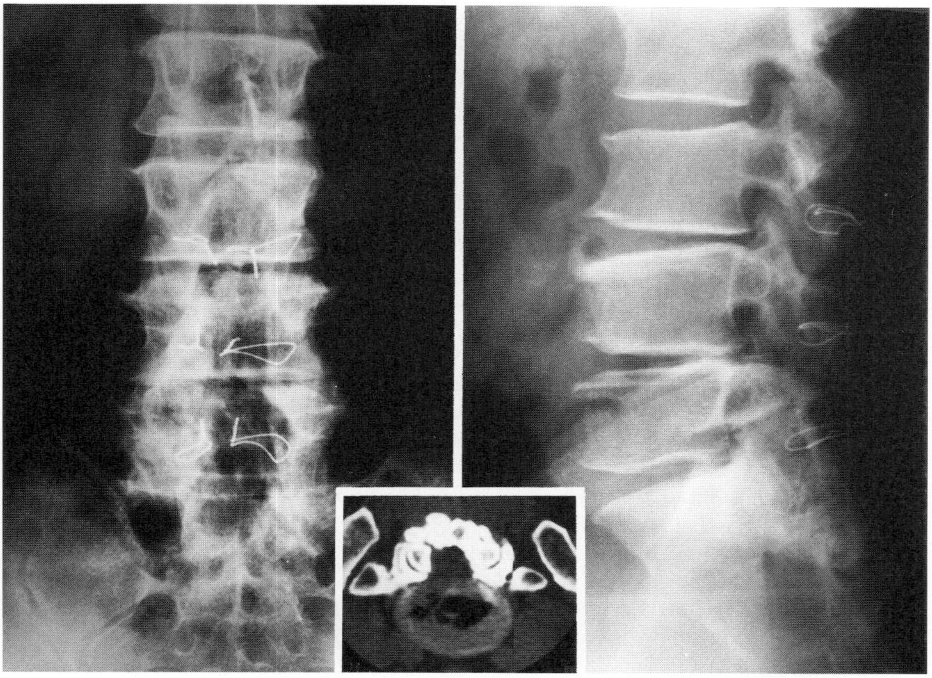

Fig. 5. A 38-year-old male with degenerative spinal stenosis from L3–L5 accompanied by postdiskal ossification at L4. Inset are shown postoperative CT of L4–L5 taken 3.5 years after operation. They demonstrate good stability and canal expansion. Symptom relief was excellent

We perform spine fusion for degenerative spine diseases under a distinct policy: huge spinal instrumentation should not be used primarily for degenerative spine diseases except for spine trauma, and permanent spinal stability is only produced by sufficient bone grafting.

The first trial of lumbar laminoplasty was reported by Raimond et al. [9], followed by Kawai et al. [10] and Tsuji et al. [2–4]. This latter decompression/stabilization technique with no use of instrumentation, as described in textbooks [2,3], provides sufficient expansion of the canal as well as reconstruction of the posterior supportive elements to prevent the postoperative spinal instability [1–4].

However, there is a technical limitation in this procedure; it does not include nerve root tunnel decompression especially at the hinged side. If lateral unroofing is necessary, decompressive laminotomy or unroofing of the nerve root tunnel should be performed before laminar rotation. In contrast, intraspinal intervention such as diskectomy and spur or tumor removal is possible because of the wide gap obtained on the open side.

In this study, the clinical results of this surgery were satisfactory, and there was no spinal instability. The reinforcement of spinal stability was semirigid and seemed to be equivalent to the Hibbs type of posterior fusion. No iatrogenic spinal stenosis was encountered in the present series, and the spinal canal was maintained wide and square-shaped in cross section.

In conclusion, the expansive laminoplasty, non-instrumentation stabilization/decompression procedure, is a useful procedure for various types of lumbar spinal stenosis with and without spinal instability.

References

1. Matsui H, Tsuji H, Sekido H, Hirano N, Katoh Y, Makiyama N (1992) Results of expansive laminoplasty for lumbar spinal stenosis in active manual workers. Spine 17:3
2. Tsuji H (1991) Comprehensive atlas of lumbar spine surgery. Mosby, St Louis, pp 102–119
3. Tsuji H (1991) Fundamental techniques and principles in lumbar spine surgery, 2nd edn. Nankodo, Tokyo, pp 152–159
4. Tsuji H, Sekido H, Itoh T, Yamada H, Katoh Y, Makiyama N (1990) Expansive laminoplasty for lumbar spinal stenosis. Int Orthop 14:309–314
5. Herron LD, Trippi AC (1989) L4–5 degenerative spondylolisthesis. The results of treatment by decompressive laminectomy without fusion. Spine 14:534–538
6. Johnsson K-E, Redlund-Johnell I, Uden A, Willner S (1989) Preoperative and postoperative instability in lumbar spinal stenosis. Spine 14:591–593
7. Johnsson K-E, Willner S, Johnsson K (1986) Postoperative instability after decompression for lumbar spinal stenosis. Spine 11:107–110
8. Lee CK (1983) Lumbar spinal instability (olisthesis) after extensive posterior spinal decompression. Spine 8:429–433
9. Raimond AJ, Gutierrez FA, Racco CD (1976) Laminoplasty and reconstruction of the posterior spinal arch for spinal canal surgery in childhood. J Neurosurg 45: 555–560
10. Kawai S, Hattori S, Oda H, Yamaguchi Y, Yoshida Y (1981) Enlargement of the lumbar vertebral canal in lumbar canal stenosis. Spine 6:381–387

PART 3

Stabilization Methods

3.1 How to Stabilize the Lumbar Spine: An Overview

Kiyoshi Hirabayashi[1]

Introduction

To restore the functions of the spinal column, i.e., its support function, its mobility, and its capacity to contain the spinal cord and cauda equina, spinal surgery has the following three strategies: decompression, reposition, and stabilization.

For permanent stabilization, spinal bony fusion is indispensable; however, it is worthwhile to note the amazing recent advances of instrumentation surgery; these have made it possible to promote such stabilization and to attain repositioning more effectively by the use of various kinds of implants.

The quality of the graft is the other decisive factor for the success or failure of bony fusion. It is well-known that, biologically speaking, autogenous bone is best; however, in this case, there are some problems, such as pain at the donor site after the removal of the bone to be grafted, and the time required for such procedures. In attempts to overcome these problems, allogeneic bone grafts, as well as substitute materials, have been the subject of research and development.

It should also be noted that the greater the degree of rigidity of stabilization of the spinal column thus acquired, the greater is the compensation made by the adjacent intervertebral levels for the loss of mobility caused by the immobilization. As a result, degeneration of the adjacent motion segment is likely to be accelerated. Furthermore, in consequence of the above, low back pain and symptoms such as radiating pain or numbness in the leg may recur with instability of the motion segment or postoperative degenerative spinal canal stenosis, as shown on the X-ray image in Fig. 1. Therefore, spinal fusion should not be carried out without careful consideration, results such as those above being the reason that we await the development of artificial discs with sufficient mobility.

In this paper, keeping the above viewpoints in mind, the author intends to clarify the consequences of and the contributions made by each symposiast

[1]Department of Orthopaedic Surgery, School of Medicine, Keio University, 35 Shinanomachi, Shinjuku-ku, Tokyo, 160 Japan

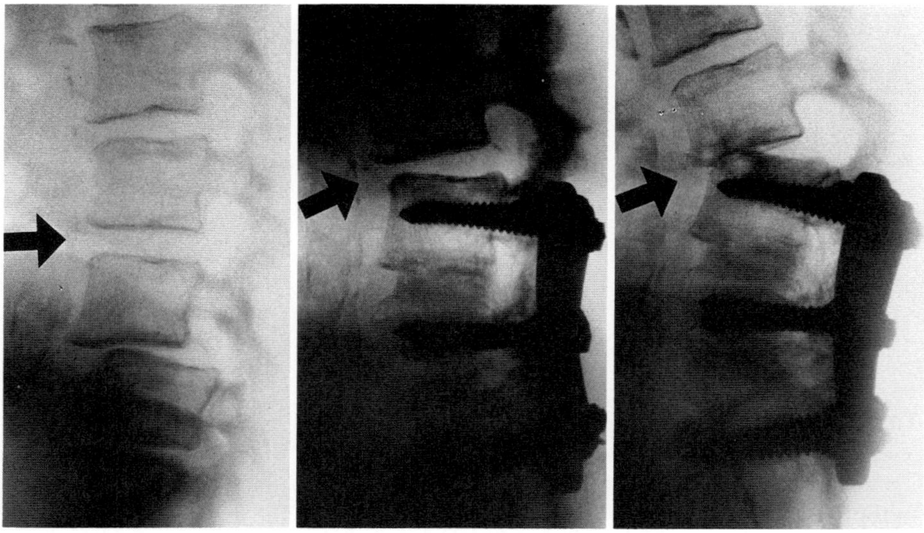

a,b c

Fig. 1. Instability of the adjacent motion segment after posterior interbody fusion with Steffee's [14,15] plating **a** preoperative image, **b** image at 1 year 4 months, and **c** image at 2 years 4 months postoperatively

regarding current strategy for stabilization of the lumbar spine. Further, the author would like to emphasize the significance of semirigid wire fixation in addition to anterior spinal body fusion, a method originated by himself, as well as emphasizing desirable perspectives regarding the stabilization of the spine.

Strategy for Stabilization of the Spine

Stabilization of the spine is permanently guaranteed only when bony union is attained at the fusion area. Accordingly, it is extremely important for spinal surgeons to determine the strategy to be employed with regard to how firmly and early bony union may be secured.

The conditions that regulate the process of bony union over time include two categories of factors: systemic factors, such as age, nutrition, etc.; and local factors, such as vascularization of the fusion area, the biological and biomechanical quality of the grafted bone or its substitute, the quality and quantity of the contact surface between the grafted bone and recipient, the compressive force applied to the contact area, and the quality and quantity of immobilization, etc.

Biologically, it is desirable for the grafted bone to have good properties for bone induction, and biomechanically, to have an appropriate calcium content. Therefore, as stated by Ramani (Chap. 3.4), it is obvious that the use of bank bone is biologically better than that of a substitute, and, further, autogenous bone is better than bank bone. However, biomechanically, the use of a substitute is advantageous since its rigidity can be adjusted. Nevertheless, there seem to be no problems clinically with the use of autogenous bone or bank bone unless the bone is porotic.

Regarding the contact surface between the grafted bone and the recipient, interbody fusion is most important biologically, as well as biomechanically, followed by posterolateral fusion and then posterior fusion, in terms of the extent and smoothness of the contact surface, and the advantageous loading effect onto the bone graft.

As reported by Nakai and Ohwada (Chap. 3.3 and 3.5), spinal instrumentation, among other procedures, plays an important role in accelerating and securing the bony union by improving immobilization [1]. Spinal instrumentation also allows the patient to become ambulatory at an early stage, due to the immediate and strong immobilization, and it not only reduces the necessity of using casts or braces but also corrects spondylolisthetic or scoliotic deformity and allows the maintenance of such a corrected position, as stated by Roy-Camille (Chap. 3.8).

However, at the same time, one should keep in mind that the role of the implant is a temporary supporting one, in which the implant itself is not to bear the burden permanently, but is to maintain repositioning until the completion of bony union and the development of biomechanical strength.

There is a limit in compensating the imperfection of the grafted bone by instrumentation; as pointed out by Panjabi [2] the construct will fail if the fracture healing rate does not keep pace with the implant fatigue rate. In the case of inappropriate bone grafting, implant failure, such as breakage or loosening of screws, may develop from loading, even if the implant material is as rigid as Steffee's plate [3–5]; this would result in failure to achieve the targeted stabilization.

On the other hand, if mechanically solid bone grafting is carried out, as observed in interbody fusion, the desired osseous union is obtainable even with the degree of immobilization that may be produced by the insertion of a ceramic block into the interspinous space, as described by Tsuji (Chap. 3.6), or by tension band wiring according to our method, as described below (Fig. 2).

Alternatives to Spinal Stabilization

Based on the above-mentioned observations, the author believes that, in order to achieve spinal stabilization as early and as securely as possible, it is necessary to select the best combination of bone grafting and instrumentation after careful consideration of the respective merits and demerits of: the fusion area (interbody, posterolateral, or posterior); the graft material (autogenous, homogenous bone, or a substitute), and the implant (pedicular screw plate or rod system, wiring system or interspinous block spacer) (Table 1).

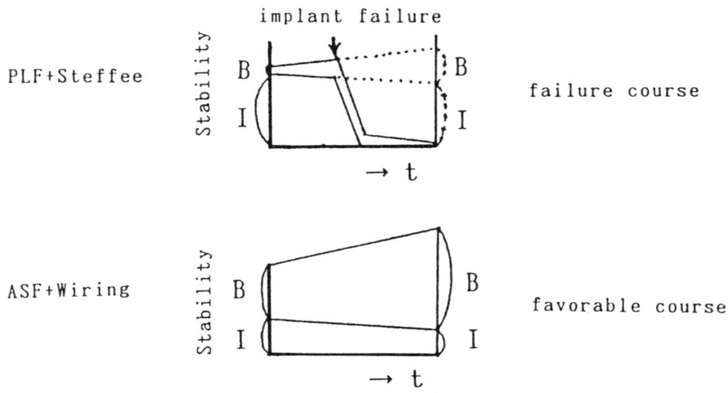

Fig. 2. Comparison between the stabilizing process following successful ASF with wiring and unsuccessful PLF with Steffee's plating [14,15]. *B*, grafted bone; *I*, implant; *ASF*, anterior body fusion; *PLF*, posterolateral fusion

In selecting the spinal fusion method, in addition to the above, it is necessary to consider certain other factors such as the method of approach to the pathogenic lesion and the extent of the fusion level.

For those cases which necessitate posterior decompression, the dorsal approach is suitable; therefore, it is natural to select one of the following: posterior lumbar interbody fusion (PLIF), posterolateral fusion (PLF), or posterior fusion (PF). However, in the above situation, one should not ignore the disadvantage of PLIF in that it necessitates intracanal exploration, which may lead to adhesion around the dural tube. Thus, it might be wise to minimize intracanal invasion.

Similar to those cases of spinal bone tumor or tuberculous spine where an approach to the vertebral body is required, for patients with failed back or disc hernia, anterior body fusion (ASF) via the extraperitoneal approach should be the first choice.

On the other hand, for those cases with a multilevel fusion area, PLF or PF ought to be selected. In the case of severe dysplastic spondylolisthesis, where slipping is likely to recur after repositioning, the combined operation of interbody fusion and PLF or PF, so-called pan-spondylodesis, is necessary, and, as stated by Roy-Camille (see Chap. 3.8), it would then be reasonable to use a strong and rigid implant.

Anterior Spinal Body Fusion with Tension Band Wiring

For the last 30 years, the author [6] has been employing anterior spinal body fusion, which is superior mechanically, in patients with spondylolytic and degenerative spondylolisthesis, with fairly good operative results being obtained. However, similar to the situation seen in PLF and PF patients, the

Table 1. Alternative factors for spinal fusion.

1) Fusion area	Vertebral body,	Facet, transverse proc.,	Lamina, spinous proc.
Contact	++	+	$\underline{++}$
Compression force	+	−	−

2) Grafting material	Autogenous		Homogenous		Substitute
	Cortex	Spongy	Cortex	Spongy	
Bone induction	+	++	±	±	±
Stiffness	++	+	++	+	+∼++

3) Spinal implants	Steffee	∼	C-D	∼	Wiring
Rigidity	+++		++		+
Compression force	++		++		+

problem that remains unsolved is how to reduce the incidence of pseudoarthrosis, which occurs in 20%–30% of all such patients.

Therefore, in addition to ASF, the author has also employed the anterior screw and wiring method, since 1982, and, since 1984, the pedicular screw and wiring method has also been added in spondylolytic cases [7,8] (Fig. 3). As a result of these additions, maintenance of the reduced position in spondylolisthesis and acceleration of bony union have been improved. Anterior and posterior tension band wiring, using 6.5-mm-diameter screws for spongy bone, was more advantageous in every respect than using anterior screws and wiring alone (Fig. 4).

Since anterior and posterior wiring provide sufficient long-lasting stability at the affected intervertebral region until the grafted bone is consolidated, a strong stabilizing instrument such as a pedicular plate or rod system is not necessarily required.

Simulation, using a rigid body spring model, supported the idea that, with the combined use of the anterior and posterior wiring method with ASF, the surface force, including both normal linear force and shearing force, was distributed evenly. As a consequence of this distribution, it is unlikely that spondylolisthetic reduction loss or collapsing of the grafted bone will occur clinically [9]. However, since the essential element of this model is a rigid body, for an actual case to conform to this model, attention must be paid to reserve clinically the osseous end plate of the fused body, and, at the time of grafting, to make the cortical portion of the iliac crest fit in line with the anterior cortex of the vertebral body.

One should also keep in mind that, even though these grafting techniques are appropriate, this system may not be applicable to porotic patients in whom

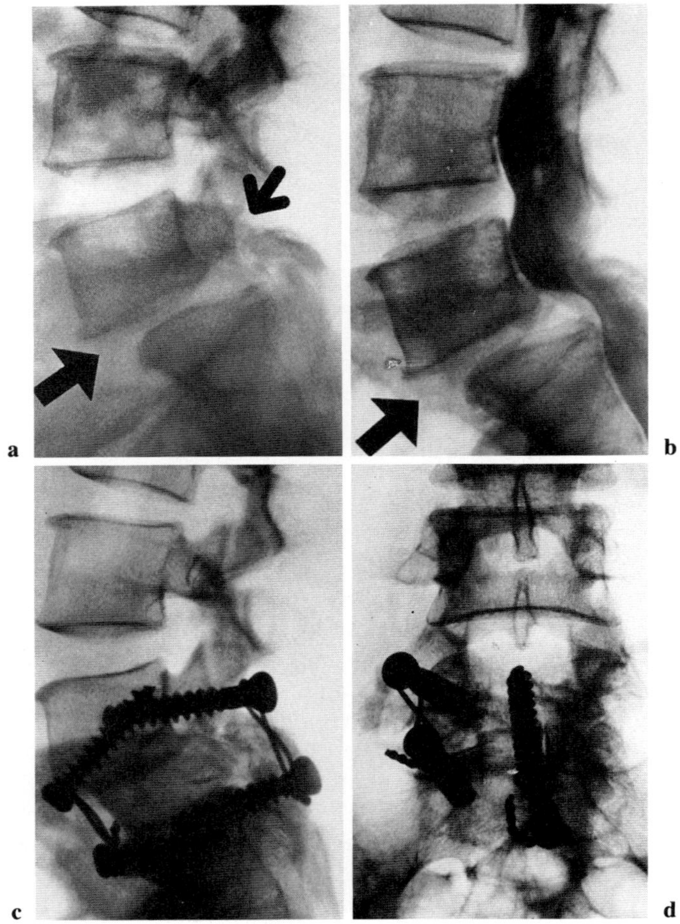

Fig. 3. Anterior spinal body fusion with anterior and posterior tension band wiring for spondylolytic spondylolisthesis. **a** and **b**, preoperative images, **c** and **d**, postoperative images

there is a possibility of causing a collapse of the iliac grafted bone or the recipient surface of the osseous end plate.

Biomechanical Analysis of Spinal Implant in Cyclic Loading

Implants may be divided roughly into two categories from the structural viewpoint: One is the rigid fixation system, such as that represented by Steffee's system [10,11], in which rigid fixation depends on the strength of the metal construct itself and the rigid fixing of the interval between the screw and the

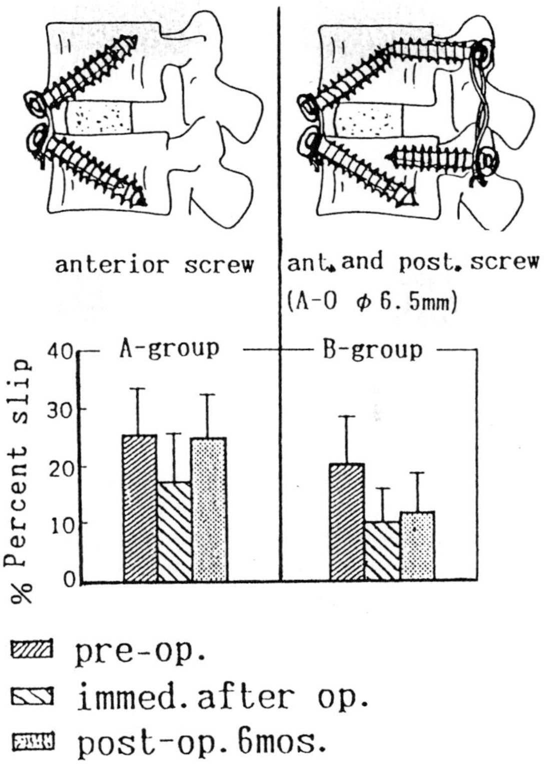

Fig. 4. Percent slip at pre- and post-operation for spondylolytic spondylolisthesis. *A-O*, Allgemeinsam Osteosynthese

plate; the other is the semirigid fixation system, where stability is maintained by the compressive force produced by tightening the interval between screws with wire, as is seen in the anterior and posterior wiring system.

The results of the experiments made by Ueno [12], using porcine vertebrae, indicated that, as might have been expected, initial stability was the best in Steffee's system [13], if the condition was such that loosening at the contact surface between the metallic device and the bone could be disregarded. However, in the case of porotic bone, where the calcium content, as well as the viscoelasticity, was low, loosening occurred suddenly at an early stage when cyclic loading was applied, as has been stated by Zindrick [3]. On the other hand, in the anterior and posterior wiring system, the figure-of-eight tightening wire, operating as if it were fixed on both ends of a seesaw, received the loading force as the tensile strength applying to it. Therefore, there was no excessive load operating on the contact area between the metallic device and the bone and, as a result, it was possible for fixation to be maintained in the porotic bone, even after cyclic loading was applied to it (Fig. 5).

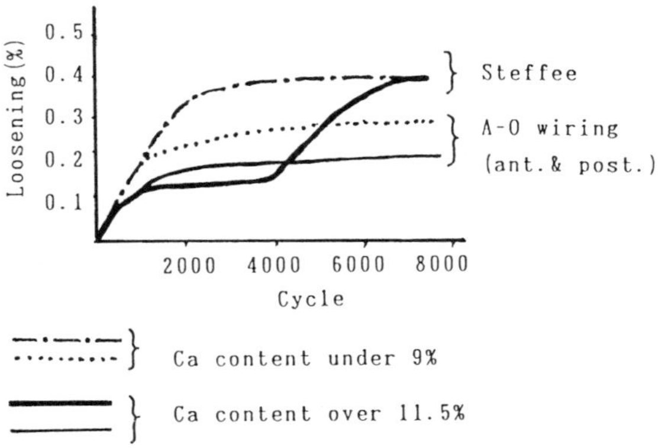

Fig. 5. Correlation between Ca content and loosening during cyclic loading

Accordingly, one must be very careful to select the appropriate operative technique or to give postoperative external fixation, keeping in mind that while the rigid fixation system, because of its excellent initial stability, allows the patient to walk at an early stage, in those patients with severe osteoporosis or multisegmental fusion, instrument failure is likely to occur biomechanically over a certain period of time.

"How to Stabilize" . . . Past, Present, and Future

Ideally, the spinal surgeon desires permanent stabilization of the spine, and, with this in mind, the surgeon attempts to obtain in situ or 100% repositioning fusion, in the belief that more rigid fusion and earlier ambulation would thus be achieved. Patients, consequently, could be released from their unpleasant casting or bracing and would be able to return to a normal life.

We all know the various efforts made by our predecessors in spinal surgery in their attempts to reach higher objectives, and our successors, we believe, will continue in the same vein in future. The author believes that the recent advances in instrumentation surgery and in bone grafts and graft substitutes are really epoch-making in the historical progress of this field.

On the other hand, as you are well aware, instrumentation surgery requires intricate and risky operative procedures and the implantation of bulky foreign substances inside the patient's body. This, of course, results in an increased possibility of local infection and metallic corrosion. In addition, this surgery consumes vast sums of money, which may be a burden to our health care budgets.

Therefore, in realizing our ideal in spinal arthrodesis, we must make careful judgments in selecting the most appropriate and minimal implants to supplement autogenous bone grafting, based on procedures developed by our predecessors and currently in use.

Conclusion

In selecting the spinal fusion technique for a given situation, some people may say that surgeons should use the technique with they are most familiar. However, basically, the most suitable fusion technique should be selected rationally, depending on the morbidity of the patient. Thus, the author believes that the best attitude for spinal surgeons to take is to exert their utmost efforts to learn and become acquainted with suitable techniques, so that they can select the optimum one, depending on the diagnosis and on the condition of the patient.

3.2 Results of Posterior Lumbar Interbody Fusion for Lytic and Degenerative Spondylolisthesis

Ralph B. Cloward[1]

Introduction

The report and discussion of results obtained from any type of surgical treatment requires a description of the pathological lesion being treated. The medical definition of spondylolisthesis is a forward slippage of the spine. The existence of this condition has been known since 1741 when Andre described an "inward warping of the spine" [1]. Neugebauer in 1834 was the first to suggest that spondylolisthesis was congenital in origin, resulting from a developmental defect in the neural ring [2].

We have come to recognize several pathological conditions which result in subluxation of one vertebral body forward on another. These include:

1. Congenital or developmental anamoly with a defect in the pars articularis and a separate neural arch (lytic spondylolisthesis) (Fig. 1A)
2. Congenital anamoly with degeneration of the articulating processes with an intact neural arch (degenerative spondylolisthesis)
3. Bilateral stress fractures of the pars articularis (traumatic spondylolisthesis)
4. Iatrogenic, due to surgical destruction of the articular facets (iatrogenic spondylolisthesis)

The cases to be described in this report will include only the first two types: lytic and degenerative spondylolistheses.

Lytic Spondylolisthesis

Etiology

The etiology of the pars defect is still controversial. Many authors still contend that the bony defect in the neural arch is acquired, i.e., a stress fracture, since

[1] Neurological Surgery, 1111 Bishop St., Suite 510, Honolulu, HI 96813, USA

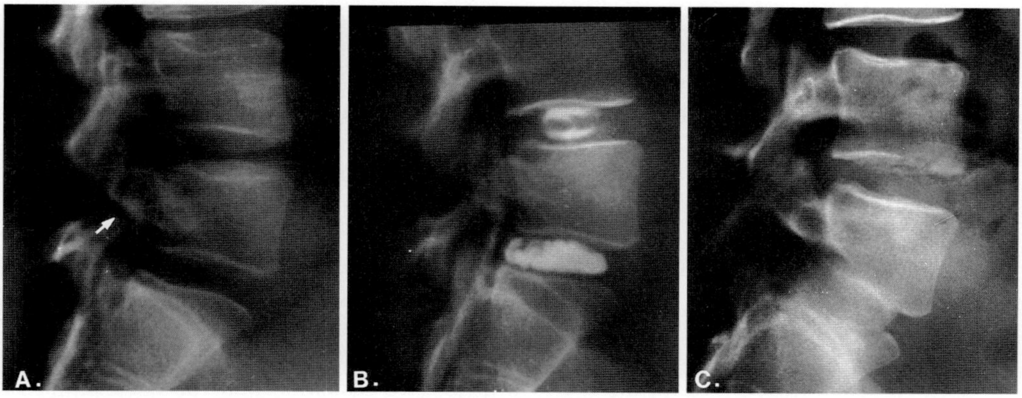

Fig. 1. A Preoperative spondylosis with pars defect and no subluxation (*arrow*). **B** Diskogram. Posterior disk protrusion with defect in posterior annulus (see epidura-gram). Normal diskogram L4–5. **C** Postoperative PLIF

X-ray evidence of the anamoly is not usually discovered until the 7th or 8th year of life.

There is stronger evidence of a developmental or congenital etiology of the anamoly. Spondylolisthesis is known to be hereditary and familial, occuring in several members of one family or in previous generations. Wiltse states that over 30% of patients with spondylolisthesis will have an immediate relative with a pars defect [3].

Additional evidence of the hereditary origin is the frequency of associated developmental anamolies of the spine, dura, dural sac, and nerve roots. These anamolies occur 13 times more frequently with a spondylolisthesis than a normal spine.

Racial predisposition is also a common factor. It occurs four times more frequently in Alaskan Indians. The percentage varies with country and race. In the United States 5%–7% of the population have this anamoly. In patients who seek medical aid for symptoms of low back pain, 10% have a pars defect.

Mechanism of Pain in Spondylolisthesis

The anterior subluxation of a vertebral body in spondylolisthesis is frequently painful and disabling. The pain is of two types: (1) musclo-skeletal, and (2) radicular.

The initial symptom is backache, described as a dull aching pain, often referred to the hips and/or posterior thighs as far as the knee. The major source of the back pain has been proven to originate in a traumatic internal ruptured intervertebral disk at the level of the spondylolysis. The pain, therefore, is diskogenic.

This source of back pain is determined by diskography. In all cases of spondylolisthesis with a narrow disk space, the diskogram (Fig. 1B) demonstrates internal rupture and degeneration of the disk. The disk is painful when injected. If a diskogram at the level of the spondylolysis shows a normal nucleus pulposus and an intact annulus fibrosus, the patient will experience no pain when a contrast material is injected. These findings indicate a functionally normal joint of the spine. If the patient has symptoms of back pain, the cause must be sought elsewhere, either an adjacent disk or another source.

If spondylolisthesis is a congenital anamoly, why does it remain asymptomatic until the second or third decade, or later? The evidence of pars defect is nearly as high in children as in adults yet symptoms are uncommon in children. The diskogram with spondylolysthesis always shows a painful, traumatic degenerated disk. Since children seldom have disk injuries, we conclude that the back pain is diskogenic.

Radicular pain is due to nerve root pressure or traction at the level of the subluxation. Pain radiates down one leg, or more often both legs with numbness and reflex changes similar to that of a herniated disk syndrome. Leg pain from nerve root impairment occurs less often in spondylolisthesis than disk herniation of traumatic or degenerative origin. Nerve root pain can be caused by:

1. Movement of the loose lamina at the isthmic cleft
2. Compression from a mass of fiber-cartilagenous tissue build-up around the pars defect
3. A frank protrusion of the disk (this is rare)

Bilateral symptoms with impaired function of the first sacral nerve roots and/or cauda equina may occur with severe subluxation (3rd or 4th degree).

Surgical Treatment

Many surgical operations have been devised to treat the pain of spondylolisthesis. These include:

1. Decompression operations: removal of the disk, or removal of the separate neural arch (the Gill procedure)
2. Spinal fusion techniques to arrest the progressive subluxation and instability.

The results of these operations have been only moderately successful. A decompression often aggravates the pain and increases the subluxation. Spinal fusion operations, either posterior fusion or transverse process posterior-lateral fusion, have a high rate of pseudarthrosis, probably due to the already unstable joint. Recently, this instability has been addressed by the use of metallic implants, that is, interpedicular screws and plates or various posterior rods and wiring. These techniques have the advantage of mechanically reducing the subluxation, but may fail if not accompanied by a bony fusion.

The ideal surgical fixation for spondylolisthesis is interbody fusion (Fig. 1c). If the intervertebral disk is removed and replaced with bone grafts and the vertebral bodies become fused, movement of the joint is eliminated and progression of the subluxation is arrested. This gives prompt and permanent relief of the low back pain.

The interbody fusion operation is performed either by an anterior or a posterior approach. The first interbody fusion recorded by Burns in late 1930s was by an anterior, transabdominal extra-peritoneal approach [4]. The first posterior interbody fusion for lumbar disk disease was performed by Cloward in 1943 [5] and the first spondylolisthesis case in 1946 [6].

Technique of PLIF for Spondylolisthesis

A transverse skin incision is made over the prominent tip of the fifth lumbar spinous process. The muscles are detached from the laminae of L4, L5, and S1, and retractor blades inserted. The separate neural arch is identified by its hypermobility. It is disarticulated by incising the ligamentum flavum above and below and the facet capsule laterally, and removed in one piece. The ligamentum flavum, attached to the margin of L4 and S1, is incised and the ligament reflected laterally in a flap. It is attached to the lateral muscle wall with a suture.

The exit of the L5 and S1 nerve roots from the spinal canal are concealed beneath overhanging bony ledges: L5 by the ledge of the mushroom, pars articularis, and S1 nerve root by the flat articular facet of S1. These bony structures are carefully removed with appropriate sharp osteotomes to give complete exposure and decompression of the nerve roots.

Epidural fat and vessels between the nerve roots and lateral to the dural sac are cauterized, incised and removed, exposing the L5–S1 disk and the drop-off of the body of L5.

The disk space is exposed and widened vertically with a vertebra spreader inserted between the L4 and S1 spinous processes in the midline, and cranked open as wide as possible. The disk space is also exposed laterally by retracting the dural sac and nerve roots to the midline with a Self-retaining Nerve Root Retractor.

Preparing the Interspace

The disk is cut out following the margins of the adjacent vertebra, beneath the dural sac and as far lateral as possible. The cartilage endplates are stripped from their attachments to the adjacent vertebral surfaces down to the anterior longitudinal ligament; all soft disk material is removed from the interspace with a large disk rongeur. The cortical bony surfaces of the adjacent vertebra are completely removed with curved osteotomes leaving a smooth, flat bleeding surface of cancellous bone.

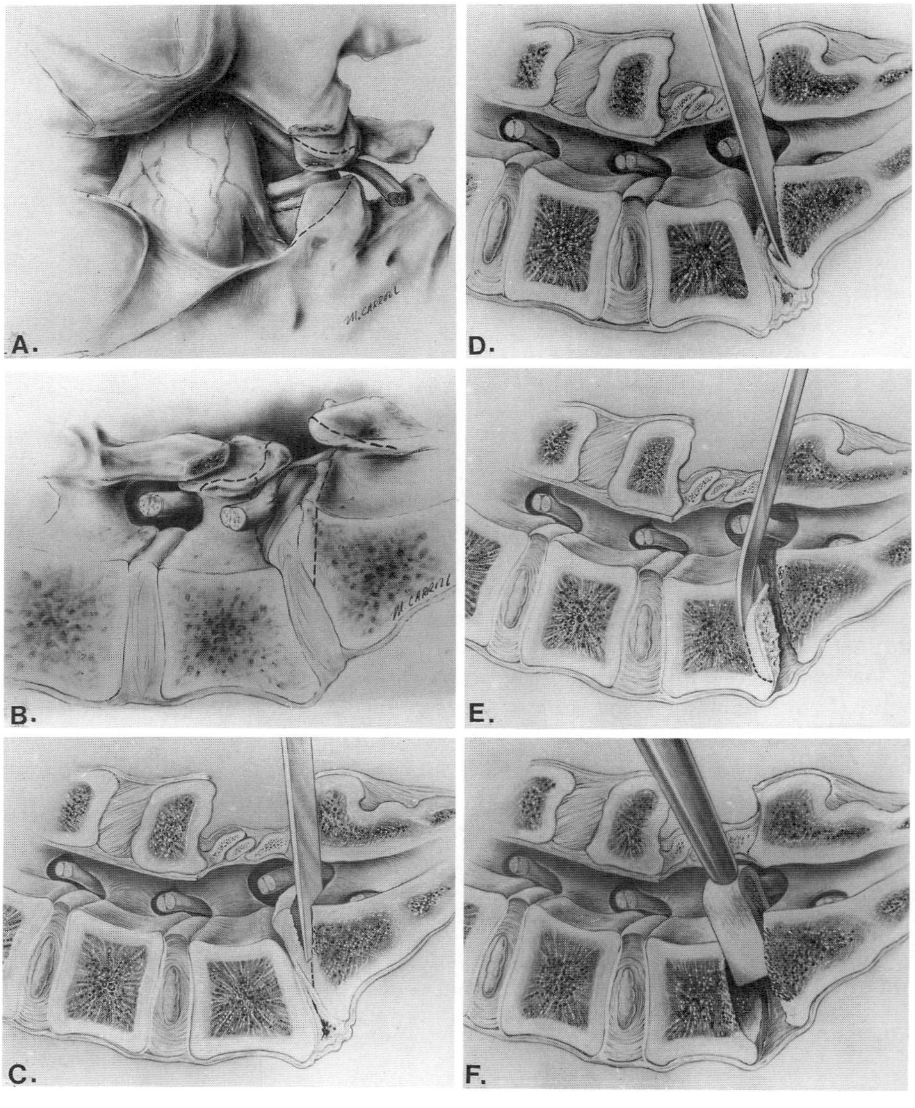

Fig. 2. **A** After laminectomy, ligamentum flavum flaps are reflected to expose the dural sac and L5. S1 nerve roots. **B** Note "mushroom" and overhanging rim of pars articularis compressing L5 nerve root. *Dotted Line* shows bone removed with osteotome including S1 facet. **C,D** Cortex removed from S1 vertebra using straight osteotome, then curved for the last 1 cm. **E** Decortication of L5 vertebral body including residual disk and cartilage plate. **F** First bone graft impacted into disk space. Note that subluxation of L5 on S1 has been reduced with a vertebra spreader

Grafting Technique (Fig. 2F)

The grafts obtained from the bone bank are full thickness, tricortical blocks of iliac bone. These are fashioned with an air drill to the exact measurements of the prepared disk space, after first widening the disk space by a few turns on the vertebra spreader. The first graft is impacted and moved medially, then a second graft inserted. If there is room for a third graft, the second graft is moved laterally and the third inserted between the two.

The same procedure is carried out bilaterally; usually four, but often five or even six grafts can be impacted to completely fill the disk space.

Postoperative Care

The patient is permitted out of bed the same day or the day following surgery and can walk to the bathroom with assistance whenever able. No casts or braces are required for first and second degree spondylolistheses. For the more rare third and fourth degree subluxation, a chair-type steel brace is used for 30 days. X-ray evidence of fusion across the disk space is often visible within 4–5 months.

Statistics on Lytic Spondylolisthesis Cases

The statistics for lytic spondylolisthesis cases are given in Table 1.

Results

X-Ray

Solid bony union was achieved in 157 cases (94%), and in 10 patients (6%) there was partial absorption of bone grafts (radiologically considered fusion failure). Strong fibrous union, however, resulted in all patients being symptom free.

Clinical

At the last follow-up report, 95% of patients were pain free and satisfied.

Degenerative Spondylolisthesis with Intact Neural Arch

This condition was first described by Junghans in 1930 [7]. He indicated that the pathology responsible for the anterior subluxation was a congenital anamoly of the articular processes. The pars articularis is intact but elongated. The facet joint at L4/L5 exhibits a more horizontal orientation which permits anterior slipping of the facet forward with subluxation of the upper vertebral body. The

Table 1. Lytic spondylolisthesis cases.

	No. of cases (n)	Remarks
Total (1946–1989)	167	Symptoms occurred in most cases between the age of 30 and 50 years
Males	106 (63%)	
Females	61 (37%)	
Symptoms		
Low back pain	167	
Accompanied by leg pain	109 (64%)	
Degree of subluxation		
1st degree, 2nd degree	156 (94%)	1st–4th degrees = pre-spondylisthesis (spondylosis)
3rd degree, 4th degree	10 (6%)	5th degree: spondyloptosis
5th degree	1	The 5th degree case was not operated
Levels operated		
L5/S1	142 (85%)	
L4/L5	20 (12%)	
Pars defect at two levels	3	
Anomalies	63	
Spine	41 (64%)	
Spina bifida	26	
Spinous process	4	
Vertebral body	8	
Sacralization	3	
Nerve roots	19 (30%)	
High take off	3	
Short root	9	
Cojoined nerve	7	
Absent dural Sac	2 (4%)	
Dural midline defect with cysts	1 (2%)	

facet has a 45° sloping angle instead of a normal vertical one. (Fig. 3A). The disk below the slipped vertebra is always narrow indicating progressive degeneration. Eventual subluxation causes nerve root compression and leg pain. This spinal disorder is found primarily in postmenopausal women and is always at the L4/L5 level. The reason for this is unknown.

Personal Cases

Details of these cases are given in Table 2.

Indications for Operation

The indications are the same as for lytic spondylolisthesis:

1. Relief of back and leg pain
2. Reduction and arrest of subluxation
3. Elimination of spinal instability

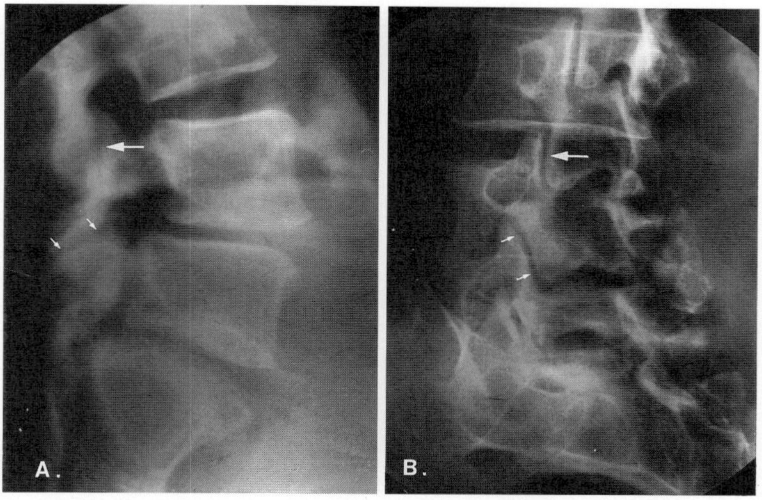

Fig. 3A,B. Degenerative spondylolisthesis L4–5. Note sloping facet, (*small arrows*) and normal vertical facet (*large arrows*)

Table 2. Degenerative spondylolisthesis.

	No. of cases (*n*)	Remarks
Total (since 1965)	31	Average age at operation was 60 years
Males	5 (16%)	
Females	26 (84%)	
Symptoms		Duration of symptons was 1–10 years
Low back pain	31	
Radiating into one leg	24 (77%)	
Radiating into both legs	16 (50%)	
Previous surgery	10	Each case averaged three operations in a 10-year period
Decompressive laminectomy	9	
Attempted interbody fusion with posterior dislocation of the bone graft	1	All previous operations resulted in "failed back"
"Virgin" cases	21 (67%)	
Fusion results	31	
Delayed	9	
Reoperation	6	
Symptom-free (final)	28 (90%)	

Technique

All cases were treated by posterior lumbar interbody fusion. It was possible to reduce the subluxation in every case (Fig. 4A,B). Six operations performed after 1981 were accompanied by spinous process wiring for added stability (Fig. 4B).

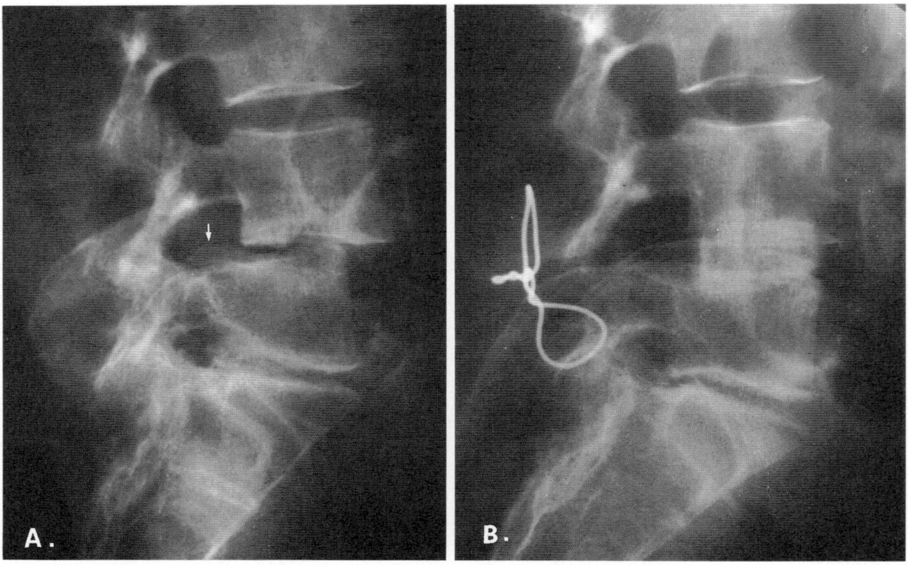

Fig. 4. **A** Anterior subluxation (*small arrow*) before operation. **B** Subluxation reduced. The spinous process at L5 was inadvertently fractured due to osteoporosis. Wire attaches the spinous process at L4 to the lamina at L5

Results

Results for these cases showed a higher rate of postoperative complications, usually a delay in the fusion. This was attributed to age, osteoporosis, and the congenital instability of the pathological joint. Fusion was delayed in nine cases. These patients became asymptomatic after 8–14 months. Six of these required reoperation (refusion).

End results for these 31 cases was very good. A final review in 1991 showed 28 (90%) patients were completely symptom free. Only 1 patient was still disabled with a lawsuit pending, and 2 patients had died of other causes.

Comment

Today, I would probably recommend the use of Steffee's plates and pedicular screws be included in the PLIF operation. This has been shown to result in a higher percentage and more rapid rate of initial fusion in degenerative spondylolisthesis.

Conclusion

The highest percentage of total permanent recovery from the symptoms of spondylolisthesis, both lytic and degenerative, can be accomplished by a posterior lumbar interbody fusion. In degenerative spondylolisthesis, the best operation is reduction and posterior lumbar interbody fusion (without laminectomy) accompanied by spinous process wiring or peduncular screws and plate fixation. The latter technique is not indicated in lytic spondylolisthesis if a proper interbody fusion is performed with ample bone grafts.

References

1. Andre N (quoted by Newman PH) (1963) The etiology of spondylolisthesis. J Bone Joint Surg [Br] 45:38
2. Neugebauer FL (1884) Fin neuer beitrag zur cauistik and aetiologie der spondylolisthesis. Arch Gynecol 22:347
3. Wiltse LL (1962) The etiology of spondylolisthesis. J Bone Joint Surg [Am] 44:539
4. Cloward RB (1952) Treatment of ruptured invertebral discs by vertebral fusion: indications, operative technique, and after care. J Neurosurg 10:154
5. Cloward RB (1981) Spondylolisthesis: Treatment by laminectomy and posterior interbody fusion, Review of 100 cases. Clin Orthop 154:74–82
6. Junghanns J, Schmorl G (1971) The human spine in health and disease, 2nd edn. Grune and Stratton, New York, pp 35–37

3.3 Posterior Lumbar Interbody Fusion: With and Without Pedicle Screw Fixation

Sadaaki Nakai, Hidezo Yoshizawa, Kazuhiko Kenmotsu, Satoshi Nishimoto, and Tomofumi Morita[1]

Introduction

We are presently using posterior lumbar interbody fusion (PLIF) [1] for posterior decompression and simultaneous interbody fusion mainly in one or two segments in the lumbar and lumbosacral areas for selected intervertebral disk hernia cases, failed back cases, and various sorts of spondylolisthesis cases. Internal fixation with pedicle screw systems is also being conducted in selected cases so as to diminish pseudarthrosis, shorten postoperative bed rest, and reduce spondylolisthesis. In this paper we compare the results of simple PLIF and PLIF with pedicle screw fixation in order to investigate the differences between these two methods based on various parameters.

Materials and Methods

PLIF was performed on 161 patients from 1978 to 1990. Of these, 2 patients died due to unrelated complications. Of the remaining 159 patients, simple PLIF was done in 103 and PLIF with pedicle screw fixation in 46. These 149 cases were analyzed. The patients included 100 males and 49 females with a mean age of 44.3 years (ranging from 12 years to 73 years). The follow-up period for the 149 patients was on average 5 years 2 months (ranging from 1 to 13 years). There were 101 cases of intervertebral disk hernia, 24 cases of degenerative spondylolisthesis, 10 of spondylolytic spondylolisthesis, 5 of spondylolysis, 4 of congenital spondylolisthesis, 2 of degenerative scoliosis, 2 of epiphyseal slipping, and 1 of iatrogenic spondylolisthesis.

We performed simple PLIF in 103 cases and PLIF with pedicle screw fixation in 46 cases. We used the Cotrel-Dubousset (C-D) pedicle screw system in all

[1] Department of Orthopaedic Surgery, School of Medicine, Fujita Health University, Toyoake, Japan

Table 1. Operative methods and segments.

	Operated segments							
	L3–L4	L4–L5	L5–L6	L5–S	L3–L4 + L4–L5	L4–L5 + L5–S	L2–L3 + L3–L4 + L4–L5	Total
Simple PLIF		88	1	11	1	2		103
PLIF + pedicle screw	2	26		13	1	3	1	46
Total (*n*)	2	114	1	24	2	5	1	149

Table 2. Operative methods and etiologies.

	Etiologies								
	LDH	DL	LL	Lysis	CL	DS	ES	IL	Total
Simple PLIF	93	3	1	4			2		103
PLIF + pedicle screw	8	21	9	1	4	2		1	46
Total (*n*)	101	24	10	5	4	2	2	1	149

LDH, lumbar intervertebral disk hernia; *DL*, degenerative spondylolisthesis; *LL*, spondylolytic spondylolisthesis; *CL*, congenital spondylolisthesis; *DS*, degenerative scoliosis; *ES*, epiphyseal slipping; *IL*, iatrogenic spondylolisthesis

but 1 case. Simple PLIF was done at the L4–L5 level in 88 cases and the L5–S1 level in 11 cases. PLIF with pedicle screw fixation was done at the L4–L5 level in 26 cases and the L5–S1 level in 13 cases (Table 1). The pedicle screw was used more frequently at the L5–S1 level, as mentioned above. The etiology seen in the patients treated with simple PLIF was mainly lumbar intervertebral disk hernia, but in those treated by PLIF with pedicle screw fixation, the etiology was mainly spondylolisthesis (Table 2).

In these cases, operating time, intraoperative blood loss, time for bone union, correction rate of the spondylolisthesis, lordosis of the fused segment, and clinical results were analyzed.

Lordosis of the fused segments was measured following Speck et al. [2]. Bone union was evaluated based on criteria by Yamamoto et al. [3] as follows: (1) a diminished line between the bone grafts and vertebrae, (2) a change in the obtuse angle between the bone grafts and vertebrae, and (3) an increase in the trabeculae of the bone grafts. Clinical results were evaluated by subjective symptoms (low back pain, 3 points; leg pain and/or tingling, 3; gait, 3) and clinical signs (straight-leg-raising test, 2 points; sensory disturbance, 2; motor disturbance, 2) based on the scoring system advocated by the Japanese Orthopaedic Association (JOA). The rate of improvement was calculated by Hirabayashi's method as follows: $\{(\text{postoperative points} - \text{preoperative points})/(\text{normal points} - \text{preoperative points})\} \times 100(\%)$.

Results

In the group treated by simple PLIF, blood loss was 456 ± 227 ml, operating time was 243 ± 50 minutes, and time for bone union was 5.1 ± 1.6 months. For PLIF with pedicle screw fixation, the values were 557 ± 213 ml, 381 ± 75 minutes, and 4.2 ± 1.1 months, respectively. Compared to PLIF with pedicle screw fixation, the blood loss was less ($P < 0.05$), and the operating time was shorter ($P < 0.01$), but the period for obtaining bone union was longer ($P < 0.01$) for simple PLIF. In addition, for simple PLIF, 3 weeks postoperative bed rest was necessitated, but for PLIF with pedicle screw fixation, 16.5 days were required on average.

Operated Segments

L4–L5 Level

Surgery was performed at the L4–L5 level in 114 cases. In these, simple PLIF was performed in 88 cases, mainly for lumbar intervertebral disk hernia cases, and PLIF with pedicle screw fixation in 26 cases, mainly for degenerative spondylolisthesis cases (Tables 1, 2). The operating time for PLIF with pedicle screw fixation was longer than for simple PLIF (354 ± 54 min > 239 ± 48 min, $P < 0.01$). No difference was seen regarding blood loss, bone union, or lordosis of fused segments.

L5–S1 Level

Surgery was performed at the L5–S1 level in 24 cases: 11 cases of simple PLIF and 13 cases of PLIF with pedicle screw fixation. Simple PLIF was done mainly for intervertebral disk hernia cases, and pedicle screw fixation mainly for spondylolytic spondylolisthesis cases (Tables 1, 2). Intraoperative blood loss for simple PLIF was less (382 ± 144 ml < 568 ± 222 ml, $P < 0.05$) and operating time shorter (253 ± 49 min < 391 ± 82 min, $P < 0.01$) than for PLIF with pedicle screw fixation. The time required for bone union was longer for simple PLIF (5.5 ± 1.7 months > 3.8 ± 0.8 months, $P < 0.05$). Lordosis of fused segments in simple PLIF was greater (27.0 ± 7.3° > 12.2 ± 7.0°, $P < 0.01$) than for PLIF with pedicle screw fixation.

Etiology

Degenerative Spondylolisthesis

There were 24 cases of degenerative spondylolisthesis (Table 3). Among them, 22 operations were performed at the L4–L5 level, 1 operation at the L3–L4 level, and 1 operation at the L4–L5 + L5–S1 levels. Simple PLIF was done in 3 cases and PLIF with pedicle screw fixation in 21 cases. With pedicle screw fixation, the period for bone union was 4.1 ± 1.0 months, lordosis of fused

Table 3. Degenerative spondylolisthesis.

	Cases (n)	Bone union (months)	Lordosis of fused segments (°)	Correction of spondylolisthesis (%)
Simple PLIF	3	5.5	12	48
PLIF + pedicle screw	21	4.1 ± 1.0	13.0 ± 7.0	40.7 ± 23.0
Total	24	4.2 ± 1.1	12.8 ± 6.9	41.8 ± 23.6

Table 4. Spondylolytic spondylolisthesis.

	Cases (n)	Bone union (months)	Lordosis of fused segments (°)	Correction of spondylolisthesis (%)
Simple PLIF	1	4	22	23
PLIF + pedicle screw	9	4.1 ± 1.0	11.5 ± 5.6	56.8 ± 32.9
Total	10	4.1 ± 0.1	12.7 ± 6.3	53.0 ± 32.8

Table 5. Lumbar intervertebral disk hernia.

	Cases (n)	Operating time (min)	Bone union (months)	Lordosis of fused segments (°)
Simple PLIF	93	239 ± 45	5.2 ± 1.6	13.2 ± 8.5
		*	**	*
PLIF + pedicle screw	8	345 ± 86	4.4 ± 1.4	5.7 ± 5.6
Total	101	246 ± 54.9	5.1 ± 1.6	12.4 ± 8.5

There were significant differences between simple PLIF and PLIF with pedicle screw system on the operating time and the lordosis of the fused segments (* $P < 0.05$)
There was no significant difference on the period for bone union between them (** n.s.)

segments was 13.0 ± 7.0°, and the correction rate of spondylolisthesis was 40.7 ± 23.0%.

Spondylolytic Spondylolisthesis

There were 10 cases of spondylolytic spondylolisthesis, in 8 cases at the L5–S1 level and in 2 cases at the L4–L5 level (Table 4). All but one case were treated by PLIF with pedicle screw fixation. The period for bone union was 4.1 ± 1.0 months, lordosis of fused segments was 11.5 ± 5.6°, and the correction rate of spondylolisthesis, 56.8 ± 32.9% for PLIF with pedicle screw fixation.

Lumbar Intervertebral Disk Hernia

There were 101 cases of intervertebral disk hernia, including 84 at the L4–L5 level, 11 at the L5–S1 level, and 3 at the L4–L5 + L5–S1 level (Table 5). Simple PLIF was performed in 93 cases and PLIF with pedicle screw fixation in 8 cases. The operating time for simple PLIF was less that than for PLIF with pedicle screw fixation (239 ± 45 min < 345 ± 86 min, $P < 0.05$), and lordosis of simple PLIF cases exceeded that of PLIF with pedicle screw cases (13.2 ± 8.5° > 5.7 ± 5.6°, $P < 0.05$).

Clinical Results

The JOA score and the rate of improvement were not correlated with either operative methods, etiologies, or correction rate of spondylolisthesis.

Complications

There were two cases of paresis due to pedicle screw insertion, one permanent and the other transient. There were also two cases of infection, one directly following simple PLIF and the other 6 months following PLIF with pedicle screw fixation. We had ten pseudarthroses, all after simple PLIF. No pseudarthrosis was seen in the PLIF with pedicle screw fixation cases.

Discussion

We had two indications for PLIF in lumbar intervertebral disk hernia cases. One indication was diffuse annular bulges [4], where the annulus fibrosus circumferentially protruded beyond the peripheral rim of the vertebral bodies. In these cases we could not extract typical intervertebral disk hernia, because the annulus fibrosus protruded circumferentially and there was no localized intervertebral disk hernia. The other indication was failed back cases with clinical symptoms in the lower limbs but without evidence of recurrent intervertebral disk hernia, which could be managed with a second herniotomy [5].

Indications for additional internal pedicle screw fixation included various sorts of spondylolisthesis, cases of insufficient postoperative bed rest due to various complications especially in the cardiorespiratory system, and osteoporosis with a high possibility of collapsing bone grafts. In the spondylolisthesis cases the bone union can be obtained in a translated position without instruments [2,6], but we would reduce the translation (spondylolisthesis) since the influence of translation on neighboring segments was not clearly analyzed, and also in order to get a wider area for bone union.

Several methods of instrumentation have been employed in the past, but recently we have favored the pedicle screw for the PLIF procedure. Analysis showed that the operating time was longer (381 ± 75 min > 243 ± 50 min) and intraoperative blood loss was greater (557 ± 213 ml > 456 ± 227 ml) for PLIF with pedicle screw fixation than for simple PLIF. Usually we provided 400 or 800 ml of autogenous blood for the operation, and homologous blood was rarely needed. Hypotensive anesthesia was also useful for reducing intraoperative blood loss. In both cases, we used only autologous bone grafts from the anterior or posterior iliac crest. For this maneuver about 1 h was necessary. Operating time could therefore be shortened by the use of banked bone.

The time for bone union was on average 4.2 months for pedicle screw fixation and 5.1 months for simple PLIF. The duration of bed rest following pedicle screw fixation was on average 16.5 days, but it could be shorter since extremely long periods of bed rest were required in some cases owing to complications. On the other hand, we consider 3 weeks bed rest adequate after simple PLIF because of the waiting time for the healing of the soft tissues.

Analysis of the L4–L5 and L5–S1 levels showed differences in operating time for simple PLIF and for pedicle screw fixation. At the L5–S1 level, significant differences in the time for bone union and the lordosis of fused segments were noted between simple PLIF and pedicle screw fixation. With spondylolisthesis, bony fusion is considered difficult to achieve, and most patients treated by pedicle screw fixation were suffering from spondylolisthesis. It is therefore justified to say that the pedicle screw fixation leads more easily to solid bone union. However, in about one half of the pedicle screw cases, oblique X-rays showed a clear zone around the screws. In addition, it was also difficult to penetrate the anterior cortex of the sacrum in all cases because of the acute angle of screw insertion due to the ilium. In such cases we used a spica cast postoperatively to compensate for the insufficient stability of screws in the sacrum.

The lumbar lordosis is usually flexible, but with fusion in one or two segments the flexibility must be restricted. Besides, the saggital balance of the spine can be changed because of compression fractures due to osteoporosis. Accordingly, it is worthwhile measuring and comparing the lordosis of fused segments in various situations. Compared to simple PLIF, there was less lordosis at the L5–S1 level in pedicle screw cases and lumbar intervertebral disk hernia with pedicle screw cases. The reasons for this are as follows: at the L5–S1 level, most cases of pedicle screw fixation were spondylolytic spondylolisthesis with a hypolumbosacral angle. In these cases, correction of translation (spondylolisthesis) was possible, but sufficient correction of the slip angle could not be achieved (Fig. 1). In the lumbar intervertebral disk hernia cases, this may have been due to a decreased lordosis of the lumbar spine on the Hall frame during surgery. The pedicle screw fixed the lumbosacral junction at the hypolordotic angle on the Hall frame. Where simple PLIF was performed, this angle changed spontaneously after surgery.

Because the influence of the anterior translation (spondylolisthesis) on neighbouring segments has not been clearly analyzed, and in order to obtain wider area for bone union, we would reduce spondylolisthesis. The correction rate of spondylolisthesis with a pedicle screw system was 40.7 ± 23.0% (n = 21) in the

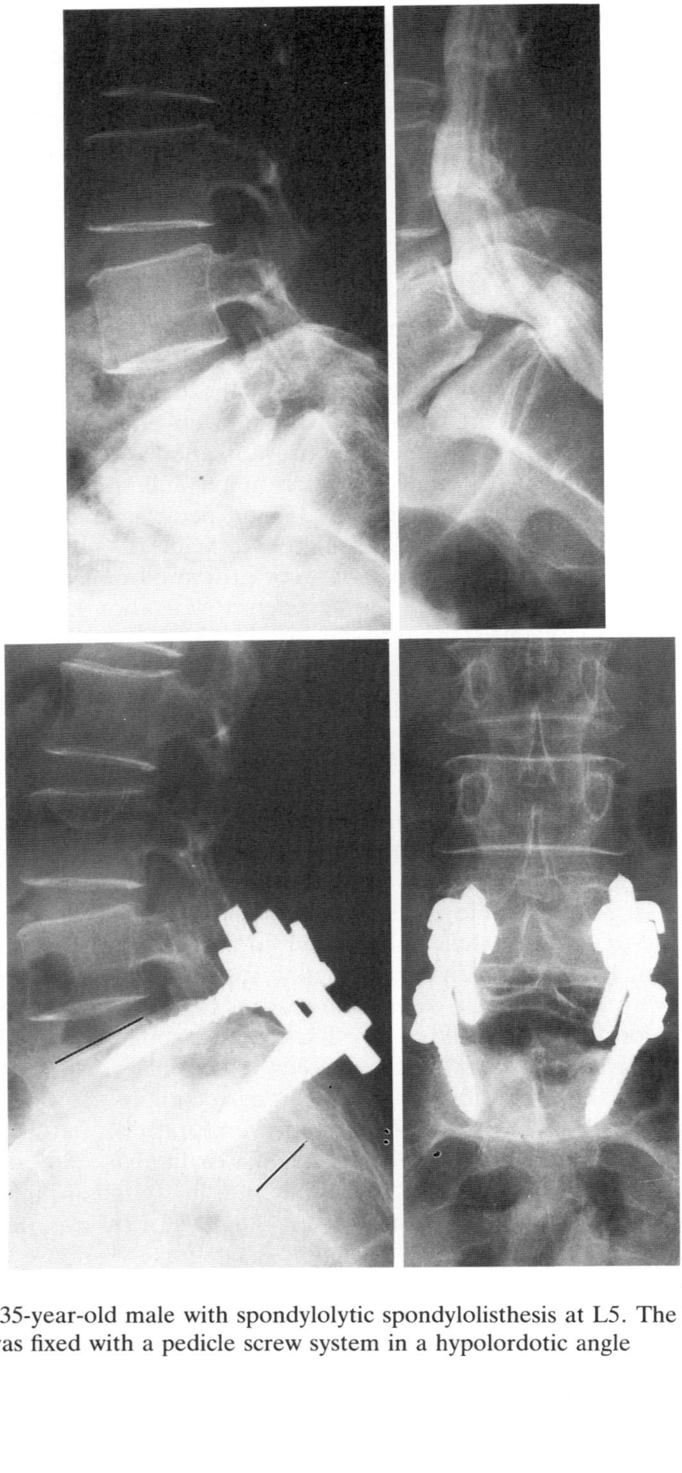

Fig. 1. A 35-year-old male with spondylolytic spondylolisthesis at L5. The lumbosacral junction was fixed with a pedicle screw system in a hypolordotic angle

degenerative spondylolisthesis cases and 56.8 ± 32.9% ($n = 9$) in the spondylolytic spondylolisthesis cases. We could not say positively that it was a satisfactory reduction, but complete reduction might not always be necessary.

There were 10 cases of pseudarthrosis among the 103 cases treated by simple PLIF (9.7%), but most of these cases were encountered in the early stages of this study. There was no pseudarthrosis in cases treated by pedicle screw fixation. Since most pedicle screw cases were spondylolisthesis, where bony fusion is thought to be difficult to obtain, pedicle screw fixation is more effective for obtaining solid fusion.

As mentioned above, the advantages of pedicle screw fixation are early bone union (especially for the spondylolisthesis cases), shorter period of postoperative bed rest, and better correction of spondylolisthesis. The problems caused by use of the pedicle screw system were excessive bleeding and prolonged operating time, but the rate of complications was not especially high. In the osteoporotic cases, pedicle screw fixation could prevent the collapse of the bone grafts, but oblique X-rays showed a clear zone around the screws in about one half of the cases.

The indications for additional pedicle screw fixation can be summarized as follows; (1) spondylolytic spondylolisthesis and degenerative spondylolisthesis, (2) osteoporosis with a high possibility of the collapse of bone grafts and adjacent vertebrae, apart from excessive cases, and (3) poor risk patients with insufficient postoperative bed rest.

Conclusions

For PLIF with pedicle screw fixation the operating time was 138 min longer and blood loss was 101 ml greater than the values for simple PLIF. However, bone union was achieved approximately 1 month earlier without pseudarthrosis. In L5–S1 cases and lumbar intervertebral disk hernia cases, lordosis of fused segments was less in PLIF with pedicle screw fixation cases than simple PLIF cases.

The correction rate of spondylolisthesis with pedicle screw fixation was 40.7% in degenerative cases, and 56.8% in spondylolytic cases, but no correlation between the correction rate and clinical results could be found.

References

1. Cloward RB (1985) The treatment of ruptured lumbar intervertebral disk by vertebral body fusion. Clin Orthop 193:5–154
2. Speck GR, McCall IW, O'Brien JP (1984) The angle of kyphosis. Spine 9:659–660
3. Yamamato M, Kadowaki T, Ota N, et al. (1990) PLIF for lumbar degenerative spondylolisthesis. Rinsho Seikeigeka 25:487–494
4. MacNab I (1977) Backache. Williams and Wilkins, Baltimore

5. Yoshizawa H, Oiwa T (1986) Pathology and treatment of failed back cases – Posterior approach as a salvage operation. J Jpn Orthop Ass 60:S54–56
6. Yoshizawa H (1988) Treatment of degenerative spondylolisthesis. Seikeigeka 39: 1815–1820

3.4 Posterior Lumbar Interbody Fusion Combined Auto- and Allograft Technique

Prem S. Ramani[1]

Introduction

The Surgical treatment of ruptured lumbar intervertebral disk with or without lumbar instability, or association of lumbar instability without prolapsed lumbar intervertebral disk is controversial in terms of the necessity of spinal fusion. Even today with more accurate diagnostic methods it has not been possible to lay down specific criteria for lumbar stabilization. The subject has been further shrouded in controversy because many patients remain asymptomatic for long periods just with excision of the prolapsed lumbar intervertebral disk. It has not been possible to differentiate rigid criteria for patients requiring fusion and those who do not need it. Cloward began performing fusion in 1943 [1], but at that time there was very little enthusiasm for the procedure, presumably due to technical difficulties and failure to duplicate the clinical results and the fusion rate. However in recent times, the painstaking and dedicated efforts of Lin and others have produced tremendous interest and enthusiasm for posterior lumbar interbody fusion (PLIF) [2–11]. Understanding of bone physiology and realization that the patient's own corticocancellous bone from the iliac crest is the best bone for osteosynthesis has further heightened interest in PLIF [12–17]. In certain cases, such as isthmic or degenerative spondylolisthesis or traumatic spondylolisthesis, the instability is anatomically obvious. However, if a large amount of disk material is removed, settlement of the disk space and instability in the motion segment definitely occurs, but it is not anatomically obvious immediately. Only when facet hypertropy, tropism, and spinal stenosis with spondylosis has occured can instability be appreciated.

I have done PLIF more liberally in (1) cases showing obvious instability, (2) cases where instability is apparent by the secondary changes described above, or (3) cases who might be suspected of developing instability in the future, such as large central disk prolapses in the young or a disk causing total myelographic block. Patients with failed backs have formed an important group in this series,

[1]Department of Neurosurgery, L.T.M.G. Hospital, Sion (West), Bombay 400 022, India

where PLIF has been uniformly carried out in all cases. A large number of patients in this series came from coastal areas where fishing is a common profession. Spondylolysis and spondylolisthesis are very common in these people and hence I am called upon to treat a large number of cases. The problem of backache is equally common in this part of the world as elsewhere, and so the number of females in this series was also quite large.

Materials and Methods

During a period of 5.5 years from January 1986 until June 1991, a total of 250 PLIF operations were performed. After an initial trial using a few techniques, I finally developed my construct of PLIF and most of the operations since then have been carried out using this construct or model.

In all there were 137 males (54.8%) and 113 (45.2%) females. The oldest patient was a male aged 74 years and the youngest patient a male aged 23 years. There were 83 patients (33.2%) aged between 31 and 40 years. The next most common age group contained 65 patients (26%) between the ages of 41 to 50 years. There were 43 patients (17.2%) between 21 and 30 years, 36 patients (14.4%) between 51 and 60 years, 19 patients (7.6%) between 61 and 70 years, and 4 patients (1.6%) between 71 and 75 years. More than half the patients in this series who underwent PLIF surgery had anatomical instability, i.e., spondylolysis or spondylolisthesis (isthmic or degenerative). A total of 128 patients (51.2%) had various grades of instability in the lumbar spine. The majority of these patients came from the state of Goa in India, which although small in size, has a large number of cases of varying grades of anatomical lumbar instability. Goa is a coastal state and fishing is an important industry. Here children are subject to stresses like walking in water, pulling fishing nets, rowing boats in rough waters, and so on. The hilly terrain of the state makes it obligatory to climb hills, and this may also contribute to the increased incidence of lumbar instability.

The other indications for lumbar stabilization in this series are outlined in Table 1.

Table 1. Indications for lumbar stabilisation.

Indication	Cases (*n*)	Percentage
Spondylolysis/listhesis	100	40.0
Failed back	41	16.4
Central PIVD in the young and PIVD in labourers	29	11.6
Facet hypertrophy	23	9.2
Total myelographic block	20	8.0
Degenerative spondylolisthesis	28	11.2
Traumatic instability	9	3.6

PIVD, prolapsed intervertebral disk

Some cases in the failed group had undergone posterolateral fusion but it had failed. Some had total settlement of the disk space with extensive degenerative changes. Most had had a laminectomy performed elsewhere which had not come up to their expectations. As a policy I believe in preservation of the posterior motion segment [14,18,19] and as far as is possible laminectomy is not performed.

In cases of spondylolisthesis with a forward slip of 40% or less, almost total reduction was achieved. In the remaining cases, fusion was carried out in the optimum reduced position. In all cases of spondylolisthesis I now include PLIF, pedicle screws and plates, and posterolateral fusion, for the following reasons. The Indian population is accustomed to sitting on the floor for many of their day-to-day activities, such as to eat, clean the floor, wash clothes, or cut vegetables. They squat on the toilet. They squat to sell fish or other merchandise, to cook food, and to work in the field. They feel most relaxed sitting on the floor leaning against a wall. I had two early cases of failed fusion in spondylolisthesis and this has resulted in extra caution being exercised with these patients. The number of cases of failed back goes on increasing day by day and at one time I treated nine cases of failed back in 6 months. PLIF is done at one or two levels, along with use of pedicle screws and plates. The operation is time consuming but the relief of symptoms makes the surgery worthwhile. In two cases where settlement of the disk was unilateral and had caused list of the lumbar spine, the PLIF was done only on one side to correct the list.

The PLIF Construct

Bone grafts for interbody fusion in the lumbar spine have been used for 48 years [1]. The principle involved in this procedure is the distraction of the vertebral bodies by placement of grafts under impaction. The procedure stabilizes the unstable segment, corrects lordosis, widens the intervertebral foramina, and decompresses the dura in the spinal canal.

Essentially the grafts placed under impaction must satisfy two basic criteria: (1) they must incorporate with the host bone to achieve true bony fusion and (2) they must have enough mechanical strength in them so that until true bony fusion is achieved, they maintain the vertebral bodies distracted and participate in the weight-bearing mechanism of the spine from the time the patient starts walking again. Thus far it has been difficult to obtain an ideal graft which is mechanically strong, potentially viable, and which will quickly incorporate with the host bone. Anatomically the graft should be tricortical with strong cortical bone on three sides placed peripherally for weight bearing and enough cancellous bone in the centre for osteosynthesis. However it is not possible to obtain such a graft from the iliac crest. Live cancellous bone is the best bone for osteosynthesis [12,16,17]. It has enough bone morphogenic protein (BMP) and osteoblastic cells [17]. Cancellous bone from the iliac crest is best suited for fusion and hence it is universally used.

Small tricortical grafts prepared by ethylene oxide sterilization have better strength and mechanical properties [20,21]. They are best suited to take the weight of the body and keep the vertebrae distracted. However, it does not have osteosynthetic capability. It merely acts as scaffolding which must eventually be replaced by live bone through creeping substitution. The process is slow and remodelling can take up to 2 years. During this period the graft may slip out of position and create complications, and this has been a point of concern among spinal surgeons interested in lumbar stabilization.

Various constructs have been used [1–3,11,22,23]. Cloward used only ethylene-oxide-sterilized allografts [20,21]. His construct is slow to fuse, the technique is difficult, and in inexperienced hands complications have occurred.

Once the bone physiology was more clear and the superiority of autogenic bone for osteosynthesis was established [16,17], Lin used only autogenic bone in his construct [24]. He used four bicortical grafts along with slivers of cancellous bone from the iliac crest. His cases achieved fusion quickly within 4 months but they were not mechanically strong. Some amount of disk settlement did occur, with the percentage of settlement varying from case to case. The other constructs have not been popularly used although Collis has vast experience in total disk replacement (TDR) using calf bone in anterior lumbar interbody fusion (ALIF) [3].

Through trial and error I became convinced that using only one type of bone was not satisfactory to encompass all the principles involved in PLIF [23]. It is essential to have enough cancellous autogenic bone to promote quick osteosynthesis and at the same time there has to be a device such as allograft with enough strength to bear the weight of the body without causing settlement until such time as true bony or anatomical fusion has occurred. Therefore a bone bank was established which gave the advantage of providing enough bone grafts of various sizes and shapes with quick availability in the operating room.

My model is constructed as follows (Fig. 1). Quasi total diskectomy is carried out and only partial decortication of the cortical end-plates is done on both sides. The anterior longitudinal ligament is exposed; a microscope is sometimes used at this stage to remove the disk tissue lying anteriorly, thus exposing the ligament. The depth, height, and width of the grafts are measured and two tricortical allografts selected and designed in the correct shape and size. Two bicortical autografts are obtained from the posterior iliac crest along the superior glueteal line through the same horizontal incision used for PLIF. Enough slivers of cancellous bone are obtained from the iliac crest, and cancellous slivers up to 5 mm thick are impacted into the bed and sides of the disk space. The two allografts are positioned in the centre of the disk space, and the two autografts are placed laterally, one on each side. Any space left behind in the disk space is filled with high density live cancellous bone chips.

With this construct the patient is allowed out of bed with a firm lumbosacral belt within 24 h of operation. The construct has proved to be very satisfactory

Fig. 1. Comined auto- and allograft technique

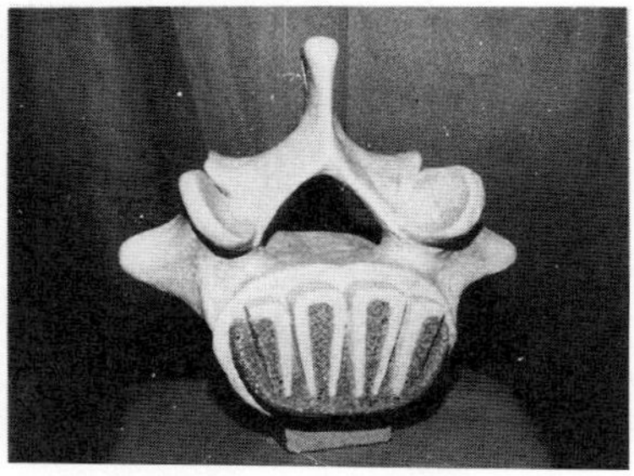

- **Dr. P.S. Ramani's Construct of PLIF**
  - **Bed and Sides Filled with Live Bone Chips**
  - **Two Central Tricortical Grafts from Bone Bank**
  - **Two Lateral Bicortical Grafts from PT's Iliac Crest**

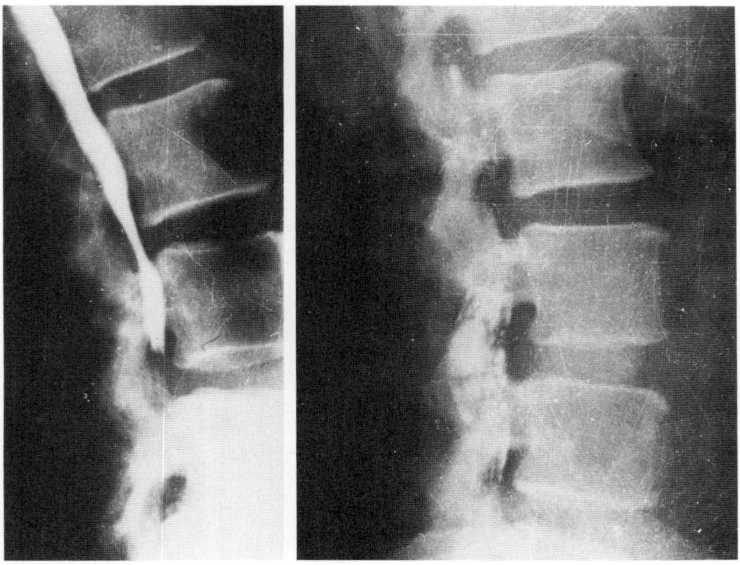

Fig. 2. Total myelographic block treated with PLIF without laminectomy

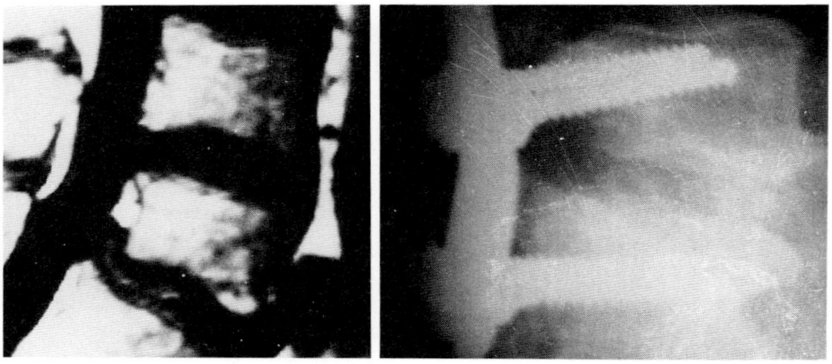

Fig. 3. A case of L5–S1 spondylolisthesis treated with PLIF and pedicle screws and plates (VSP)

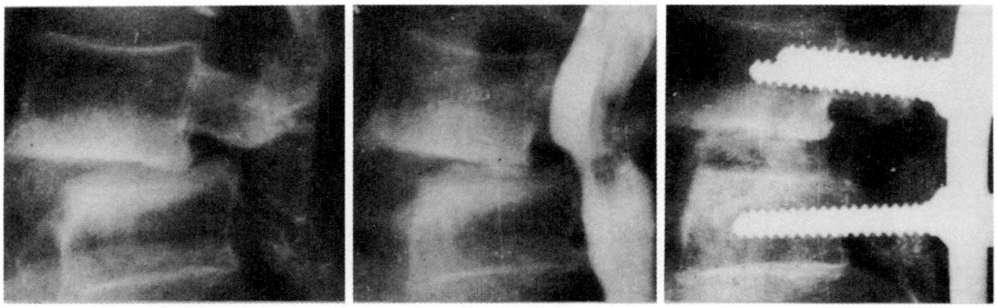

Fig. 4. Adequate decompression and stabilization in a case of failed back following laminectomy

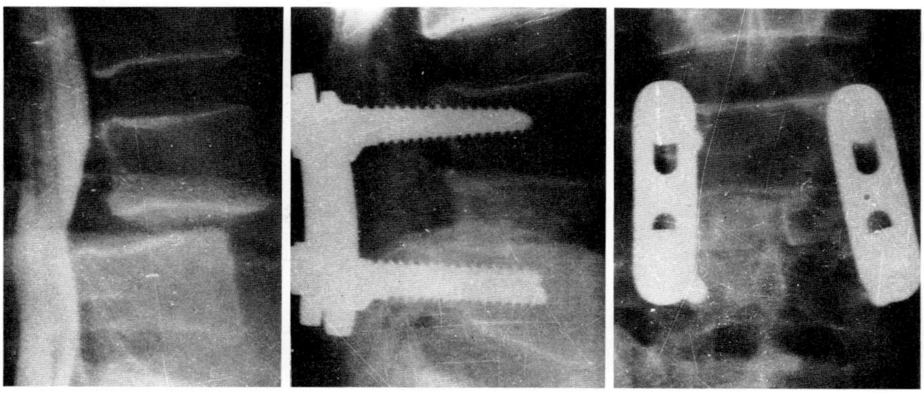

Fig. 5. A case of failed back with spondylolisthesis. Correction, decompression, and stabilization done with PLIF and implants

(Fig. 2). It has enough bone, and it has enough osteogenic potential to stand the axial loads of the spine until remodelling takes place. Significant absorption of autografts has not been seen as the bank bones provide mechanical stability. Functionally the model has worked well.

The metallic implants are the Steffee-type variable screw placement (VSP) system [25] made of stainless steel manufactured locally. The screws are 5.5 mm wide and have a 38-mm long cancellous portion. Since spinal plates and screws provide a high degree of stability, the system has been utilized in all cases of spondylolisthesis and has helped in particular in early mobilization of the patient (Fig. 3). Extensive destabilization for adequate decompression of the neural elements is now possible. The pedicle screw and plates system is used extensively in the treatment of failed backs with remarkable relief of pain and neurological symptoms (Fig. 4). With this system of implants and PLIF it has been possible to obtain most effective reduction, destraction, and stability in most cases of varying grades of lumbar instability (Fig. 5).

Clinical Results

The significant pointer for a successful clinical result in this type of surgery is the return of patient to his original job. Some patients had no motivation to return to work and others were entertaining ideas of compensation. However, results in terms of symptom relief and bony fusion have been extremely good. Lin's classification has been used to analyze the results [26]. The excellent and good categories were grouped together and simply labelled as good. Good clinical results with relief of pain were obtained in 209 patients (83.6%). The results were fair in 34 patients (13.6%) and 7 patients (2.8%) were included into the category of poor results as the relief of pain in them was not satisfactory. A total of 165 patients (66%) have returned to their original jobs within a maximum of 1 year from the date of operation. As mentioned earlier, many of these patients are labourers working in the fishing industry in coastal areas. Some of them just did not want to return to work in the sea although there was relief of pain, and they preferred sedentary work on land. Industrial workers aiming for compensation also showed unsatisfactory results in terms of return to work. Most housewifes agreed they had benefited from the operation. A total of 46 patients (18.4%) are not doing any work although 27 of them (10.8%) are satisfied with the operation. Infection developed in 5 patients. In 2 patients the grafts were removed and after 2 months they were reoperated on using PLIF, pedicle screw and plates. One of these has gone back to his original job as a goldsmith, and the other, a 74-year-old diabetic patient, lives in an old people's home. The remaining 3 patients were treated conservatively in consultation with a bacteriology expert and they have shown satisfactory fusion. One of them, a grocer, can even lift 50 kg in weight, an other can ride his motorcycle, and the third is a watchman on sedentary duty.

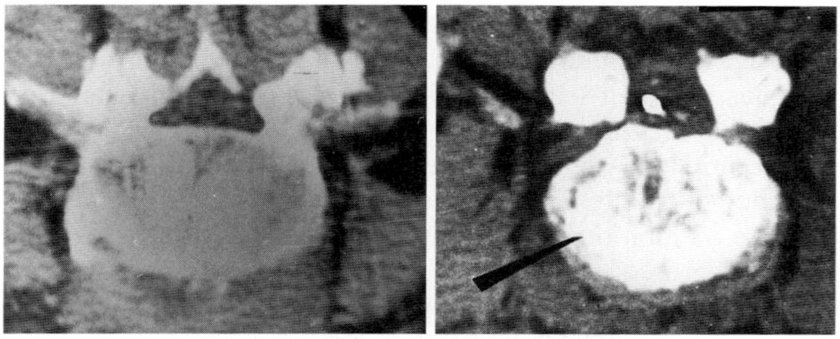

Fig. 6. CT scan 4 months after surgery (*left*). Two central allografts can be clearly identified. Two lateral autografts are seen remodeling. At 18 months after surgery there is complete remodeling with thick bone organised at the periphery (ring formation: evidence of true bony fusion) and cancellous bone at the centre (*right*). The anterior longitudinal ligament is seen developing calcification (second ring formation)

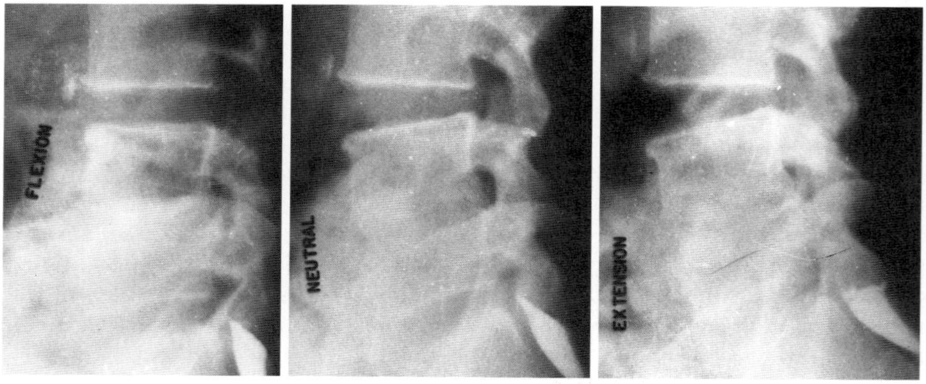

Fig. 7. Plain roentgenograms taken 18 months after PLIF surgery in neutral, flexion, and extension positions show solid fusion between L4 and L5

There was no neurological damage in this series although the dura was torn on a few occasions. In these cases, the dura could be sutured, and it was not felt necessary to underrun the stitch or insert a fat graft as described by Lin [24].

PLIF failed in 3 patients with spondylolithesis treated without metallic implants. I reoperated with implants on 1 patient, but the 2 other patients have not agreed to reoperation although clinically they are not happy. Patients above the age of 60 years have shown a higher percentage of unsatisfactory clinical results.

Discussion

It is now certain that one type of material cannot satisfy the two principles involved in PLIF, namely quick osteosynthesis and mechanical stability. For quick osteosynthesis live bone is essential, and the posterior part of the iliac crest is best suited for this. Along the superior gluteal line the bone is quite thick, and it can be obtained through the same horizontal incision used for PLIF. Many bicortical grafts and enough cancellous chips can be obtained from this site. The morbidity is minimum and if incision is not extended laterally too far one can avoid cutting the cluneal nerve (superior gluteal) and the resultant numbness over the buttock. Iliac bone has enough cancellous bone and osteosynthesis can be quickly achieved. To maintain mechanical stability two tricortical allografts are used in this construct. Bank bone is much stronger than live bone [21]. Two tricortical grafts of 8 mm in width are enough to provide sufficient mechanical stability until such time as remodelling has occurred. Bank bone also has other advantages. Sufficient quantities of various graft shapes and sizes are easily available in the operating room and ethylene-oxide-sterilized bone can be stored at room temperature.

Strong stability in the centre surrounded by bone with strong osteogenic potential, along with sufficient stability, is the concept of the construct that I have used, based on the flagpole concept of biomechanics of the spine advocated by Evans [27]. There is enough strength in this construct for the patient to get up after 24 h and start walking without an extremely rigid external support. Since this model incorporates the basic principles involved in PLIF it should prove very useful.

The rate of fusion was assessed with the help of serial CT scans taken at 4-month intervals for up to 2 years. Excellent fusion seen in 92.5% of patients suggests that the construct is good. Only CT scans can allow the study of true bony fusion (Fig. 6). Fibrous ankylosis can give good clinical results without true bony fusion and this cannot be correctly assessed with either roentgenograms in flexion or extension or with polytomograms. Results based on these studies need to be more critically evaluated (Fig. 7).

Allografts are slow to fuse. They are lacking in BMP which is so essential for osteosynthesis [16,17]. The greater the number of cells containing this protein, the quicker the osteosynthesis. The cancellous bone of the iliac crest contains the largest number of these cells as compared to any other cancellous bone in the body. Cancellous bone of the femur and tibia contains more fatty cells and has less osteoinductive properties.

For better stability, the use of metallic implants (the Steffee-type VSP System [25]), especially in cases with anatomical instability, is a welcome adjunct to PLIF. Along with a crossbar, the whole construct provides three-dimensional stability to the spine so that the construct should prove useful even in obese patients.

References

1. Cloward RB (1953) The treatment of ruptured intervertebral disk by vertebral body fusion. J Neurosurg 10:154–168
2. Blume HG (1982) Unilateral lumbar interbody fusion by posterior approach with dowel grafts. In: Lin PM (ed) Posterior lumbar interbody fusion Charles C. Thomas, Springfield, pp 252–275
3. Collis JS (1985) Total disk replacement: A modified posterior lumbar interbody fusion; Report of 750 cases. Clin Orthop 193:64–67
4. Leong JCY (1989) Anterior interbody fusion. In: Lin PM, Gill K (eds) Lumbar interbody fusion. Aspen, Maryland, pp 133–148
5. Lin PM (1977) Posterior lumbar interbody fusion. In: Sweer WH, Schmidek HH (eds) Current techniques in operative neurosurgery, 2nd edn. Grune and Stratton, New York, pp 1339–1364
6. Ramani PS (1986) Posterior lumbar interbody fusion. In: Sinha KK, Chandra P (eds) Progress in clinical neurosciences, I. Neurological Society of India, pp 33–42
7. Ramani PS (1988) Posterior lumbar interbody fusion. Clin Orthop India 2:95–103
8. Ramani PS (1988) Spondylolysis and spondylolisthesis: Its recognition and management. In: Sinha KK, Chandra P (eds) Progress in clinical neurosciences, I. Neurological Society of India, pp 101–114
9. Ramani PS (1989) Posterior lumbar interbody fusion. Review of 100 cases. Neurology India 37:607–618
10. Ramani PS (1989) Posterior lumbar interbody fusion. Associated Personnel Services Publication, Bombay, pp 103–131
11. Takeda M (1985) Experience in posterior lumbar interbody fusion. Unicortical versus bicortical autologus grafts. Clin Orthop 193:1201–126
12. Burwell RG (1985) The function of bone marrow in the incorporation of a bone graft. Clinical Orthopaedics 200:125–141
13. Frost HM (1985) The pathomechanics of osteoporosis. Clinical Orthopaedics 200: 198–225
14. Gordon GS (1985) Estrogen and bone. Clinical Orthopaedics 200:174–180
15. Nachemson AL (1985) Advances in low back pain. Clinical Orthopaedics 200: 266–278
16. Prolo DJ, Rodrigo JJ (1985) Contemporary bone graft physiology and surgery. Clinical Orthopaedics 200:322–342
17. Urist MR (1980) Bone transplantation. In: Urist MR (ed) Fundamentals and clinical bone physiology. Lippincott, Philadelphia, pp 331–368
18. Junghans J, Schmorl G (1977) The human spine in health and disease. Grune and Stratton, New York, pp 357–385
19. White AA, Panjabi MM (1978) Clinical biomechanics of spine. Lippincot, Philadelphia
20. Cloward RB (1957) Ten years' experience with a one man bone bank. J Int Col Surg 23:110–117
21. Cloward RB (1980) Gas-sterilized cadaver bone graft for fusion. A simplified bone bank. Spine 5(1):4–7
22. Ma GWC (1985) Posterior lumbar interbody fusion with specialized instruments. Clin Orthop 193:57–63
23. Ramani PS (1989) A new model for posterior lumbar interbody fusion. In: Ramani PS (eds) Posterior lumbar interbody fusion. Associated personnel services, Bombay, pp 89–96

24. Lin PM (1982) Technique of PLIF. In: Lin PM (ed) Posterior lumbar interbody fusion. Charles C. Thomas, Springfield, pp 94–139
25. Lin PM (1982) Evaluation of clinical results. In: Lin PM (ed) Posterior lumbar interbody fusion. Charles C. Thomas Springfield, pp 154–160
26. Steffee A (1989) The variable screw placement system with posterior lumbar interbody fusion. In: Ramani PS (ed) Posterior lumbar interbody fusion. Associated Personnel Services, Bombay, pp 212–226
27. Evans JH (1985) Biomechanics of lumbar spine. Clin Orthop 193:38–44

3.5 Posterior Lumbar Interbody Fusion with Allograft and Plates

Tetsuo Ohwada, Tomio Yamamoto, Kazumasa Nose,
Masahiro Inaoka[1], and Masaaki Kakiuchi[2]

Introduction

Since 1979, we have applied posterior lumbar interbody fusion (PLIF) with autologous iliac bone grafts in fusion surgery for degenerative conditions of the lumbar spine, such as degenerative spondylolisthesis (DS), spondylolytic spondylolisthesis (SO), prolapsed intervertebral disk (PID) with marked instability, and degenerative lumbar canal stenosis (LCS) with instability. In these conditions, decompression of all the involved neural elements and stabilization of the affected segments are indicated. PLIF is biomechanically the best fusion method available and also provides wide visualization of the neural elements posteriorly [1–3].

Review of 371 cases of PLIF operations, however, revealed a high rate of problems with bony union, such as collapse of the iliac autograft, delayed union or nonunion of the autograft (Table 1). These problems were also associated with an unsatisfactory clinical outcome [4]. It was suggested that some reinforcement procedure was needed to obtain more successful fusion and better clinical results.

Since 1987, we have used a pedicle screw and plate system for reinforcement to obtain more rigid segmental stability. We tried the Roy-Camille plate and screw system first [5], and then used Steffee's VSP system as a supporting method of PLIF [6,7]. The superior mechanical strength of these pedicle screw fixation systems combined with PLIF has been well demonstrated [7], so we have applied this method in all the PLIF operations.

However, even with rigid fixation devices, the collapse of the iliac bone autograft still occurs sometimes [4]. Actually, even though the incidence of delayed union or nonunion has decreased with the adoption of these fixation devices (especially with the VSP system), the incidence of autograft collapse

[1] Division of Orthopaedic Surgery, Osaka Koseinenkin Hospital, 4-2-78 Fukushima, Fukushima-ku, Osaka, 553 Japan
[2] Department of Orthopaedic Surgery, Osaka Police Hospital, Osaka, Japan

Table 1. Fusion results of PLIF in patients with degenerative lumbar diseases.

	L-PID	L-DS	L-SO	Total	
Union in situ	206	19	30	255	
Collapsed union	24	16	4	44	31.3%
Delayed union	17	6	11	34	
Collapsed nonunion	14	2	5	21	
Nonunion	14		3	17	
Total	275	43	53	371 cases	

L-PID, lumbar prolapsed intervertebral disk; L-DS, lumbar degenerative spondylolisthesis; L-SO, lumbar spondylolytic spondylolisthesis

Table 2. PLIF with allograft and the VSP system.

	No. of cases (n)	Average age (years)
Total	35	55 (18–77)
Males	16	
Females	19	
L-PID	15	51
L-DS	11	59
L-SO	2	66
L-CS	7	62
PLIF		
One segment	30	
Two segments	4	
Three segments	1	

Postoperative follow-up periods 12–30 months, average 16.7 months
L-CS, lumbar caual stenosis; PLIF, posterior lumbar interbody fusion

has not been reduced much. This appears to be due to the inherent mechanical weakness of iliac bone graft [4].

Since May 1989, we have started to use solid cortical bone allografts combined with iliac bone autografts. The purpose of the introduction of cortical bone allografts was to preserve the disk space height and avoid collapse of the iliac bone autografts. It also decreases postoperative discomfort at the iliac donor site, which mostly occurs because of dissection of the cruneal nerves. The purpose of this paper is to discuss the clinical utility of bone allografts combined with autografts and the VSP system in the PLIF procedure.

Materials and Methods

Thirty-five patients with degenerative lumbar disease were operated on using PLIF with cortical bone allografts combined with iliac bone autografts and the VSP system. There were 16 males and 19 females, aged from 18 to 77 years old (55 years on average). Fifteen patients had prolapsed intervertebral disk (L-PID), 11 had degenerative spondylolisthesis (DS), 2 had spondylolytic olisthesis (SO), and 7 had degenerative lumbar canal stenosis (LCS) (Table 2). PLIF was performed at a single spinal level in 30 cases, at two levels in 4 cases, and at three levels in 1 case. Postoperative follow-up ranged from 12 months to 30 months (16.7 months on average).

Operative Procedure

The operation was performed in Cloward's original manner [2,8]. Two to four pieces of cortical bone allografts were packed into the central portion of the intervertebral space, and two or three pieces of iliac bone autografts were then inserted around the allografts (Fig. 1). Cancellous bone chips were also used in a few cases. The cortical endplates of the vertebrae were preserved in recent cases to avoid migration of the solid cortical bone allografts into the vertebral body. A VSP screw and plate system was added in all cases and compression force was applied to stabilize the operated spinal segments. Patients were kept

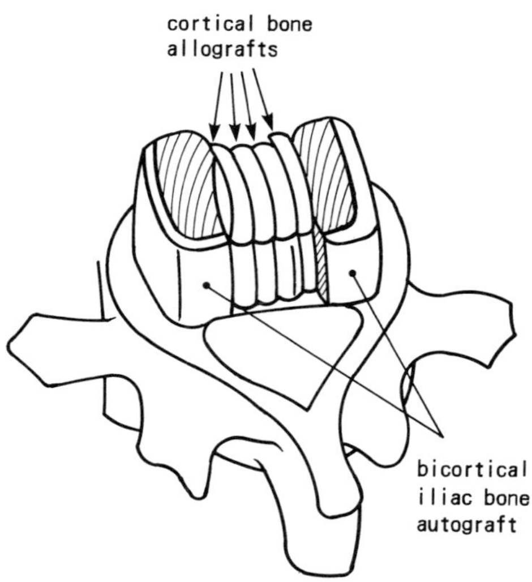

Fig. 1. Diagram showing the operative method for PLIF with cortical bone allografts combined with iliac bone autografts. Two to four pieces of cortical bone allograft are packed into the central portion of the intervertebral space and two or three bicortical iliac bone autografts are inserted around the allografts. The cortical endplates of the vertebral bodies should be preserved to avoid migration of the solid cortical bone allograft

in bed for 7–10 days postoperatively, and then allowed to walk with a soft brace.

Bone Allograft

The method of preparation of the cortical bone allografts was developed by one of the authors (K.M.) [9]. Allografts were prepared from human tibial bone shafts taken from amputated lower limbs. Donor bone must be free from viral infections such as hepatitis or AIDS. Grafts were usually obtained from limbs amputated for ischemic necrosis caused by arteriosclerosis obliterans. The bones were cleaned of soft tissue and cartilage, stored by freezing, and thawed by immersion in deionized water just before preparation. For preparation, the bones were defatted in a mixture of chloroform and methanol for 24h at room temperature, and the cortical bone was then cut into grafts suitable for the intervertebral spaces using a mechanical saw. The defatted bone was freeze-dried in a vacuum at −80°C for about 1 week. The defatted and freeze-dried bone was then exposed to ethylene oxide gas for sterilization. After chloroform-methanol treatment and ethylene-oxide-gas sterilization, the bone allografts, cut into sizes suitable for the intervertebral spaces, were stored in air at room temperature, and then transferred to the operating theater for clinical use [9].

Clinical Evaluation

All patients were examined by one of the authors and classified into four categories according to Inoue's criteria [10], on the basis of symptoms, daily life, and occupational activities:

- Excellent: Full recovery of symptoms and no restriction of occupational or daily activities
- Good: Residual or occasional symptoms, but able to continue all normal activities
- Fair: Partial recovery of symptoms, and unable or difficult to continue working
- Poor: No recovery or worsening of symptoms

Roentogenological Evaluation and Classification

Fusion was judged by plain X ray films and tomograms. Usually, roentgenological evaluation was done monthly after surgery until fusion was confirmed. Fusion was judged to be definitely achieved when we saw any of the following findings on X ray films:

1. Decrease or disappearance of the border between the autologous iliac bone and the vertebral body
2. Loss of sharpness of the outer corners of the border between the vertebral body and the bone autograft, indicating early bone formation at the junction
3. An increase of the density of the trabeculae of the autograft

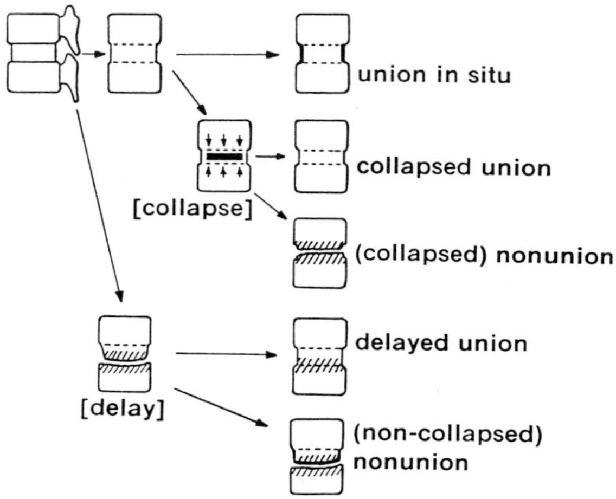

Fig. 2. Classification of the fusion results. Roentogenological fusion results were classified into five categories

Table 3. PLIF with iliac bone autograft.

	L-PID	L-DS	L-SO	Total
PLIF	275	43	53	371
PLIF + R-C	18	13	13	44
PLIF + VSP	50	13	24	87
Total	343	69	90	502

R-C, Roy-Camille plate and screw system; VSP, Steffee's VSP system

A clear zone or marginal sclerosis around the cortical bone allograft was commonly seen on X ray films even though bony fusion of the autograft was confirmed, so it did not indicate delayed union or nonunion.

Classification of the fusion results is shown in Fig. 2. When primary fusion was confirmed at both junctions within 6 months postoperatively and the original shape and height of the grafts was maintained, we designated it as union in situ. Union which was confirmed more than 6 months postoperatively with preservation of the height and shape of the grafts was delayed union. This is one of the common complications of bone union. Collapse of the graft is the second commonest complication. There is an abrupt loss of graft height with absorption of the central part of the graft, and this usually occurs at 2–4 months postoperatively. Union of a collapsed graft was called collapsed union and nonunion was called collapsed nonunion. Nonunion was defined by a persistent clear zone at one junction of the graft with marginal sclerosis at the edges.

Roentgenological results were evaluated at the final follow-up in all cases.

Roentgenological outcome of the PLIF with allografts and the VSP system was compared with that of PLIF with iliac bone autografts (PLIF, 371 cases;

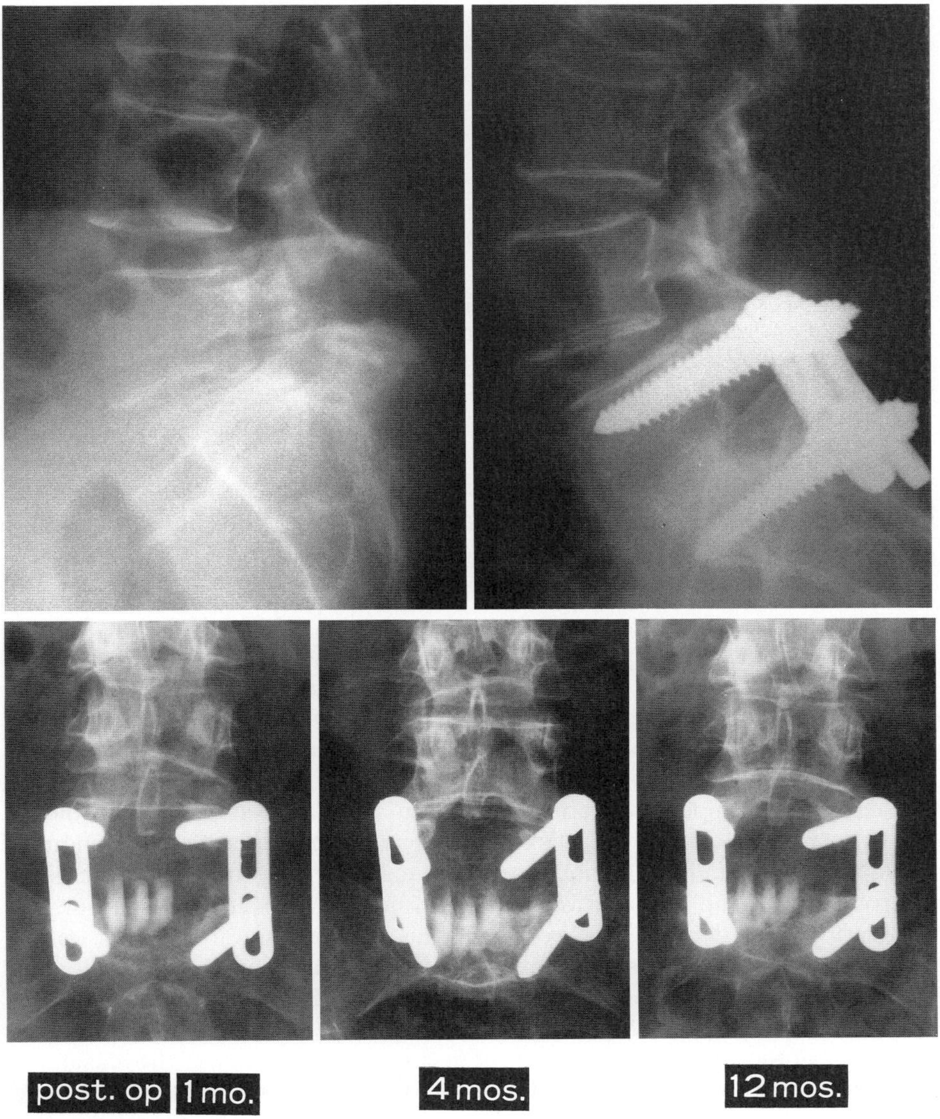

a b

c d e

Fig. 3a–e. A 58-year-old female with L5 spondylolytic olisthesis **a** Preoperative and **b** post-operative lateral X ray films. **c–e** Anterioposterior X rays showing the gradual incorporation of the solid cortical bone allografts. The margin of the bone allograft was clear 1 month post-operatively (**c**). After 4 months (**d**), the clear zone had disappeared and the margin of the allograft became vague. After 1 year (**e**), the allograft had also been incorporated and its contour was unclear

PLIF with Roy-Camille's plate, 44 cases; PLIF with Steffee's VSP system, 87 cases). The total number of these subjects was 502 cases (Table 3).

Results

Clinical Results

An excellent clinical outcome was achived in 18 patients (51.4%), a good outcome in 12 patients (34.3%), fair in 3 patients, and poor in 2 patients. The sum of the excellent and good results was 85.7%. PID patients had an excellent result in ten cases and a good result in five cases. DS patients had an excellent result in seven cases, a good result in three cases, and a fair outcome in one. For L-CS, an excellent result was achieved in only one patient, a good result in four, a fair result in one, and a poor result in one. Of the SO cases, one each had a fair and poor outcome. The proportion of excellent and good results was nearly equivalent in the PLIF series, and the PLIF with transpedicular screw fixation and autograft series.

Roentgenological Results

Thirty-one cases (88.6%) out of 35 patients having PLIF with cortical bone allograft and the VSP system showed sound bony union within 6 months postoperatively and were judged as union in situ. In all cases, the iliac bone autograft surrounding the cortical bone allograft fused 2–6 months after the operation. The average period until sound bony union of the iliac bone autograft was 3.7 months after the operation. The clear zone around the allograft subsequently disappeared gradually and the allograft was eventually incorporated (Fig. 3). Disappearance of the clear zone was seen 4–15 months postoperatively, and at 10 months on average. In only one case, marginal sclerosis around the allograft was persistent, but the iliac autograft outside the allograft was fused solidly and we judged this case as union in situ (Fig. 4).

Collapse of the autograft and axial migration of the cortical bone allograft was seen in only one case (Fig. 5). Collapse occurred 6 months postoperatively when the cortical bone allograft migrated into the vertebral body. The cortical endplates of the vertebrae had been cut in this case, and this was the reason for axial migration of the allograft. Once this migration had occurred, the iliac bone autograft was so weak that it collapsed. Fusion eventually occurred in this case and we judged it as collapsed union.

Delayed union was seen in three cases. In all three cases, partial absorption and sclerosis of the iliac autografts occurred without a decrease in height. The cortical bone allografts thus worked as stable interbody spacers with the aid of the VSP system, and fusion was seen 9–12 months after the operation. There were no cases of nonunion in this series. There were also no complications related to the allografts: no infection, no toxic or immune reaction, and no collapse or absorption of the allografts.

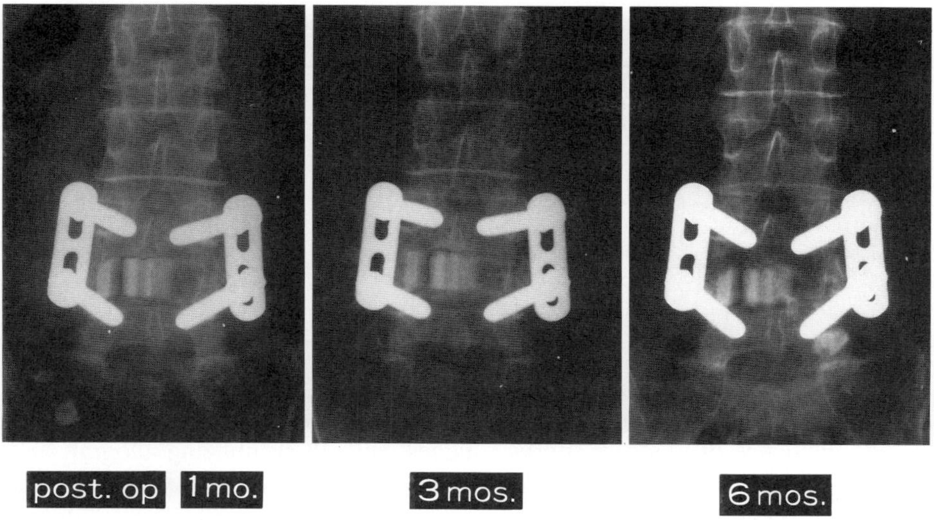

a b,c

Fig. 4a–c. A 68-year-old female with L4 degenerative spondylolisthesis. **a** After 1 month. **b** After 3 months, a clear zone was obvious around the allograft. **c** After 6 months, the clear zone around the allograft surrounded by marginal sclerosis was still evident. The iliac bone autograft eventually fused, and the classification was union in situ

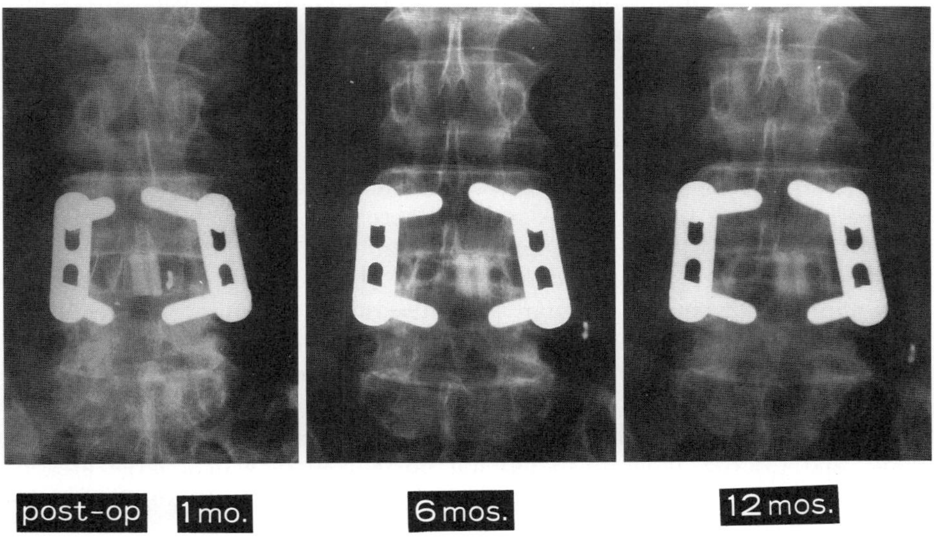

a b,c

Fig. 5a–c. A 63-year-old male with L4/5 prolapsed intervertebral disk. **a** After 1 month. **b** At 6 months postoperatively, collapse of the iliac bone autograft was seen and the cortical bone allograft had migrated into the vertebral body. Loss of intervertebral space height was evident on the anterioposterior X ray. Once such allograft migration has occurred, collapse of the autograft is inevitable. **c** After 12 months

Table 4. Correlation between different operation methods and roentogenological results.

Results \ Operation	PLIF	PLIF + R-C	PLIF + VSP (autograft)	PLIF + VSP (allograft)
Union in situ	255 (68.7%)	31 (70.5%)	74 (85.1%)	31 (88.6%)
Collapsed union	44 (11.8%)	7 (15.9%)	8 (9.2%)	1 (2.8%)
Delayed union	34 (9.2%)	2 (4.5%)	4 (4.6%)	3 (8.6%)
Collapsed nonunion	21 (5.7%)	4 (9.1%)	1 (1.1%)	
Nonunion	17 (4.6%)			
Total	371	44	87	35

Roentgenological results were compared for each operation method in Table 4. The incidence of union in situ was highest with PLIF utilizing allograft and the VSP system. The incidence of bone union problems decreased from 31.3% to 14.9% with application of the VSP system, and then to 11.4% with combined use of cortical bone allografts and iliac bone autografts. Nonunion was very rare when the VSP system was used for reinforcement, and most importantly the incidence of graft collapse was markedly reduced by using cortical bone allografts. Even though the incidence of delayed union increased in this series, the solid allografts prevented the collapse and absorption of the iliac autografts and so promoted bony union at the initial intervertebral height even after some delay.

Discussion

In the early 1940s, Cloward developed the technique of PLIF [8]. He used bone allografts for interbody fusion, and there have been many reports published on PLIF with bone allografts. In Japan, however, the use of cadaver bone is illegal and therefore the development of bone allografts has been very slow and did not become popular. Recently, one of the authors developed a new technique of preparing bone allograft and began using such graft for spinal fusion surgery [9]. The principles of the clinical application of bone allograft are as follows: (1) the allograft should be kept in contact with a wide area of the recipient bone, (2) the allograft should be fixed firmly to the recipient bone, and (3) the allograft should not be in contact with a large area of nonskeletal bone. Therefore, PLIF is the best method of utilizing bone allografts in spinal surgery.

The introduction of cortical bone allografts to PLIF has three advantages. Firstly, and this is the main reason for the introduction of the bone allografts, the cortical bone allograft acts as a solid intervertebral spacer and preserves the disk space height. Thus, it avoids collapse of the iliac bone autograft that has been inserted around the allograft. Iliac bone autografts go through a stage of

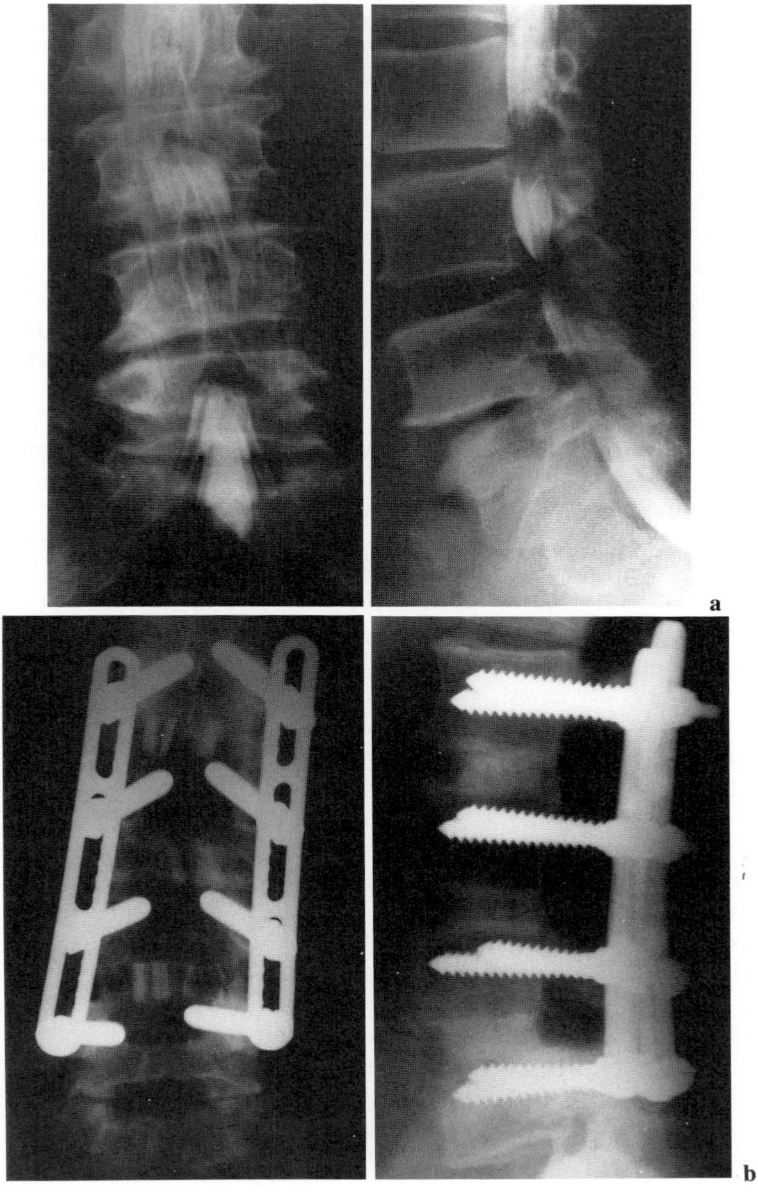

Fig. 6a,b. A 64-year-old male with multisegmental canal stenosis. **a** Myelogram showing multisegmental canal stenosis with slippage at L4/5. **b** PLIF was performed for three intervertebral segments with bone allografts and autografts, supported by the VSP system mechanical weakness due to the biological reactions occurring during their incorporation, and sometimes they collapse a few months postoperatively, especially in patients with osteoporosis. The solid and slowly reabsorbed cortical bone allograft can maintain the disk space height for at least a few years, while the autograft is incorporated and gains strength by new bone apposition. Thus, the cortical bone allograft provides a superior biomechanical stability when the VSP system is also applied. Preservation of the cortical endplates of the surrounding vertebral bodies is also important, since the cancellous bone of the vertebral body is not solid enough to prevent the axial migration of a hard cortical allograft. Once axial migration of the cortical allograft occurs, collapse of the autograft inevitably followes. We had only one case of autograft collapse after migration of the allograft (Fig. 5). Another three cases with delayed union showed partial absorption and sclerosis in the center of the bone autograft. Unless a solid cortical bone allograft had been applied to support the intervertebral space, these patients would also have suffered graft collapse. Their bones eventually fused after several months, and the cortical bone allografts thus promoted bony union even in complicated cases.

A second advantage of application of bone allografts is prevention of postoperative discomfort at the donor site. We usually take four pieces of bicortical iliac bone autograft from the posterior iliac spine, and dissection of the cruneal nerves is necessary. Some patients subsequently complain of disabling discomfort at the donor site, even though the initial pain in the back and lower limbs has been completely cured. When bone allografts are used, we only have to take two pieces of autograft and do not have to dissect the cruneal nerves. It also reduces the operating time.

Thirdly, bone allografts can provide sufficient bone stock when multisegmental fusion is indicated. We have used the PLIF method for multisegmental lumbar fusion surgery (Fig. 6), although only in a few cases. The iliac bone autograft stock available for PLIF is limited, so the introduction of the allografts is very beneficial in such cases.

Fusion results of PLIF with cortical bone allograft was compared with other methods of PLIF (Table 4), and the clinical utility of cortical bone allografts was demonstrated. Application of the bone allografts increased the incidence of sound bony union. Graft collapse significantly decreased because the cortical bone allografts acted as a solid intervertebral spacer. The combination of the VSP system and such a solid interbody spacer provides superior biomechanical stability, better fusion, and better clinical results.

References

1. Cautilli RA (1982) Theoretical superiority of PLIF. In: Lin PM (ed) Posterior lumbar interbody fusion. Charles C Thomas, Springfield, pp 82–93
2. Cloward RB (1982) Modification of PLIF for spinal stenosis. In: Lin PM (ed) Posterior lumbar interbody fusion. Charles C Thomas, Springfield, pp 219–226
3. Lin PM (1980) Posterior lumbar interbody fusion. Clin Orthop 180:154–168

4. Yamamoto T, Ohta N, Ohwada T (1989) Posterior lumbar interbody fusion for degenerative spondylolisthesis. In: Ramani PS (ed) Posterior lumbar interbody fusion. Kisher Aras, Bombay, pp 177–186
5. Roy-Camille R, Saillant G, Mazel C (1986) Internal fixation of the lumbar spine with pedicle screw plating. Clin Orthop 203:7–17
6. Steffee AD, Sitkowski DJ (1988) Posterior lumbar interbody fusion and plates. Clin Orthop 227:99–102
7. Steffee AD (1988) Segmental fixation of the spine with VSP plates and screws. In: Cawthen JC (ed) Lumbar spine surgery, 2nd edn. Williams and Wilkins, Baltimore, pp 379–397
8. Cloward RB (1953) The treatment of ruptured lumbar intervertebral disc by vertebral body fusion. J Neurosurg 10:154–168
9. Kakiuchi M, Ono K (1989) Chloroform-methanol-treated, ethylene-oxide-gas-sterilized bone allografts as bank bone. In: Ramani PS (ed) Posterior lumbar interbody fusion. Kisher Aras, Bombay, pp 132–141
10. Inoue S, Matsui N (1975) Anterior lumbar interbody fusion for lumbar disc herniation (in Japanese). Saigai Igaku 18:76–89

3.6 Effects of Ceramic Interspinous Block on Anterior Lumbar Interbody Fusion

Haruo Tsuji, Norikazu Hirano, Hisao Matsui, Hiroshi Ohshima, Hirokazu Ishihara, and Yoshiharu Katoh[1]

Introduction

Anterior interbody fusion (AIF) for degenerative lumbar disk and/or infectious diseases promises the most stable long-term performance for patients. However, this type of surgery necessitates long periods of rest and abstention from work to obtain a sound bony union, and the union failure rate is relatively high. Results of lumbar AIF using autogenous bone grafts have been reported by many authors, but the fusion rate varied from 56% to 94% [1–9].

The possible causes of nonunion may be related to bone graft technique and variation of the postoperative care system. Nonunion may also be due to biomechanical faults attributable to anterior longitudinal ligament insufficiency, which results in backward displacement of the instantaneous axis of rotation [10,11], following increase in lumbar lordosis after postoperative ambulation.

The present article describes the efficacy of ceramic interspinous block (CISB) for AIF of the lumbar spine based on the results of 153 consecutive cases.

Patients and Methods

Between February 1984 and June 1991, we performed extraperitoneal lumbar AIF combined with CISB implementation on 153 patients with disk herniation/symptomatic disk degeneration (95 cases), spondylolisthesis (45 cases), iatrogenic diskitis (6 cases), and CISB implementation for anterior union failure (7 cases). In addition, 67 patients received anterior fusion with no use of CISB (CISB-unassisted) between 1981 and 1983. Thereafter, CISB-assisted anterior fusion was employed. The patients consisted of 115 males and 38 females, and the average age was 41 ± 12 years, ranging from 14 to 66 years. In terms of

[1] Department of Orthopaedic Surgery, Faculty of Medicine, Toyama Medical and Pharmaceutical University, Toyama, 930-01 Japan

the patients' occupation, there were 28 sedentary workers or housewives, 54 moderate manual workers, 66 heavy manual workers, and 8 patients with no difinite job. Follow-up averaged 3 years and 1 month, ranging from 4 months to 7 years.

In contrast, the 67 patients with CISB-unassisted anterior fusion included 50 men and 17 women, and the average age was 43 years. Of these, 14 cases (21%) resulted in nonunion. Thus the remaining 53 patients were used in the comparison as a control.

Follow-up was performed by serial interviews and radiologic examination, and the results were evaluated using our 100-point full scale evaluation system for low back pain syndrome [12].

The types of CISB-assisted surgery used for the 153 patients consisted of 121 cases of anterior fusion and CISB implementation, 13 anterior fusion with CISB and extraperitoneal antero-lateral diskectomy [13,14] at another level, 7 anterior/posterior combined surgery with CISB, 7 cases of salvage by CISB implementation alone for interbody fusion failure, and 5 cases of H-graft with CISB.

Design of the Interspinous Block

In most patients, a side-wall type of interspinous block made from alumina ceramic (Kyocera Co., Kyoto) was used, but recently this has been changed to blocks made from high-density polyethylene (HDP) which is more elastic than alumina ceramics (Fig. 1 inset). The following four heights were used in both series: 11 mm, 13 mm, 15 mm, and 18 mm.

Concept of Interspinous Blocking in AIF

AIF impairs the mechanical integrity of the anterior supportive structure, such as by causing anterior longitudinal ligament and anterior/anterolateral annulus fibrosus, and this results in an acceleration of spinal instability after surgery. One concept for spinal stabilization is use of a tripod system [15] (Fig. 1), but breakdown of the anterior supportive structure following anterior total diskectomy impairs the tripod support system. When lumbar lordosis increases or the spine extends backwards in CISB-unassisted fusion, a distraction force is produced at the anterior part of the vertebral body (Fig. 2, left inset). In contrast, in CISB-assisted fusion with an extended spine position, the compression force is distributed evenly on the graft-vertebra interface (Fig. 2, right inset). The mechanical drawback of AIF has prompted the idea of anterior fusion combined with a Harrington or transpedicular screw-plate system [16–18].

Thus, the interspinous block, as a rule, should be implemented at the same functional spinal unit in which interbody fusion was performed (Fig. 2A,B). If

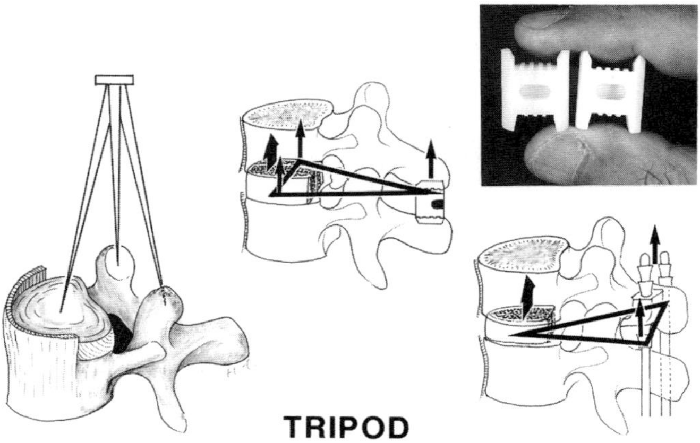

Fig. 1. Schematic drawing of the tripod support system and the concept of reconstruction of the system in anterior interbody fusion. *Inset,* samples of CISB (*right*) and HDP-SB (*left*)

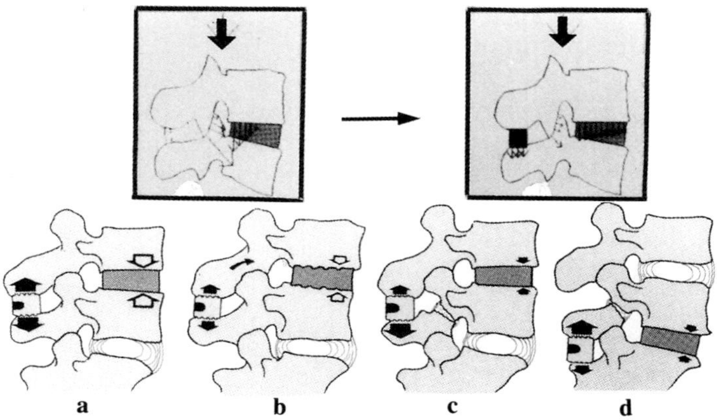

Fig. 2. Equalization of compression stress on the graft-vertebral interfaces for fusion in deranged disk (**a** and **b**), and in deranged disk with spondylolysis (**c** and **d**). Computer simulations in slightly extended position with (*right inset*) and without (*left inset*) ceramic interspinous block (CISB) are shown

Table 1. Results of 153 patients.

Score range		Number	Percent
Excellent	(100-90)	123	81.5
Good	(89-80)	25	16.7
Fair	(79-60)	2	1.3
Poor	(59-)	1	0.6

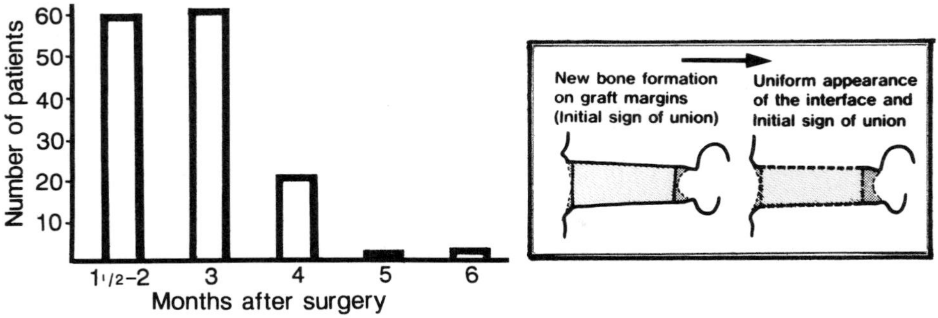

Fig. 3 Incidence of radiological manifestation of initial sign of bone union by time. Criteria is shown in the inset

spondylolysis or spondylolisthesis coexists with disk lesion in adjacent vertebra, CISB can also provide stability for the loose lamina. (Fig. 2C,D).

Aftercare

A standard aftercare protocol for CISB-assisted anterior fusion is as follows: walking with soft lumbar support or short body cast at 2 weeks, hospital discharge at 3 weeks, sedentary work with brace at 5 weeks, and moderate/heavy manual work and sports activity at 12 and 16 weeks after surgery, respectively. The postoperative time for cast application is 5 weeks on average.

Results

All clinical results were satisfactory except for three cases with fair and poor results (Table 1). Average symptom scores on the 100-point full scale were 52.0 ± 13.7 points before surgery and 95.7 ± 5.1 points after surgery. The recovery ratio was 90.8 ± 11.1%.

Initial signs of radiological bone union, evaluated using criteria shown in Fig. 3 (inset), had appeared in most cases by 4 months after surgery, and complete bony union was achieved by 8 months on average (Table 2). Union failure judged at 6–8 months after surgery was seen in three spondylolisthesis cases (2.0%). Thus the union rate in the present study was 100% for disk lesions (Fig. 4) and 93% for spondylolisthesis. The results of CISB-assisted AIF showed statistically significant differences as compared to those of CISB-unassisted fusion (Table 2). In seven cases of CISB implementation for salvaging anterior union failure, bony union was achieved within 6 months.

Complications were encountered in eight cases (4.5%): there were three cases of CISB dislocation, treated by replacement with the prototype CISB (cylindrical shape without side-wall); three cases of thrombophlebitis; one case

Table 2. Comparison of postoperative time of bone union.

	CISB-assisted (n = 148)[a]	CISB-unassisted (n = 53)
Initial sign of bone union (months)	2.6	4.6
Complete union (months)	8.0	15.0
Union failure rate (%)	2.0	21.0

[a] Excludes 5 cases that underwent H-graft and CISB

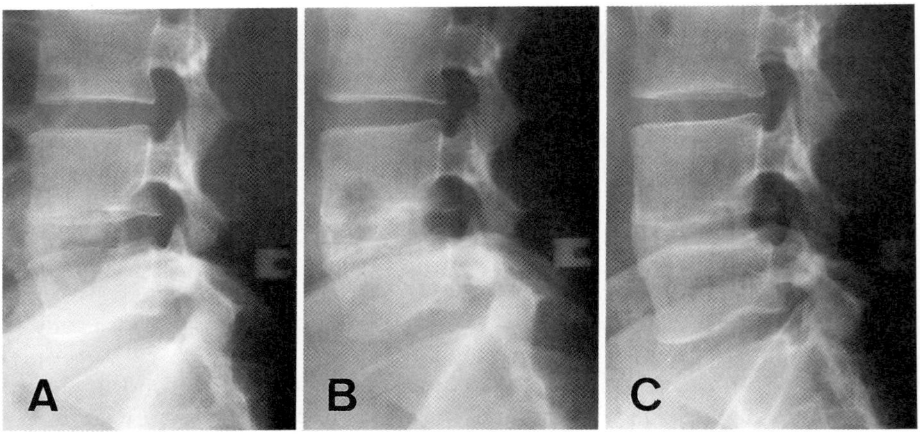

Fig. 4 A case showing the radiological course of bone union 10 days (**A**), 3 months (**B**), and 6 months after surgery (**C**)

of transient leg palsy in a patient with severe spondylolisthesis at L4 accompanied by a large posterior spur; and one case of nerve root irritation due to excessive rotation of the lysis lamina following CISB implementation.

Discussion

A major drawback of lumbar AIF fusion is the high possibility of nonunion. Accordingly, internal fixation has recently been used [16–18], but we think that huge instrumentation is rather non-physiological and too aggressive for elderly patients.

The biomechanical breakdown of the anterior supportive structure produced by the anterior approach and computer simulation of the CISB-unassisted fusion model suggest that pressurization of the graft-vertebra interface is impossible to maintain when the patient stands and walks, and therefore the bone union may fail. In 1990, we further improved the diskectomy bone graft

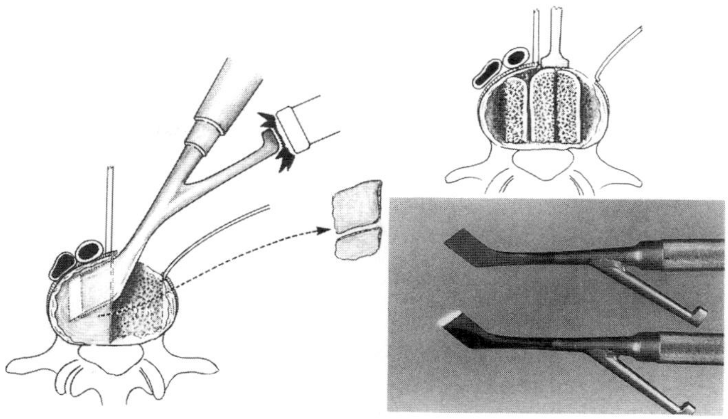

Fig. 5 Schemes of improved anterior diskectomy/cartilagenous plate removal and bone grafting for preservation of anterior ligamentous function. *Inset*, flag chisels

technique to preserve the anterior longitudinal ligament function as much as possible; through very limited exposure of the anterior disk, complete removal of the disk and cartilagenous plate is performed using a specially designed flag chisel [19] (Fig. 5).

Conclusion

The interspinous block in AIF provides immediate reinforcement of spinal stability and early body union and early ambulation of the patient due to mechanical reconstruction of a tripod support system of the lumbar spine.

References

1. Chow SP, Leong JCY, Yau ACB (1980) Anterior spinal fusion for deranged lumbar intervertebral disk. Spine 5:452–458
2. Flynn JC, Hoque A (1979) Anterior fusion of the lumbar spine, end result study with long-term follow-up. J Bone Joint Surg [AM] 61:1143–1150
3. Freebody R, Bendall R, Taylor RD (1971) Anterior transperitoneal lumbar fusion. J Bone Joint Surg [Br] 53:617–627
4. Harmon PH (1963) Anterior excision and vertebral body fusion operation for intervertebral disk syndromes of the lower lumbar spine. Three to five-year results in 244 cases. Clin Orthop 26:107–127
5. Hodgson AR, Wong SK (1986) A description of a technic and evaluation of results in anterior spinal fusion for deranged intervertebral disk and spondylolisthesis. Clin Orthop 56:133–162
6. Hoover NW (1968) Methods of lumbar fusion. J Bone Joint Surg [Am] 50:194–210
7. Inoue SI, Watanabe T, Hirose A, Tanaka T, Matsui N, Saegusa O, Sho E (1984) Anterior diskectomy and interbody fusion for lumbar disk herniation. A review of 350 cases. Clin Orthop 183:22–31

8. Inoue SI, Watanabe T, Goto S, Takahashi K, Takata K, Sho E (1988) Degenerative spondylolisthesis. Pathology and results of anterior interbody fusion. Clin Orthop 227:90–98
9. Stauffer RN, Coventry MB (1972) Anterior interbody lumbar spine fusion. Analysis of Mayo clinic series. J Bone Joint surg [Am] 54:756–768
10. White AA, Panjabi MM (1987) Clinical biomechanics of the lumbar spine. Lippincott, Philadelphia
11. Yoshioka T, Tsuji H, Hirano N, Sainoh S (1990) Motion characteristic of the normal lumbar spine in young adults: Instantaneous axis of rotation and vertebral center motion analysis. J Spin Dis 3:103–113
12. Tsuji H, Hirano N, Katoh Y, Ohshima H, Ishihara H, Matsui H, Hayashi Y (1990) Ceramic interspinous block (CISB) assisted anterior interbody fusion. J Spin Dis 3:77–86
13. Tsuji H (1984) Extraperitoneal anterolateral diskectomy (EPALD) for herniated nucleus pulposus of the lumbar spine (in Japanese). Orthop Surg 35:795–803
14. Tsuji H (1991) Comprehensive atlas of lumbar spine surgery. Mosby, St Louis
15. Evans JH (1985) Biomechanics of lumbar fusion. Clin Orthop 193:38–46
16. Kostuik JP, Errico TJ, Gleason TF (1986) Techniques of the internal fixation for degenerative conditions of the lumbar spine. Clin Orthop 203:219–231
17. O'Brien JP, Dawson MHD, Heard CW, Momberger G, Speck G, Weatherly CR (1986) Simultaneous combined anterior and posterior fusion. A surgical solution for failed spinal surgery with a brief review of the first 150 patients. Clin Orthop 203:191–195
18. Ryan MD, Taylor TKF, Sherwood AA (1986) Bolt-plate fixation for anterior spinal fusion. Clin Orthop 203:196–202
19. Tsuji H (1991) Fundamental technique and principles in lumbar spine surgery. Nankodo, Tokyo

3.7 Boucher Screw Fixation of the Spine: A Translaminar Pedicle Screw Technique

C. Edmund Graham[1]

Introduction

In the 1940s the celebrated Canadian spinal surgeon Boucher [1] conceived the notion of the translaminar pedicle screw to immobilize lumbar spinal segments, thus promoting a higher rate of spinal fusion and permitting earlier unrestrained postoperative patient mobilization (Fig. 1). In this way, rigid immobilization was obtained for the 10 weeks required for graft taking. In 1948, King [2] described a method of internal fixation of the facet joints using short screws placed almost transversely across the lateral articulations. However, a year later, Thompson and Ralston [3] reported a high incidence of failure using the short screw technique. Bosworth [4] was of the opinion that the presence of screws would produce a psychologically damaging effect. Considering the amount of metal placed in patients nowadays the psychological effect has proved to be of no consequence. In 1951, Barr [5] felt that the incidence of failure with spinal fusion was too high, and in 1952, Watson-Jones [6] felt that the screw fixation would be temporary because the screws would loosen. In fact the screws rarely loosen and if they do, as indicated by the presence of a rarefaction zone, then the graft has probably failed to take. In 1953, Young [7] postulated that if there was a fusing operation available that offered a higher prospect of union with a shorter period of hospitalization, a larger proportion of patients would opt for surgery. In 1953, Scott [8]. In an editorial, stressed the need for a spinal fusion technique that would reduce postoperative hospital stay. In 1954, Boucher [1] read a paper at the annual meeting of the Canadian Orthopaedic Association in which he described the use of longer screws, passing from the lamina down the pedicle into the body below, as a more rigid form of internal fixation for spinal fusion. In 1959, he presented a full report in the Journal of Bone and Joint Surgery and this is the method described herein. Boucher reported no known failures in 130 cases.

[1] Prince of Wales Hospital, Randwick, 253 Oxford Street, Bondi Junction, Sydney, NSW 2022, Australia

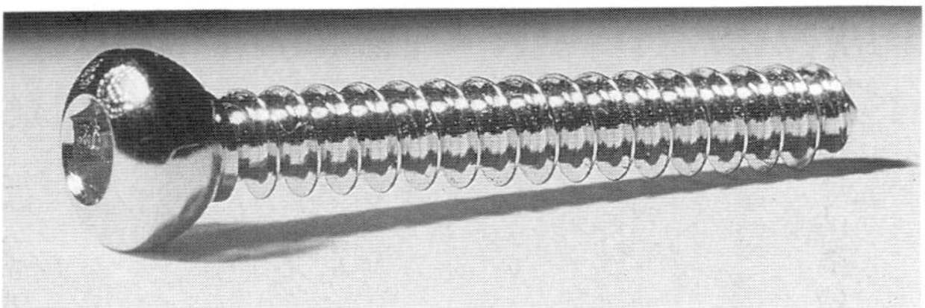

Fig. 1. The AO screw is used in translamina intrapedicular screw fixation. The usual length, 30 or 36 mm, can be calculated from radiographs thus avoiding the use of a depth gauge

Indications

Spinal fusion is recommended for patients whose relentless low back pain has failed to respond to an adequate period of conservative treatment and in whom there is objective evidence of diskogenic or facetal pain. Fusion is indicated for patients with protracted low back pain or intermittent episodes of disabling discomfort associated with tenderness at the appropriate level together with diskographic evidence of disruption at that same area. The diskogram is of considerable importance: obtaining precise pain reproduction at the time of diskography predisposes a good result. Abnormalities of volume, pressure, and disk anatomy at the time of diskography together with precise pain reproduction are of inestimable value in patient selection.

When making the final decision on surgery one must consider the patient's age, sex, temperament, physique, occupation, and habits. The best results are obtained in young or middle-aged patients who are seeking surgery. Their inability to take part in sport, sleep comfortably, drive a car, or sit or stand for any period of time constitutes a permanent distraction and they are eager for relief. CT scanning and myelography are useful aids to diagnosis and of late MRI has proven to be the most effective non-invasive investigative technique for disk pathology. However, there is no substitute for the pain reproduction ability of the diskogram.

Contraindications

Many patients with low back pain have a compensation claim of one sort or another and since they have a vested interest in not recovering from surgery, their results are not as satisfactory as with non-litigious patients. Psychologically disturbed patients, heavy drinkers and smokers, and obese patients, or those who suffer from osteoporosis or generalized spondylosis are also not ideal candidates for spinal fusion. In addition, back patients that have undergone multiple back operations fare poorly.

Surgical Technique

The patient is prone on an adjustable pelvic rest that enables free abdominal movements (Fig. 2). The hips and knees are flexed approximately to 90°, the back is horizontal, and the bony prominences are well padded. Positive anesthesia reduces extradural venous pressure and so lessens operative bleeding. Blood loss may be constrained by the preoperative intramural and subcutaneous injection of a vasopressin such as ornipressin (Sandoz, Sydney,

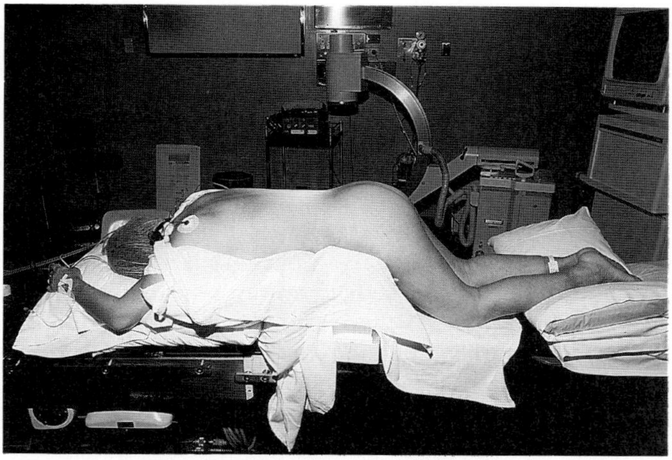

2

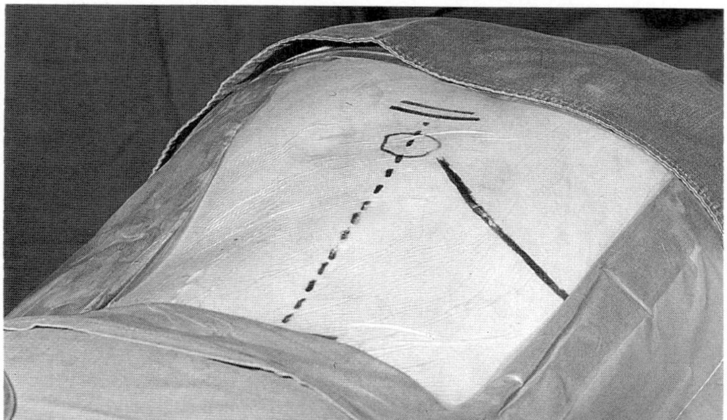

3

Fig. 2. Patient prone over the pelvic rest with hips and knees semi-flexed. Some surgeons prefer complete flexion of the hips and knees

Fig. 3. Midline incision. The *dotted lines* indicate the line of incision, the *circle*, the tender area, and the *oblique line* to the right indicates the position of the iliac crest incision. Sometimes the iliac graft may be taken through the midline incision

Australia). This vasoconstrictor is injected into the region of the midline incision. Blood transfusion is usually not necessary if attention is paid to hemostasis.

Through a midline incision (Fig. 3), soft tissue is removed from the dorsum of the upper sacrum and lower lumbar spine and laminae. The stripping process is facilitated by the use of an osteotome and gauze sponges. Interlamina lumbosacral diskectomy may be performed, if indicated, at this stage. Excision of the fatty tissue immediately lateral to the ligamentum flavum exposes a bowl-like cavity, bounded superiorly by the lamina of the 5th lumbar vertebrum, laterally by the sacral pedicle, and inferiorly by the first sacral lamina which also forms the floor of the cavity, The medial boundary is the ligamentum flavum. Tight packing of this decorticated bowl with cancellous bone graft adds strength to the fusion.

Screw Insertion

A 3.2-mm drill is powered down from the lamina into the pedicle below, being aligned with the posterior inferior angle of the third lumbar spinous process in most cases (Fig. 4). The precise screw direction is readily ascertained by drawing lines on the preoperative radiographs: a line is projected dorsally and superiorly from the centre of the pedicle upwards to the spinous process and that part of the spinous process is then used for the starting point of the drill. Drilling is performed in this direction on each side medial to the lateral articulation in an anterior, inferior, and lateral direction (Fig. 5). The drill

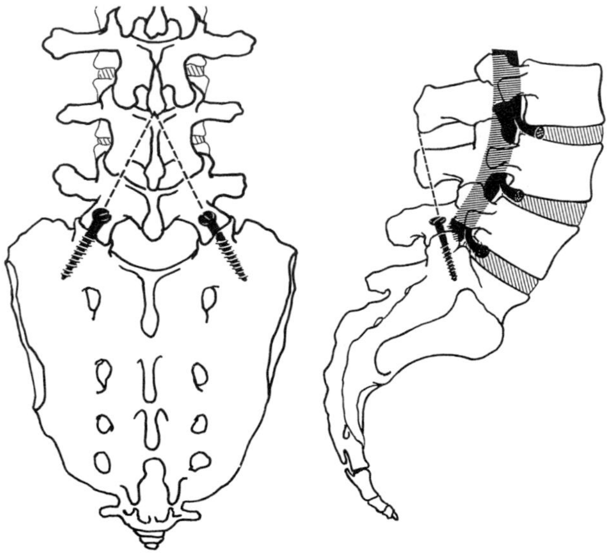

Fig. 4. Screw direction in anteroposterior and lateral views. The screws are aligned with the posterior, inferior angle of the third lumbar spinous process in both planes. For higher levels such as an L4–L5 fusion, optimum screw position is obtained by delineating the desired direction on the preoperative radiographs

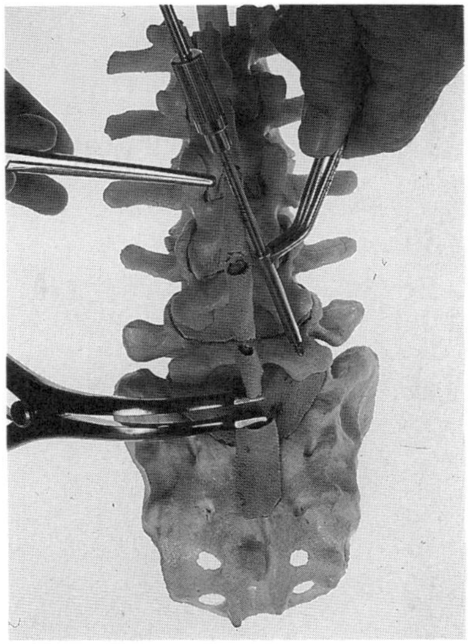

Fig. 5. An anteroposterior view indicating the lamina spreader between the fifth lumbar and first sacral spinous processes and a hole being drilled from the fifth lumbar lamina into the ALA of the sacrum, the drill being held in the correct position with a drill shield. The third lumbar spinous process is indicated by the forceps top left

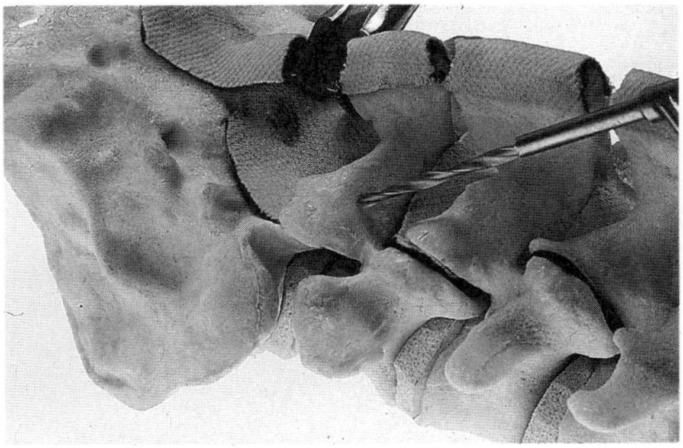

Fig. 6. Lateral view showing the drill about to penetrate the lamina and pass safely int the ALA of the sacrum

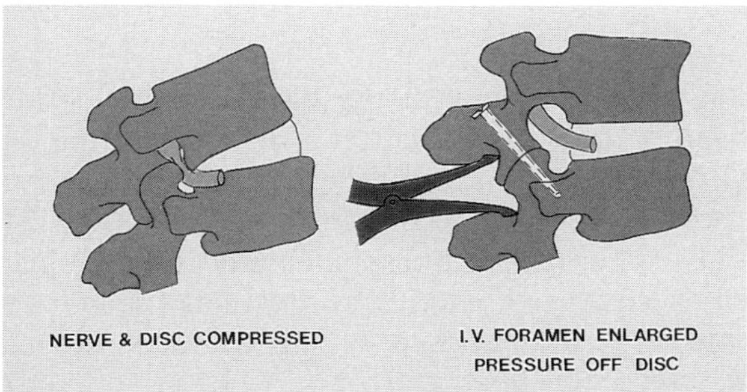

Fig. 7. The effect of the lamina spreader on the disk and nerve root. The intervertebral foramen is enlarged and held open with the aid of the lamina spreader before the screws are inserted, thus taking pressure off the nerve root and off the posterior painful part of the annulus

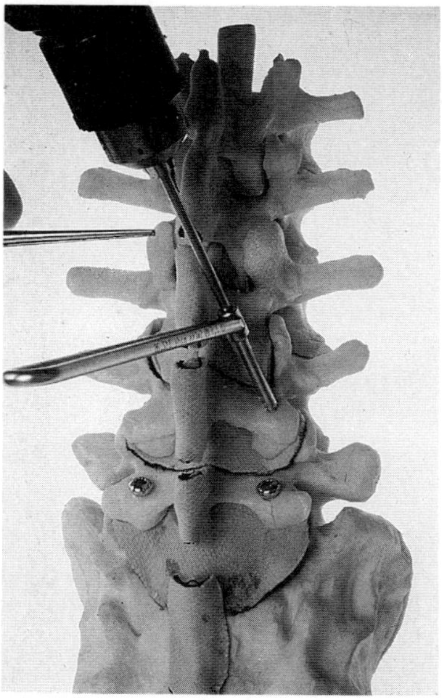

Fig. 8. Anteroposterior view showing two screw at the lumbosacral level and the drill about to penetrate the fourth lumbar lamina

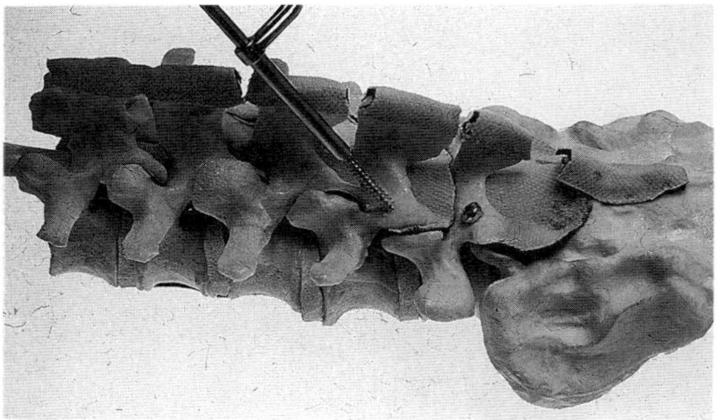

Fig. 9. Lateral view showing the drill aligned correctly with pedicle and with the superior posterior angle of the third lumbar spinous process

passes lateral to the sacral canal at the base of the superior process of the sacrum and traverses the posterior/anterior diameter of the anterior lip of the acetabulum (ALA) (Fig. 6). Note that the laminar spreader is used to separate the spinous processes at the time of screw insertion (Fig. 7) and this has a twofold effect: (1) by separating the spinous processes the load on the painful part of the annulus is reduced, and (2) by enlarging the intervertebral foramen more room is made for the nerve root. This distraction is maintained by the presence of the screws and bone graft. For a fusion between the 4th and 5th lumbar levels (Fig. 8), the screws pass from the lamina into the pedicle and body of the 5th lumbar vertebrae. In most cases the screws are aligned with the inferior posterior angle of the 3rd lumbar spinous process (Fig. 9).

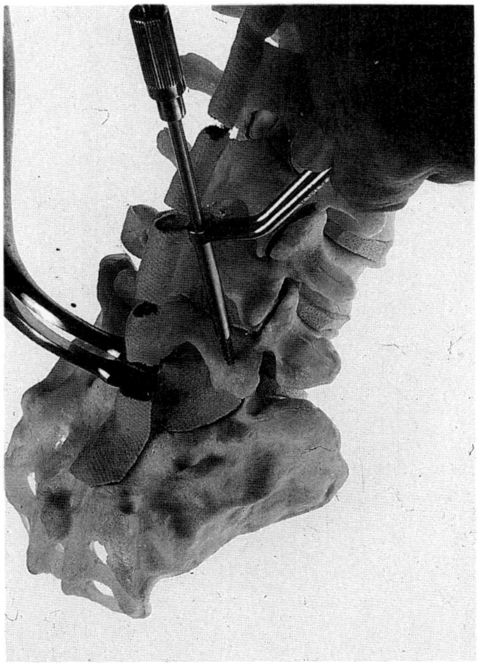

10

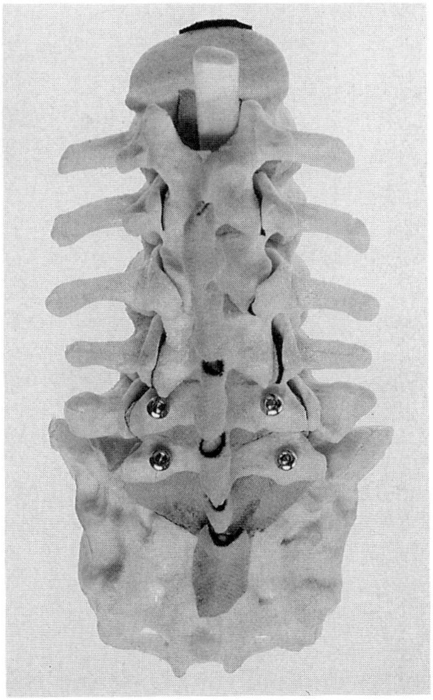

11

Fig. 10. The drill hole is tapped with the lamina spreader in situ

Fig. 11. Anteroposterior view showing all four screws in position

Tapping of Holes

The drilled holes are then tapped (Fig. 10). With the lamina spreader still in situ, a 30- or 36-mm AO screw is driven from the lamina down the pedicle into the ALA of the sacrum or the body of the 5th lumbar vertebra depending on the level being fused (Fig. 11). The degree of rigidity of the two levels can be assessed by endeavouring to separate the spinous processes with the aid of Kocher's forceps (Fig. 12). whereas before screw insertion there is a centimeter or so of movement, after even one screw has been inserted there is no detectable movement if the screw has been correctly placed. It is better to accept the imperfectly placed screw than to attempt to drill a second hole. Radiographic control is not necessary if the screws have been aligned in the method described above. Once the first screw has been correctly inserted using the alignment of the 3rd lumbar spinous process, the second screw is placed in a similar fashion at the lumbosacral level or if need be in a similar way at a higher level.

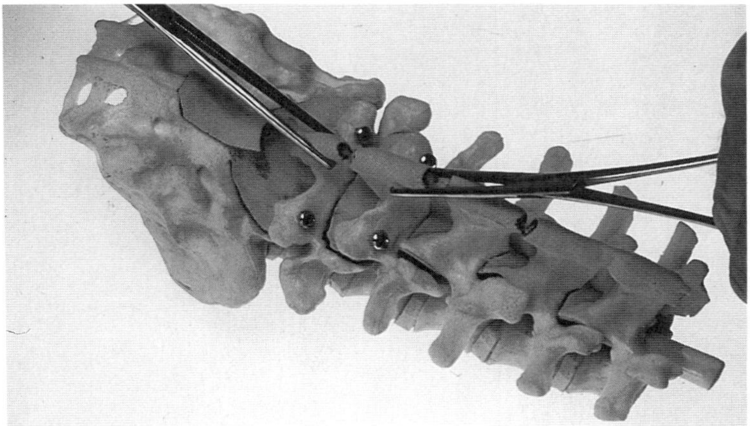

Fig. 12. Attempted separation of the spinous processes between the fourth lumbar and fifth lumbar vertebrae. With correctly placed screws no movement is possible

Preparation of the Graft and Bed

Through the main vertical incision it is possible to remove an iliac bone graft in such a way that the crest of the ilium is left intact. Cancellous bone with one cortical layer is obtained from the posterior superior spine of the ilium closest to the surgeon. It is readily obtained by subcutaneous reflection of the original midline incision. The overlying deeper fascia is incised and the roof of the iliac crest is elevated by a broad razor-sharp osteotome. Spongy bone is removed with a large curette and rectangles of bone are excised, sparing the inner plate of the ilium and thus avoiding entry into the retroperitoneal space with the attendant risk of bleeding that may cause paralytic ileus. The rectangle of bone is thoroughly cleaned, fashioned into an H-shape, and firmly slotted into the gap between the decorticated spinous processes for a posterior spinal fusion (Fig. 13). Alternatively, rectangles or squares of bone may be used for an interbody fusion (Fig. 14) or for intertransverse fusions (Fig. 15). Occasionally, when the spinous processes are large and the gap between them is small, the spinous process from the 3rd lumbar vertebra may be excised and fashioned into an H-shaped graft to be slotted between the spinous processes between the 5th lumbar vertebra and the 1st sacral vertebra (Fig. 16). In this way the iliac crest is spared. Very occasionally in patients who refuse transfusion, cement may be used to stabilize a spine in conjunction with the screws and Kirschner wires as indicated (Figs. 17, 18). This avoids the blood loss associated with removal of donor iliac bone. Cement fusion gives great rigidity, but it is not always of a permanent nature. It is felt that this procedure provides reduced movement at the painful disk area rather than permanent immobilization.

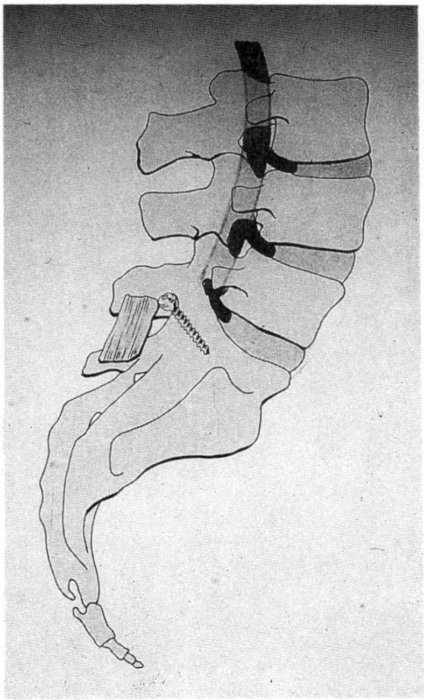

13

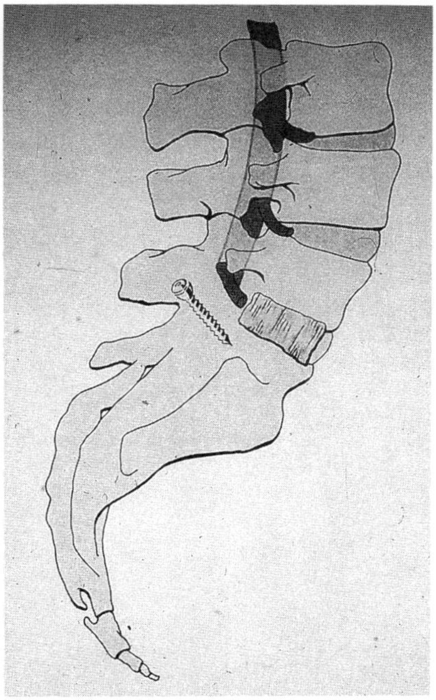

14

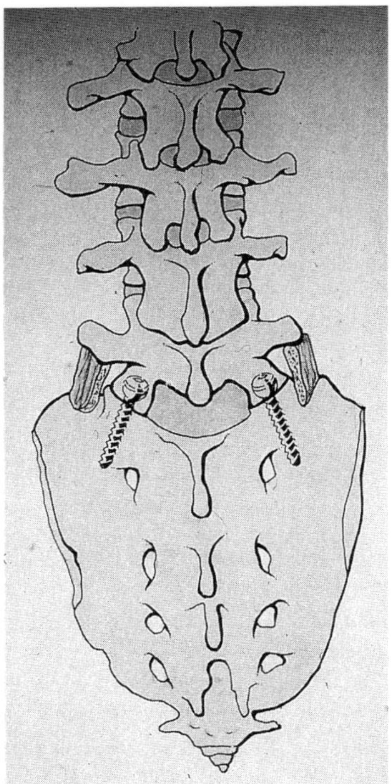

15

Fig. 13. Posterior spinal fusion at the fifth lumbar and first sacral level with the screws in position

Fig. 14. Interbody fusion with the screws in position

Fig. 15. Intertransverse fusion with the screws in position

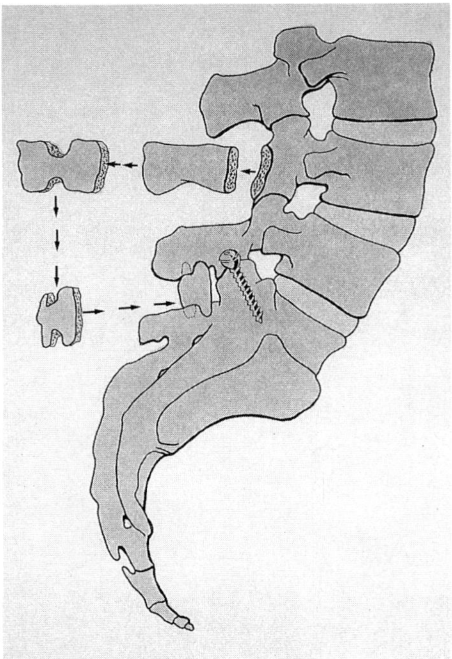

16

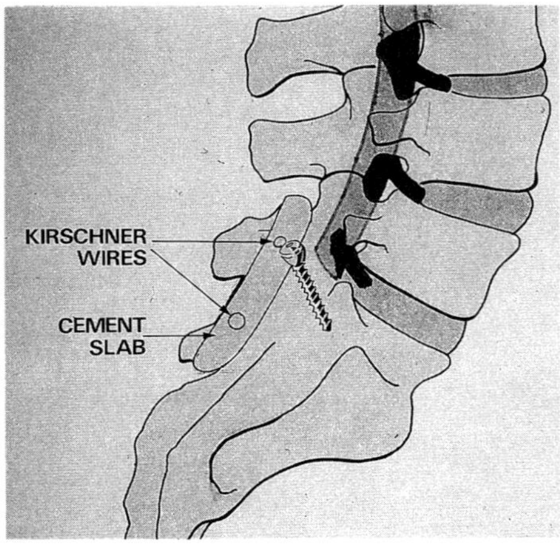

18

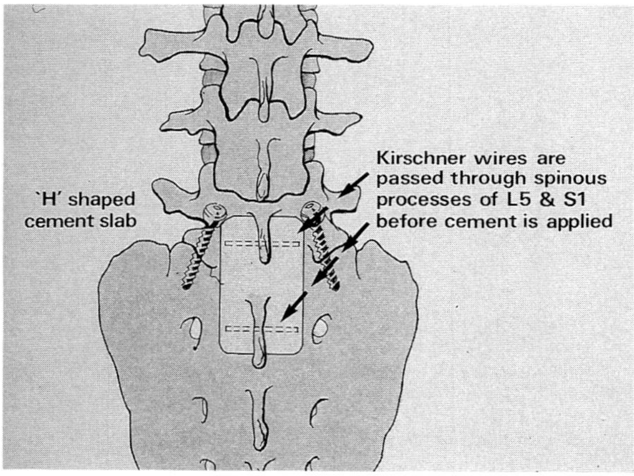

17

Fig. 16. Spinous process fusion. The spine of the third lumbar vertebrae has been removed, fashioned into an H-shape and slotted between the narrow gap between the fifth lumbar and the first sacral spinous processes

Fig. 17. Anterioposterior view of cement fusion. Screws and Kirschner wires running through the spinous processes reinforce the cement that is applied in a putty form

Fig. 18. Lateral view of cement fusion with screws in position and Kirschner wires reinforcing the cement

Before applying the H-shaped graft or intertransverse graft, razor-sharp osteotomes are used to remove all soft tissue from the spinous processes and laminae. Periosteum is cleaned away from the bones and from the dorsal aspect of the sacrum. Spongy bone is packed into the area of the bowl-like cavity after cortical bone has been elevated using a narrow osteotome. Spongy bone is placed over the decorticated laminae and the back of the sacrum as far as the facet joints which are not disrupted. When the harvesting has been completed the "LID" of the iliac crest is replaced, making a snug fit. Vacuum drainage is instituted before closure, one for the donor site and another for the main midline incision.

Postoperative Management

The patient is encouraged to move about actively in bed and is mobilized 24–48 h postoperatively. The patient is nursed in an ordinary bed without a fracture board and analgesics are given for the first 24 h. The drains are removed 24 h postoperatively. Occasionally night sedation is necessary. No external support of any kind is worn for lumbosacral fusions and it is seldom necessary for double level fusions. Activity is restricted to walking for 12–16 weeks and the patient refrains from bending or lifting and is taught to flex the knees and hips rather than to bend forward. Anteroposterior and lateral bending radiographs are taken about 4 months after operation to assess the degree of fusion. Measurements are made between the tips of the transverse processes or the spinous processes to see if movement has indeed been completely eradicated at the appropriate level. A more accurate way of assessing fusion is to use the CT scan. In this way the presence of a gap between the bone graft and the host is readily seen if fusion has failed.

Fusion at Higher Levels

The same technique has been used at higher levels in the lumbar spine and above the lumbosacral level. A screw is placed so as to pass from the lamina of the vertebrae above into the body of the vertebrae below in much the same way as described above. The drill points placed well laterally will bypass the vertebral canal and enter the upper part of the body of the vertebrae below, if directed forward and inferiorly and laterally. If there is any doubt regarding drill direction one may use guidewires and biplanar fluoroscopy to aid direction finding.

Spondylolisthesis

In patients with spondylolisthesis, the body of the 4th lumbar vertebra is attached to the body of the 5th by translamina pedicle screws. If the loose posterior element is not removed it is fixed to the sacrum by screws. With a two-level fusion in a spondylolisthetic it is imperative that the pars interarticularis defect be thoroughly decorticated and bone grafted, applying chips not only to the defect but also to the transverse processes and over the backs of the laminae and spinous processes.

Complications

Nerve Root Irritation

Minor nerve root irritation has been observed in a small percentage of patients. There has never been a complete loss of motor or sensory function in any one nerve root. Postoperative sciatica may be due to a poorly placed screw and is detectable on plain radiography or myelography. If the screw is seen to be occupying the superior part of the intervertebral foramen instead of being in the pedicle, then it could well be irritating the nerve root. The commonest error is to have the screw passing vertically or in an inward direction rather than being laterally angled. It seems that there is sufficient margin for error to allow elimination of this complication using greater care.

Infection

The risk of infection is always present but with modern techniques using laminar flow theatres and personalized exhaust systems, and double gloving, infection is reduced to less than 1%. Vacuum pressure drainage of the wound for 24 h also reduces the incidence of infection. Recent animal research indicates that one large dose of intravenous broad spectrum antibiotic administered 15 min preoperatively gives excellent protection against infection.

Screw Fracture

Since the use of AO screws, a fracture has not occurred. Before their advent, screw fracture occasionally occurred due to abnormal strain in the early postoperative days. It did not necessarily preclude a sound fusion from developing. screw removal for fracture is difficult and rarely indicated.

Deep Venous Thrombosis and Embolus Formation

Subcutaneous administration of heparin for 5 days commencing with a premedication dose has reduced the incidence of deep venous thrombosis to a great extent. In addition, an aspirin a day for 5 days may be given. Subcutaneous administration of an ergot derivative is said to further reduce the incident of deep venous thrombosis, as is intermittent pneumatic calf compression. By applying a compression force using a pneumatic device alternatively to each calf the likelihood of clot formation during the operative procedure is considerably reduced.

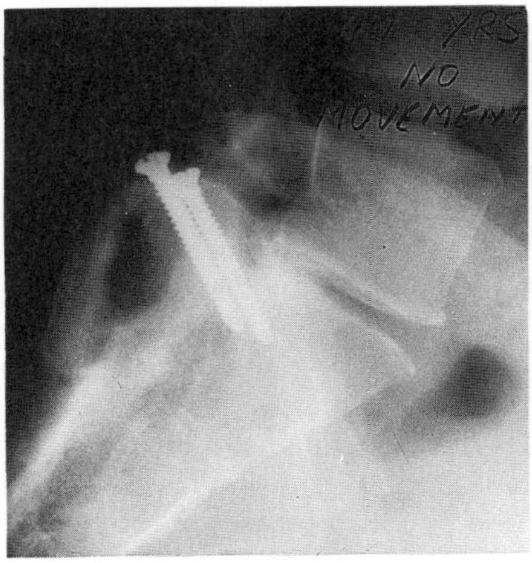

19

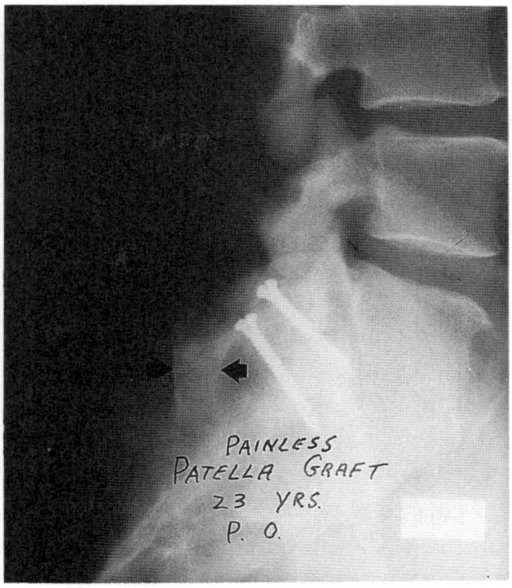

20

Fig. 19. Lateral view of a 17-year-old one-level fusion. The patient is without pain and functional radiographs demonstrate that the fusion is complete

Fig. 20. Lateral view of a one-level fusion. That graft that is located between the *arrows* was derived from a bone bank patella. At 23 years post operation, the clinical and radiological results were excellent

Results

Since 1961, I have performed 2,000 lumbar spinal fusions using this method. An independent observer randomly selected 100 of these patients whose follow-up ranged from 5 to 15 years. The fusion rate was assessed by radiologists making functional films and the clinical results were assessed using the Stauffer and Coventry method. The series consisted of 36 compensation and 54 private patients. The average age was 37 years, the average duration of symptoms was $2\frac{1}{2}$ years. Seventy-five of the patients had a one-level fusion (Figs. 19,20) and the remainder had a two-level fusion. All had failed to respond to conservative measures. Most patients were home by the 5th post-operative day. Clinical results showed that 85% had a combined good and fair result and 15% were unimproved. The radiological assessment was such that 95% of the one-level procedures had a strong fusion, whereas with double-level fusions the rate was 88%. Interestingly enough all the single level pseudarthrosis patients reported a good result. Of the single-level successful fusion patients, 82% had a good result. Double-level pseudarthrosis patients had a clinical result of 75% good and fair. Complications in this series demonstrated one patient had an L5 spinal nerve sensory injury resulting in screw removal giving rise to a satisfactory result. There was no motor loss in this case but only temporary sensory loss. Since using the AO screws there has not been any case of screw fracture.

Conclusions

We should ask ourselves three questions pertaining to this operation: (1) Is it safe? (2) Is it effective? (3) Is it worthwhile? In over 2,000 screw insertions only 4 screws had to be removed for partial nerve root injury and therefore one feels that it is a safe procedure. As to whether it is effective, the AO pedicle screw situated well down the pedicle into the body gives complete rigidity. There is a high fusion rate permiting early mobilization plus a shortened hospital stay with great financial benefit to the patient. Further, this type of internal fixation allows many weeks in a rotor bed to be reduced to a week or so in hospital, so can be considered worthwhile. This relatively simple method of spinal fusion achieves a high success rate. The CT scanning of the fused area and functional radiography are used to establish that the fusion is complete. It would seem that the adequate immobilization obtained by the use of the long well-placed screws, careful preparation of the fusion site, and the addition of well-packed cancellous bone allows early activity and reduces the incidence of failure of spinal fusion. However, in a small percentage of patients with low back problems, firm fusion of the appropriate level is not always associated with symptom relief and the opposite is also true. In these cases one suspects that the psychological work up has been inadequate.

References

1. Boucher HH (1959) A method of spinal fusion. J Bone Joint Surg [Br] 41(2): 248–259
2. King D (1948) Internal fixation for lumbosacral fusion. J Bone Joint Surg [Am] 30:560
3. Thompson WAL, Ralston EK (1949) Pseudarthrosis following spine fusion. J Bone Joint Surg [Am] 31:400
4. Bosworth DM (1957) Surgery of the spine. American academy of orthopaedic surgeons instructional course lectures, vol 14. p 9
5. Barr JS (1951) Low-back and sciatica pain. J Bone Joint Surg [Am] 33:633
6. Watson-Jones R (1952) Reactions of bone to metal. In: Fractures and joint injuries, 4th edn. Livingstone, Edinburgh; (1953) Williams and Wilkins, Baltimore, vol 1, pp 205–226
7. Young RH (1953) Observations on the results of operation for low back pain and sciatica. In: Proceedings of Cinquieme Congres International de Chirurgie Orthopedique. Imprimerie Lielens, Brussels, p 126
8. Scott JC (1953) Spinal fusion. J Bone Joint Surg [Br] 35:169

3.8 Reduction and Stabilization of High Grade Spondylolisthesis: A Study of 29 Patients Using a Posterior Approach

R. Roy-Camille, J.Y. Lazennec, C.H. Garreau, G. Saillant, and J.-P. Benazet[1]

Introduction

Patients with spondylolisthésis of grade III or more, present with a unique association of local and régional dysplasia [1–8]. Some authors have criticized the need to obtain an anatomic reduction, arguing that neurological risk is increased. There are operative difficulties, and surgery is often overly aggressive [9–24]. Our experience is based on three therapeutic objectives that can be realized in a single surgical procedure:

1. Exploration of the spinal canal and root liberation
2. Reduction which permits a restoration of normal anatomy
3. Fixation which stabilizes the spine and allows for graft incorporation

Surgical Technique

We use special plates with oblong holes superiorly for the L4 and L5 pedicles. Inferiorly, five holes are present for the sacrum. The last three holes are oblique, providing for better screw purchase.

To complete the reduction of spondylolisthesis, we use pedicle screws with threaded shanks at L4 and L5. The L4 and L5 screws are first implanted in the pedicles. Then, the plate is anchored to the sacrum, the shanks of each pedicular screw being passed through the plate's proximal holes. The nuts are then applied to the pedicular screws. With progressive turning, a reduction of the slipped vertebra occurs (Figs. 1–5).

Two points are very important:

1. Positioning the patient on a special disk hernia table which allows control of the position of the sacrum
2. Distraction between L4 and S1 which starts the reduction of the slip

[1] Orthopedic Surgery Department, Pitié-Salpetriere Hospital, 83, Boulevard de l'Hôpital, 75651 Paris Cédex 13, France

1 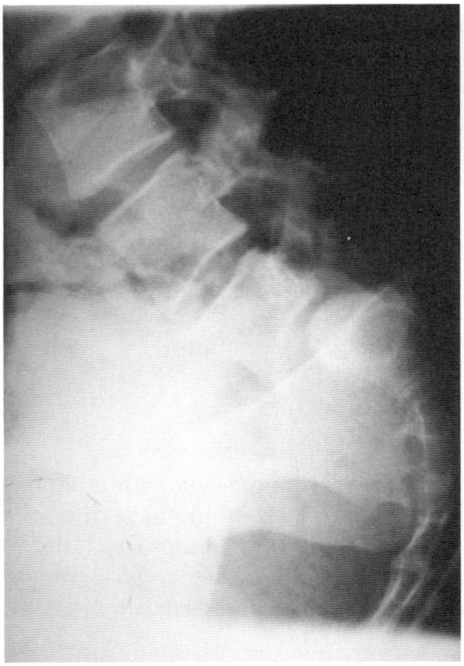

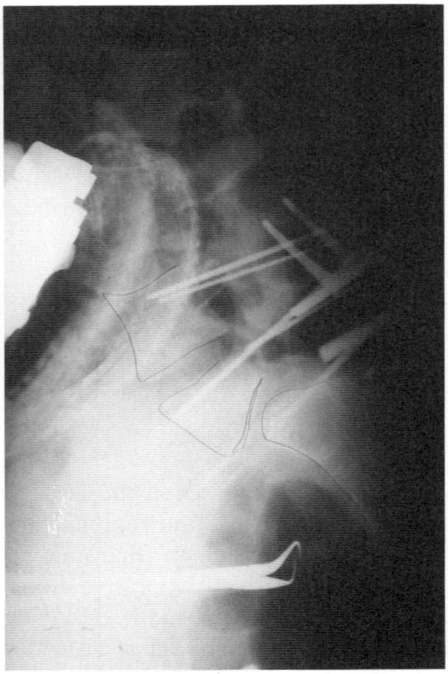 2

3 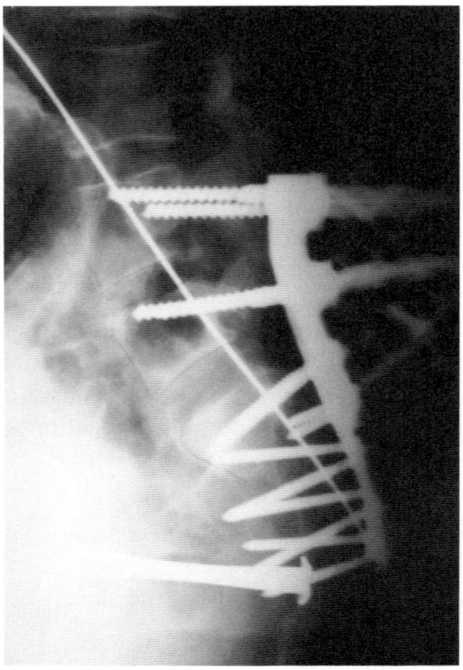

Fig. 1. High grade spondylolisthesis. Note the L5–S1 dysplasia and sacral verticalization associated with pelvic retroversion

Fig. 2. Perioperative lateral X-ray before reduction. Note the sacral retroversion

Fig. 3. Perioperative lateral X-ray. Note the positioning of pedicle screws with threaded shanks for L4 and L5

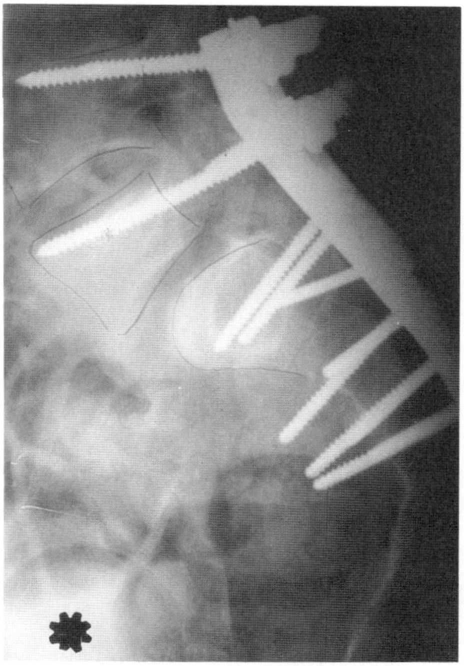

Fig. 4. Postoperative lateral X-ray. Note the reduction after distraction and applying the nuts onto the plates

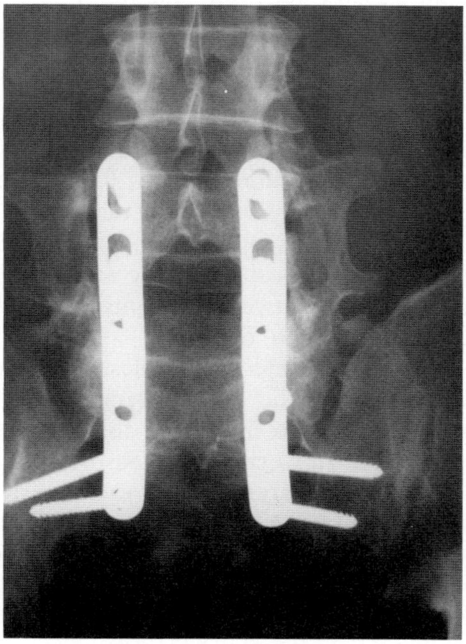

Fig. 5. Postoperative anteroposterior view. Note posterolateral bone graft

After the removal of the L5 posterial arch, a distractor is placed between the articular facets of L4 and S1 on the opposite side of the spine which is to be plated first. Then, after the plate has been applied, the distractor is repositioned between the spinous process of L4 and posterior arch of S1. This allows the second side to be plated. A posterolateral grafting is then performed.

Materials and Methods

We operated on 29 patients (17 females, 12 males; average age, 21.5 years) between 1978 and 1988. The average postoperative follow-up was 4.5 years. The patients included 19 with grade III and 8 with grade IV spondylothesis, and 2 with spondyloptosis. Preoperative evaluation revealed a high percentage of low back pain (24 patients), as well as lower limb radiculopathy (21 patients). Two patients were felt to have neurologic disorders preoperatively. One patient had an L5 deficit and the other presented with a severe hamstring contracture that was seemingly neurologic in origin.

Radiologic Evaluation

Our preoperative radiologic evaluation consisted of standard X-rays of the lumbo-sacral junction and of X-rays taken on scoliosis plates in order to evaluate the trunk position on anteroposterior and lateral views (Figs. 6–8). Several indices have been described to evaluate spondylolisthesis preoperatively and postoperatively [25–31].

We have described a dysplasia index which makes clearly visible the short anteroposterior dimension of the L5 vertebral body. Because of this short anteroposterior dimension of L5, measuring posterior wall alignment does not provide accurate criteria for reduction.

Instead of the classical Boxall's index, we have proposed an index based on measuring the position of the anterior wall. This index is calculated by dividing the distance between the anterior walls of L5 and S1 by the length of the inferior end-plate of L5.

The second regional dysplastic parameter to appreciate is the slippage angle calculated by the line tangent to the inferior end-plate of L5 and the line perpendicular to the rim of the posterior aspect of S1, tangent to its superior end-plate. However, the measurement of the slip and the slippage angle are not the only parameters to evaluate. The verticalization of the sacrum is an important factor to identify as well. The sacral angle is measured between a vertical line and a line tangent to the posterior wall of S1. Sometimes, however, there is a bend in the sacrum and this creates an inaccurate measurement. Therefore, the so-called hinge torque index was developed, calculated by first drawing a horizontal line through the center of S2. Then, a perpendicular is dropped from the middle of the inferior end-plate of L5. D1 is the length of the horizontal line between the center of S2 and the intersection of the perpendicu-

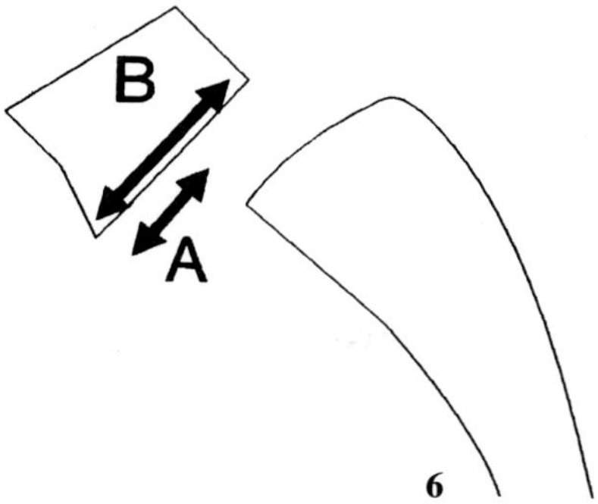

6

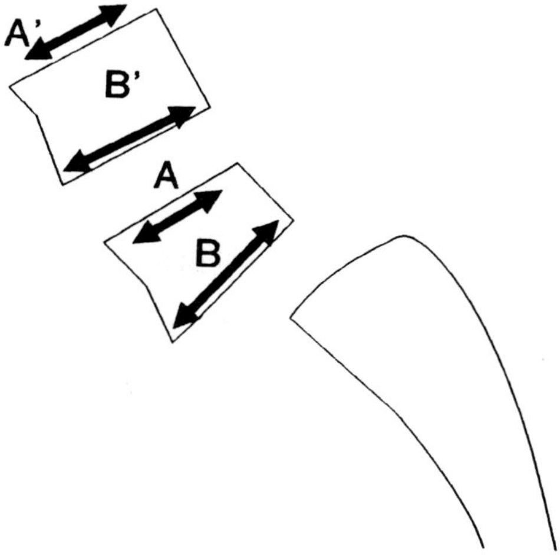

7

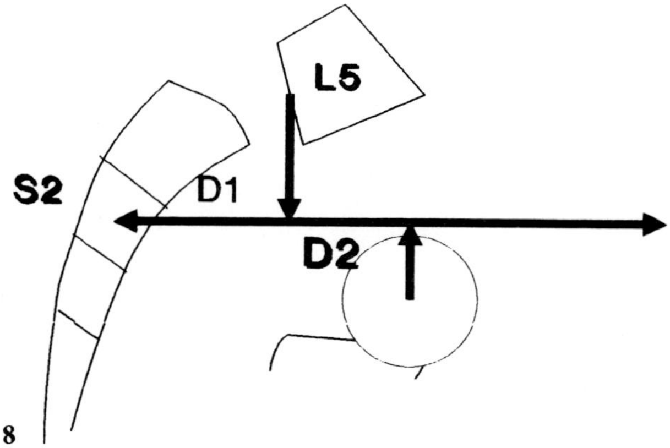

8

Fig. 6. Slipping index = A/B (normal = 0)

Fig. 7. Dysplasia index = $\frac{A + B}{A' + B'}$ (normal = 0.9)

Fig. 8. Hinge torque index (normal = D1/D2 = 80–100%)

lar. Next, a perpendicular is dropped from the horizontal line to the center of the femoral head. D2 is the length of the horizontal line from the center of S2 to the intersection with this latter perpendicular. Dividing D1 by D2 gives a normal hinge torque index between 80% and 100% [32].

This index appreciates the exact position of the sacrum, which is a very important point because the sacrum becomes retroverted in anterior slip of L5.

Clinical Results

The clinical results demonstrated a decrease in low back pain as for sciatica. Only one patient developed radiculopathy postoperatively after a very important reduction, and this neuralgia was not dermatomal but diffuse.

Peri- and Postoperative Complications

Four patients presented with postoperative hematomas, two required revisions. Two cutaneous problems occured in thin patients; these problems were treated with local wound care and were resolved easily.

The neurologic risk of high grade spondylolisthesis is well known even without reduction. In this series, there were five cases of neurologic complication: one cruralgia, one tibialis anterior deficit, one uncomplete S1, and one uncomplete L5–S1 deficit. All of the above were resolved. The fifth patient, who postoperatively presented with a severe L5 and S1 deficit, recovered incompletely.

It should be noted that all the neurologic problems occured after reduction of grade IV spondylolisthesis; each one required extensive liberation of the nerve roots.

Radiological Results

The improvement in the degree of slip averaged 36%. We noted a gain of 45% on the slipping index associated with an improvement of 36% in the slippage angle.

Out of 29 patients, 10 had complete reductions, 12 had reductions between 25% and 100%, but only 4 had reductions of less than 25%.

Critical analysis of the patients X-rays revealed a few technical problems. Three technical points are very important: (1) The position of the screws in the pedicles of L4 and L5 must not be angulated too cephalade, since they must have sufficent strength to provide for a reduction; (2) sufficient distraction of L4 must be obtained; and (3) the sacrum must be positioned as anteverted as possible in order to allow an easy reduction of L5.

Fusion has been obtained in 28 out of 29 cases after the first surgery. One case of pseudarthrosis was revised with success. At the end of the follow-up, none of the patients had lost correction.

Conclusions

The arguments for reduction are both morphological and biomechanical. Reduction of the spondylolisthesis improves the aspect of the lumbosacral junction as well as visual esthetics or the patient's body posture. Biomechanically, in theory, the reduction decreases the slip, corrects the L5–S1 angle, and suppresses pelvic retroversion, so as to improve the hinge torque value. This technique allows for a short lumbosacral fusion, unlike the length required when using Harrington instrumentation. Furthermore, one can resconstitute a more normal lordosis through a simple posterior approach [33–38].

Finally, it should be stressed that through this one stage surgery, all surgical aspects including liberation, reduction, fixation, and grafting, are under direct visual control, thus increasing the possibility of a good surgical outcome. One may stop the reduction at anytime if excessive tension is being applied to the nerve. In our series, it is important to know that all of our neurologic complications have been completely regressive except one partial recovery.

We now think that the mechanical behaviour of the instrumentation can still be improved by using posterior lumbar interbody fusion (PLIF) with cages in some cases and we have already started to incorporate this into our technique.

References

1. Bohlmann HH (1982) One stage decompression and posterolateral and interbody fusion for lumbosacral spondyloptosis through a posterior approach. Report of 2 cases. J Bone Joint Surg [Am] 64:415–418
2. Boxall DW, Bradford DS, Moe JH, Winter RB (1979) Management of severe spondylolisthesis (Grade III and Grade IV) in children and adolescents. J Bone Joint Surg [Am] 61:479
3. Harrington PR, Dickson JS (1976) Spinal instrumentation in the treatment of severe progressive spondylolisthesis. Clin Orthop 117:157–162
4. Harris IE, Weinstein SL (1987) Long-term follow up of patients with grade III and IV spondylolisthesis. J Bone Joint Surg [Am] 69:960–969
5. Louis R (1971) Les spondylolisthesis: bases antomopathologiques. Rev Chir Orthop 57 (suppl 1):99–105
6. Picault C (1971) Symposium sur le spondylolisthésis lombo sacré. XLVè réunion de la SOFCOT, 1970. Rev Chir Orthop [Suppl] 57(1):87–162
7. Roy-Camille R, Saillant G, Beurier J (1979) Spondylolisthésis L5–S1. Facteurs étiologiques et indications thérapeutiques. Rev Chir Orthop [Suppl] 65(2):84
8. Roy-Camille R, Saillant G, Veurier J, et al. (1983) Tumeurs du rachis. Spondylolisthésis L4–L5 et L5–S1. Rachis traumatique neurologique. In: Troisièmes Journées d'Orthopédie de la Pitié. Masson, Paris, pp 90–146
9. Bradford DS (1979) Treatment of severe spondylolisthesis. A combined approach for reduction and stabilization. Spine 4(5):423–429
10. Freeman B, Donati N (1989) Spinal arthrodesis for severe spondylolisthesis in children and adolescents. A long-term follow-up study. J Bone Surg [Am] 71: 594–598
11. Gill GG, White HL (1965) Surgical treatment of spondylolisthesis without spine fusion. A long follow-up of operated cases. Acta Orthop Scand [Suppl] 85:112–134
12. Goutallier D (1976) Arthrodèse antérieure dans le spondylolisthésis. Symposium SOFCOT. Rev Chir Orthop [Suppl] 2(62):125–131
13. Johnson RX, MacGuire EJ (1981) Urogenital complications of anterior approaches to the lumbar spine. Clin Orthop 154:114–118
14. Lord G (1977) Stabilisation des spondylolisthésis de plus de 50% et des spondyloloptoses. Rev Chir Orthop 1:215–225
15. Louis R, Maresca C (1977) Stabilisation chirurgicale avec réduction des spondylolyses et des spondylolisthésis. Int Orthop 1:215–225
16. Scaglietti O, Frontino G, Bartolozzi P (1976). Technique of anatomical reduction of lumbar spondylolisthésis and its surgical stabilization. Clin Orthop 117:164–165

17. Louis R (1971) Les arthrodèses stables de la charnière lombo-sacrée. Rev Chir Orthop [Suppl] 2:70
18. MacQueen M, Court-Brown C, Scott JHS (1986) Stabilisation of spondylolisthesis using Dwyer instrumentation. J Bone Joint Surg [Br] 68:185–188
19. Michel CR (1971) Réduction et fixation des spondylolisthésis et des spondyloptoses. Rev Chir Orthop [Suppl] 57(1):148–157
20. Michel CR, Caton J (1981) La réduction des grands spondylolisthésis de L5 chez l'enfant par la méthode de Harrington. Acta Orthop Belg 47:479–83
21. Munzinger U, Louis R (1981) Les arthrodèses stables de la charnière lombo-sacrée dans le traitement des spondylolisthésis. Acta Orthop Belg 47:468–78
22. Peek RD, Wiltse LL, Reynolds JB, et al. (1989) In situ arthrodesis without decompression for Grade III or IV isthmic spondylolisthesis in adults who have severe sciatica. J Bone Joint Surg [Am] 71:62–68
23. Transfeldt EE, Dendrinos GK, Bradford DS (1989) Paresis of proximal lumbar roots after reduction of L5–S1 spondylolisthesis. Spine 14:884–887
24. Vidal J (1971) Possibilités de réduction des spondylolisthésis et de la spondyloptose par le matériel de Harrington. Rev Chir Orthop 57(3):254
25. Maldague BE, Malghem JJ (1981) Aspects radiologiques dynamiques de la spondylolyse lombaire. Acta Orthop Belg 47:441
26. Meyerding HW (1941) Low-backache and sciatic pain associated with spondylolisthesis and protruted intervertebral disc. J Bone Joint Surg [Am] 23:461–470
27. Tailard W (1957) Les spondylolisthésis. Masson Paris
28. Wilson NJ (1955) Review of results of the treatment of 100 cases of spondylolisthesis. J Bone Joint Surg [Am] 37:406
29. Wiltse LL (1983) Classification and treatment of spondylolisthesis. In: Evarts CM (ed) Surgery of the musculoskeletal system, vol 2. Churchill Livingstone, New York, Chap. 19, pp 414–415
30. Wiltse LL (1962) The etiology of spondylolisthesis. J Bone Joint Surg [Am] 44: 539–560
31. Wiltse LL, Winter RB (1983) Terminology and measurement of spondylolisthesis. J Bone Joint Surg [Am] 65(6):768–72
32. Vidal J, Marnay T (1983) La morphologie et l'équilibre antéro-postérieur dans le spondylolisthesis L5–S1. Rev Chir Orthop 69:17–28
33. Sijbrandij S (1983) Reduction and stabilization of severe spondylolisthesis. J Bone Joint Surg [Br] 65(1):40–43
34. Smith MD, Bohlmann HH (1990) Spondylolisthesis treated by a single-stage operation combining decompression with in situ posterolateral and anterior fusion. J Bone Joint Surg [Am] 72:415–421
35. Snidjer JGN, Seroo JU, Snidjer CJ (1976) Therapy of spondylolisthesis by repositioning and fixation of the olisthetic vertebra. Clin Orthop 117:149–56
35. Vercauteren M, DE Groote W, Van Nuffle J, Vincent A (1981) Reduction du spondylolisthésis à grand glissement. Acta Orthop Belg 47(4–5):502–11
37. Vidal J, Fassio B, Buscayret C, Melka J (1981) Le traitement chirurgical du spondylolisthésis L5–S1. Douze and d'expérience de réduction instrumentée selon la technique de Harrington. Acta Orthop Belg 154:156–65
38. Vidal J, Fassio B, Buscayret C, Allieu Y (1981) Surgical reduction of spondylolisthesis using a posterior approach. Clin Orthop 154:156–65

3.9 Lumbar Diskectomy, Facetectomy, and Laminectomy of L4–L5 and L5–S1 Levels: Experimental Approach and Biomechanical Consequences of Practical Application

J.Y. Lazennec[1], R. Desjardins[2], R. Roy-Camille[3], C.G. Laudet[1], A. Lazennec[1], and B. Roger[1]

Introduction

Despite many experimental investigations, a lot of questions remain about the concept of lumbar instability, both degenerative and postoperative [1–5]. The purpose of this study is to analyze the possible deterioration of physiologic behavior at L4–L5 and L5–S1 levels. From the experimental point of view, these results allow one to reflect on the influence of some anatomic details on the intimate biomechanic relationships of these functional units [6,7].

One functional unit can be defined by the association of two adjacent vertebrae, the anterior and posterior longitudinal ligaments, and the interposed disk and ligaments. The important anatomical structures are the disk, the articular process, the ligamentum flavum, and the interspinous and supraspinous ligaments [4,8–12]. Lordosis and muscle activity are very influential, but unfortunately, difficult to evaluate.

How can we define the stability and instability of a functional unit? When we speak about traumatology, stability means, most of the time, stiffness. When we speak about the biomechanics and the pathophysiology of degenerative or postoperative instability, however, dynamics should be emphasized [12–14].

Materials and Methods

Eight cadavers were tested with an Adamel Lhomargy loading machine (DY.26 Adamel Lhomargy, Ivry, France) using the framework as defined by Panjabi. We respected classical loads as previously described in the literature [15–19] and conservation methods for fresh vertebrae, disks, and ligaments. In this

[1] Service d'Anatomie, Faculté Pitie-Salpetriere, 105, Bd de l'Hôpital, 75013 Paris, France
[2] Service d'Orthopédie, Hôpital Maisonneuve, 5414 Bd de l'Assomption, HIT2MA Montreal, Canada
[3] Service d'Orthopédie, Hôpital Pitie-Salpetriere, 83, Bd de l'Hôpital, 75013 Paris, France

1 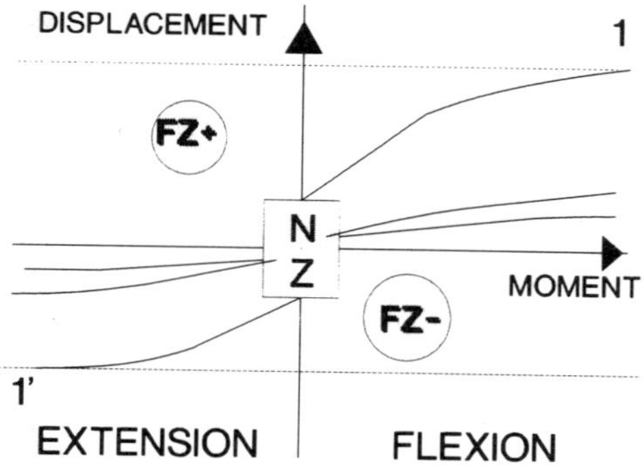

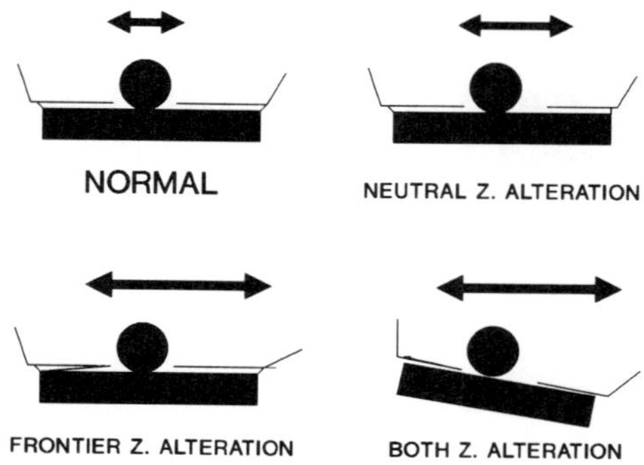 2

3 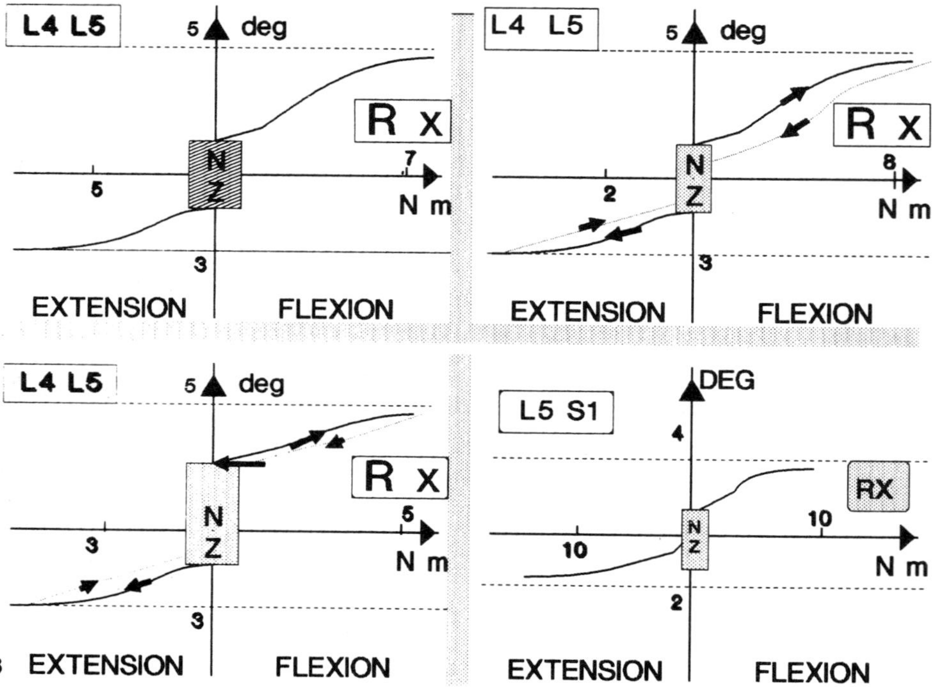

Fig. 1. Results of displacements for L4–L5 and L5–S1 units during flexion and extension

Fig. 2. Schematic representation of alterations about the neutral zone, the frontier zone, and the limits of the frontier zone

Fig. 3. Comparison between the L4–L5 neutral zone and the L5–S1 neutral zone study, we only analyzed displacements for L4–L5 and L5–S1 units during flexion and extension. To create bending modes of loading in those two directions, we used an off-center pushrod connected with the mobile upper load frame. This moving upper frame of the Adamel tester applied the load at a constant speed; continue evaluation of applied loads was performed using an Adamel strain gauge load cell. Functional unit displacement was continuously evaluated with gauges placed on the vertebrae.

We shall discuss only translation and rotation along the X and Z axes, as defined in the classic three coordinate system.

Applied moments were 5–10 NM.

Results

All of the results can be demonstrated on a single kind of curve, as seen in Fig. 1.

As previously suggested by Panjabi, we defined two zones along the curves defined by the moment displacement coordinates. First, Panjabi's neutral zone is defined by the position of the functional unit when minimal moments are applied. Successive loadings with minimal moment show that the starting point of the curve is contingent inside a neutral zone area. This neutral zone, or area about the zero point, has a variable size and every functional unit returns to this neutral zone when moment application ceases. This suggests that for each functional unit, the point of equilibrium is dynamic; thus, it is not necessarilly just a point, but an area.

The second zone, referred to as the Frontier Zone, demonstrates displacement when a significant moment is applied. This displacement has a limit for flexion and extension: dislocation or irreversible lesions occur if this limit is transgressed. We can see that the displacement curve resembles an asymptote as long as the maximum moment is not transgressed. As far as flexion and extension are concerned, maximum translation occurs along the Z axis and axial rotation along the X axis. However, small displacements occur along the other axes. These latter displacements are not very important, and we have chosen to express only translation and rotation along the axes for flexion and extension.

Alterations can occur about the neutral zone, the frontier zone and the limits of the frontier zone. Biomechanically, instability means the inability to return to a steady state; it is different from hypermobility. These concepts can be expressed simply and schematically. Imagine a ball in a small dish with an oblique rim and a central depression (Fig. 2). The equilibrium of the ball in the dish may change either by changing the size of the central depression (neutral zone), the slope of the rim (frontier zone), or the inclination of the dish (both zones).

A very important difference must be noticed between L4–L5 and L5–S1. The L4–L5 neutral zone is larger than L5–S1 neutral zone (Fig. 3). This indicates the mobility of the last space is comparatively reduced; this is secondary to the position of the articular processes. L4–L5 neutral zone altérations may be very significant. Either decreasing or increasing the zone may have grave clinical consequences especially in anterior displacement. When insignificant moments are applied to this functional unit, a physiologic tendency is noticed for anterior slipping. This depends on the lordosis and the sagittal disposition of the articular processes.

In pathologic processes, neutral zone reduction is demonstrated when facet joints and disk space narrow. This is in contrast to neutral zone increases with some diskal degeneration, articular decoaptation, and posterior ligamentous lesions.

The frontier zone is more difficult to study. Two points must be emphasized: firstly, the effects of excessive loads, with regards to the limit previously defined, and the inability to return to the neutral zone after these loads are applied, and secondly, with some pathologic conditions, other associated motions can occur.

The mode of loading is very important; the values obtained and the evaluation of the limit are largely load dependant. On the contrary, the contours of the curve do not seem to be affected. Ligamentous lesions and articular lesions are extremely important. By analyzing simple experimentally created lesions, one

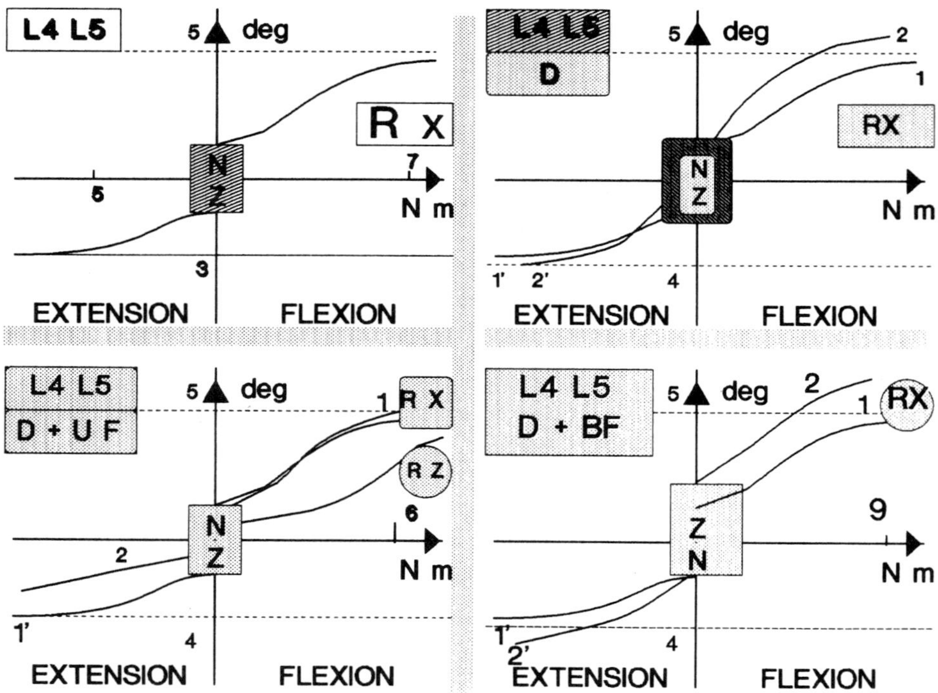

Fig. 4. The effect on axial rotation following diskectomy (*D*), unilateral facetectomy (*UF*), and bilateral facetectomy (*BF*)

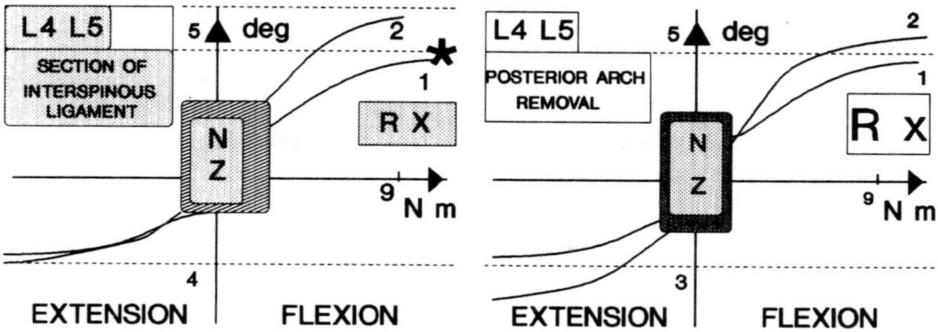

Fig. 5. Alteration of the posterior arch

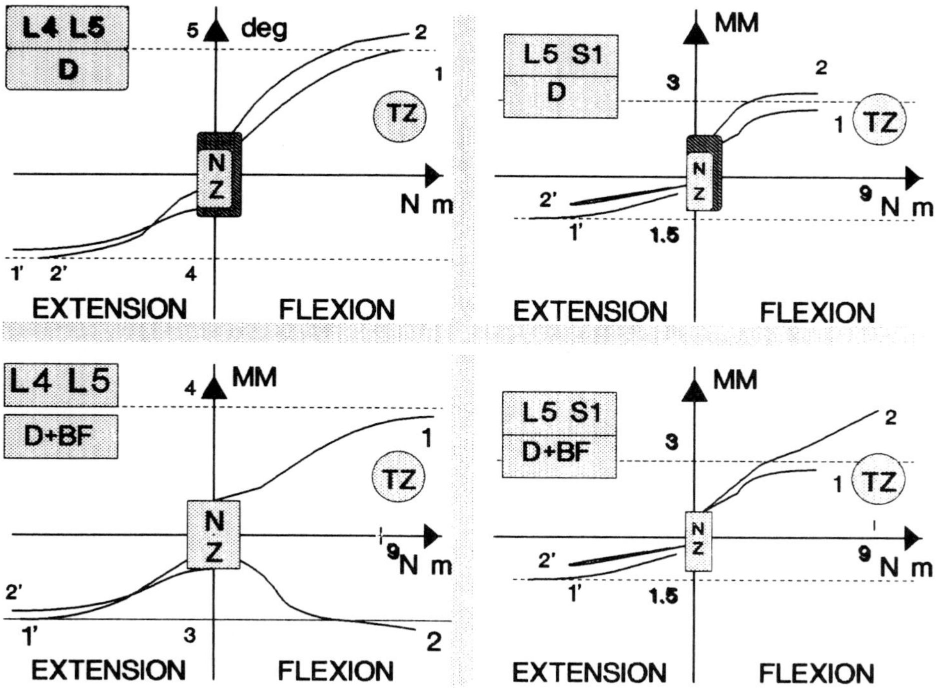

Fig. 6. The effect on translation following diskectomy (*D*) and bilateral facetectomy (*BF*)

can better comprehend the affects of surgical procedure on the functional unit.

L4–L5 diskectomy influences the neutrol zone area and the limits of the frontier zone. The modification for L5–S1 is less important for rotation along the X axis.

Unilateral facetectomy only seems to increase axial rotation along the Z axis and does not affect axial rotation along the X axis. Bilateral facetectomy increases both axial rotation along that Z axis and X axis. The contour of the curve is relatively unchanged (Fig. 4).

Lesions of the interspinous and supraspinous ligaments are also important because they modify the neutral zone and also the limits of the frontier zone. Rotation along this axis is modified as well, creating rotational instability not unlike bilateral facetectomy.

Posterior arch removal essentially affects extension movements. In our experience, only a few cases were affected as far as the neutral zone is concerned. Once this neutral zone was modified, motion disturbances were very small and the area of this zone was relatively unchanged (Fig. 5).

Translation was examined as well as rotation. With L5–S1, bilateral facetectomy and spinous ligament section had influences.

At the L4–L5 level, diskectomy has quite the same effects as for rotational movements. We studied the effect of unilateral and bilateral facetectomy on the L4–L5 level. Unilateral facetectomy slightly increases anterior displacement of L4. This lesion does not affect neutral zone dynamics and only increases the displacement of the anterior limit of the frontier zone. L4–L5 is as appropriate for diskectomy as for bilateral facetectomy. As far as translation is concerned, bilateral facetectomy enlarges the limits of frontier zone with a tendency for rétrolisthésis (Fig. 6).

From the analysis of displacement along all axes, we have concluded that the apparent tendency for anterior displacement comes from a rotational movement caused by asymmetric loading of the functional unit. Bilateral facetectomy is interesting because it does not provide the slightest tendancy for anterior displacement, but on the contrary, initiates posterior displacement of L4 on L5. This phenomenon substantiates the clinical observation of retrolisthesis at the L4–L5 level. Translation is slightly affected by bilateral facetectomy at the L5–S1 level. If the disk remains, anterior displacement in flexion is minimal. The limits of the frontier zone for anterior displacement in flexion are only slightly affected. On the other hand, extension limits remain the same.

Conclusion

This study emphasizes the need to study the biomechanics of lumbar instability. Displacement curves show very clearly the behavior of the functional unit. Defining the instability concept from these curves permits the study of two different zones: firstly, the neutral zone of Panjabi, the variations of which we have emphasized, and secondly, the frontier zone, the limits of which can be affected by elementary surgical lesions, and whose curve can be largely modified by the level studied, the mechanism of loading, and the anatomy of the functional unit.

This study has pointed out many difficultes for those involved in biomechanical work, mainly with spatial orientation and muscle function. It must also be enphasized that this study was performed on fresh cadavers, of elderly people, and without muscle simulation. This fact may affect the values for displacement, but, in all cases, the contours of the curves are comparable.

References

1. Posner I, White AA III, Edwards TW, Hayes WC (1982) A biomechanical analysis of the clinical stability of the lumbar and lumbosacral spine. Spine 7:374–389
2. Smith TJ, Fernie GR (1991) Functional biomechanics of the spine. Spine 16(10): 1197–1203
3. Tencer AF, Ahmed AM, Burke DL (1982) Some static mechanical properties of the lumbar intervertebral joint intact and injured. J Biomech Eng 104:193–201
4. Tkaczuk H (1968) Tensile properties of human lumbar longitudinal ligaments Acta Orthop Scand [Suppl] 115
5. White AA III, Panjabi MM (1978) The basic kinematics of the human spine. Spine 3(1):12–20
6. Schultz AB, Warnick DN, Berkson MH, Nachemson AL (1982) Mechanical properties of human lumbar spine motion segments. Part 1: Response in flexion extension, lateral bending and torsion. J Biomech Eng 104:193–201
7. Yang SW, Langrana NA, Lee CK (1986) Biomechanics of lumbosacral spine fusion in combined compression torsion loads. Spine 11:937–941
8. Broberg KB (1983) On the mechanical behavior of intervertebral discs. Spine 8:151–165
9. Skalli W, Lavaste F, Barraco A, Bisserie M, Saillant G, Roy-Camille R (1982) Etude "in vitro" d'un segment vertébral lombaire humain. Comportement expérimental et modélisation mécanique. J Biophys Méd Nucl 6(4):193–199
10. Haher TR, Bergman M, O'Brien M, Tallman Felmly W, Choueka J, Welin D, Chow G, Vassiliou A (1991) The effect of the three columns of the spine on the instantaneous axis or rotation in flexion and extension. Spine 16(10):312–318
11. Tibrewal SB, Pearcy MJ, Portek I, Spivey J (1985) A prospective study of lumbar spinal movements before and after discectomy using biplanar radiography, correlation of clinical radiographic findings.
12. Edwards WT (1983) A biomechanical analysis of the lumbar and lumbosacral spine in the sagittal spine. Doctoral thesis, Massachusetts Institude of Technology. Cambridge, MA
13. Goel VK, Goyal S, Clark C, Nishiyama K, Nye T (1985) Kinematics of the whole lumbar spine: effect of discectomy. Spine 10:543–554
14. Goel VK, Nishiyama K, Weinstein JN, Liu YK (1986) Mechanical properties of lumbar spinal motion segments as affected by partial disc removal. Spine 11: 1008–12
15. Guyer DW, Yuan HA, Werner FW, Frederickson BE, Murphy D (1987) Biomechanical comparison of seven internal fixation devices for the lumbosacral junction. Spine 12(6):569–573
16. Lavaste F, Asselineau A, Diop A, Grandjean JL, Laurain JM, Skalli W, Roy-Camille R (1990) Experimental procedure for mechanical evaluation of dorsolumbar segments and osteosynthesis devices. Rachis 2(6):435–446
17. Panjabi MM, Krag MH, Goel VK (1981) A technique for measurement and description of three-dimensional six degree-of-freedom motion of a body with an application to the human spine. J Biomech 14:447–460

18. Panjabi MM, Takata K, Goel VK (1983) Kinematics of intervertebral foramen. Spine 8:348–357
19. Edwards TW (1991) Biomechanics of posterior lumbar fixation: Analysis of testing methodologies. Spine 16(10):1224–1232

PART 4

Spinal Instrumentation

SECTION I Biomechanics

4.1 Biomechanical Analysis of Lumbosacral Fixation

David H. McCord[1], Bryan W. Cunningham, Yasuhiro Shono, Jordan J. Myers, and Paul C. McAfee[2]

Introduction

The lumbosacral junction is perhaps the most difficult portion of the spine in which to obtain a solid fusion [1–11]. This is particularly true following reductions of spondylolisthesis [12]. Lumbar spine fusion techniques have continued to evolve since Hibbs and Albee first described their fusion methods for tuberculosis spine infections [13,14]. At present, instrumentation systems run a wide range of design to confer desirable biomechanical properties in hopes of increasing the success of spinal fusion while obviating the need for a postsurgical orthosis.

Although multiple studies have been performed comparing one or a few lumbosacral spine fixation systems, these were often performed in a nonstandard manner or were limited in scope [6,15–19]. We analyzed ten lumbosacral instrumentation systems, each differing mainly in design of fixation at the lumbosacral junction with comparison to an uninstrumented specimen as a control.

The goals of the study were threefold:

1. we aimed to determine whether the newer transpedicular type of lumbosacral fixation offers biomechanical advantages over traditional Harrington and Luque fixation methods
2. aside from comparing implant X to implant Y, we wished to derive generic differences in fixation determined by the location of screw fixation: control (Group 4); S1 pedicle fixation only (Group 3); fixation extending inferiorly to the S2 pedicle (Group 2); and fixation bridging the sacroiliac joint and into the ilium (Group 1)
3. we hoped to determine if all devices crossing the sacroiliac joint were equivalent in stability, and whether this bony area of purchase is more

[1] Tennessee Spine Center, 329 22nd Avenue, North Nashville, TN 37203, USA
[2] Department of Orthopaedic Surgery, The Johns Hopkins University School of Medicine and Biomechanics Laboratory, Union Memorial Hospital, Baltimore, Maryland, USA

favorable than the superior acetabular bone utilized in diverging iliac crest rods (Isola Galveston) or screws (Isola iliac screws)

Materials and Methods

Sixty-six specimens were obtained from 1-month-old bull calves weighing 490–520 N. The entire vertebral column and adjoining pelvis were harvested and immediately frozen at −20°C in double wrapped freezer bags. Approximately 2 h prior to testing, the spines were removed from the freezer and immediately transversely sectioned, using a 3/4-inch osteotome at the T13–L1 disk space. Using a number 21 blade scalpel, forceps, and Cobb elevator, the remaining lumbosacral spine material was cleaned of all residual musculature. Care was taken, however, to preserve all ligamentous structures supporting the lumbosacral column. Once cleaned and thawed to room temperature, 2-mm steinmann pins were placed into the vertebral body parallel to the disk space, anteriorly in the midline of the vertebral body, and posteriorly in the spinous process at L6 and S1.

Once cleaned and thawed to room temperature, the instrumentation system under evaluation was applied. The instrumented lumbosacral spine was then mounted in a rectangular metal foundation and transfixed with the posterior elements upwards. They were transfixed with a 3⁄16-inch-diameter Steinmann pin at the following two locations: (1) the superior acetabular rim through the posterior column, and (2) the anterior ischium. The fixation mechanism surrounded the ventral pelvis, leaving the lumbar spine extending beyond the container edge. Attention was directed to keeping the iliac wings elevated off the container during transfixation. By doing this, the lumbosacral and iliosacral junctions remained unrestricted during analysis. Transfixation provided the necessary stability for accurate biomechanical analysis of each spinal system. This fixation method follows the principles of White and Panjabi in that the lumbar spine was free to move (unconstrained) with no bias as to the flexural axis of rotation or bending [20]. The total time for preparation and testing never exceeded 2 h, and all specimens were kept moistened during this period with a 0.9% saline solution. The efficacy of bovine spine as a experimental model has been well documented [20–23].

Biomechanical Parameters

All biomechanical testing was performed on a servo-controlled MTS 858 Bionix hydraulic materials-testing device (M.T.S., Minneapolis, Minn.) configured with a biaxial load cell. All transducer outputs (axial load, displacement, torque, rotation, and strain) were recorded through a high speed analog-to-digital converter (DASH 16; Metrobyte, Taunton, Mass.) to an IBM AT computer. Data acquisition was performed at a sampling frequency of 5 Hz.

Parameters for testing included a 22-cm (0.22 m) lever arm applied at a loading rate of 4.4 Nm/s. The induced load on the S1–S2 junction was measured at the load cell, and the flexion moment was calculated. Anatomically, the applied lever arm originated at the S1–S2 disk space and extended to the L1 spinous process (Fig. 1). In some cases, due to small amounts of interspecimen variability, the location of transfixation was adjusted to maintain a constant lever arm. The flexion moment was applied at a constant rate until visual failure of either the bone or bone-metal interface occurred. Final failure points, noted by an abrupt increase in strain per load and corroborated visually, were characterized in terms of applied moment, degrees of flexion, strain, mode of failure, and purchase sites of the lumbosacral fixation device. Furthermore, extensiometric values were obtained utilizing a 632.12C–20 M.T.S. extensometer, gauge length 25 ± 0.05 mm with a strain range of +50% / −10% (M.T.S., Minneapolis, Minn.). The knife edges were inserted precisely at the S1 proximal end-plate and L5 distal end-plate anteriorly, thereby calculating displacements over a range of two disk spaces, L5–L6 and L6–S1, and one vertebral body, L6, in order to take full advantage of the extensometer's range. All biomechanical testing was performed in the load control mode.

Statistical analysis was performed using a one way analysis of variance (ANOVA). The Student-Newman-Keuls (SNK) multiple comparison test was used to analyze differences between groups. Additionally, a Global Analysis of Variance was performed [24,25].

Instrumentation Constructs

We tested ten lumbosacral fixation constructs with the following components:

1. ISOLA Galveston technique with a ¼-inch rod extending from L4 to the ilium [26]
2. ISOLA iliac screw design with ¼-inch rods extending from L4 to S1
3. C-D iliosacral screw with ¼-inch rods from L4 to S1
4. Kirschner sacral plates which permit three points of fixation: S1, S2, and the iliac wing
5. C-D Chopin block system
6. C-D butterfly construct
7. Isola sacral hook design
8. Harrington distraction instrumentation
9. Luque rectangular ¼-inch rods [27]
10. Steffee plate system with a plate extending from L4 to S1 and 6.5 mm diameter by 40 mm pedicle screws
11. Control specimen with no instrumentation

All Isola and Steffee systems were supplied by AcroMed Corporation (Cleveland, Ohio); all C-D systems by Cotrel-Dubousset (Sofamor, Berck-Plage, France); all Kirschner systems by Kirschner Medical (Baltimore, Md.); and all

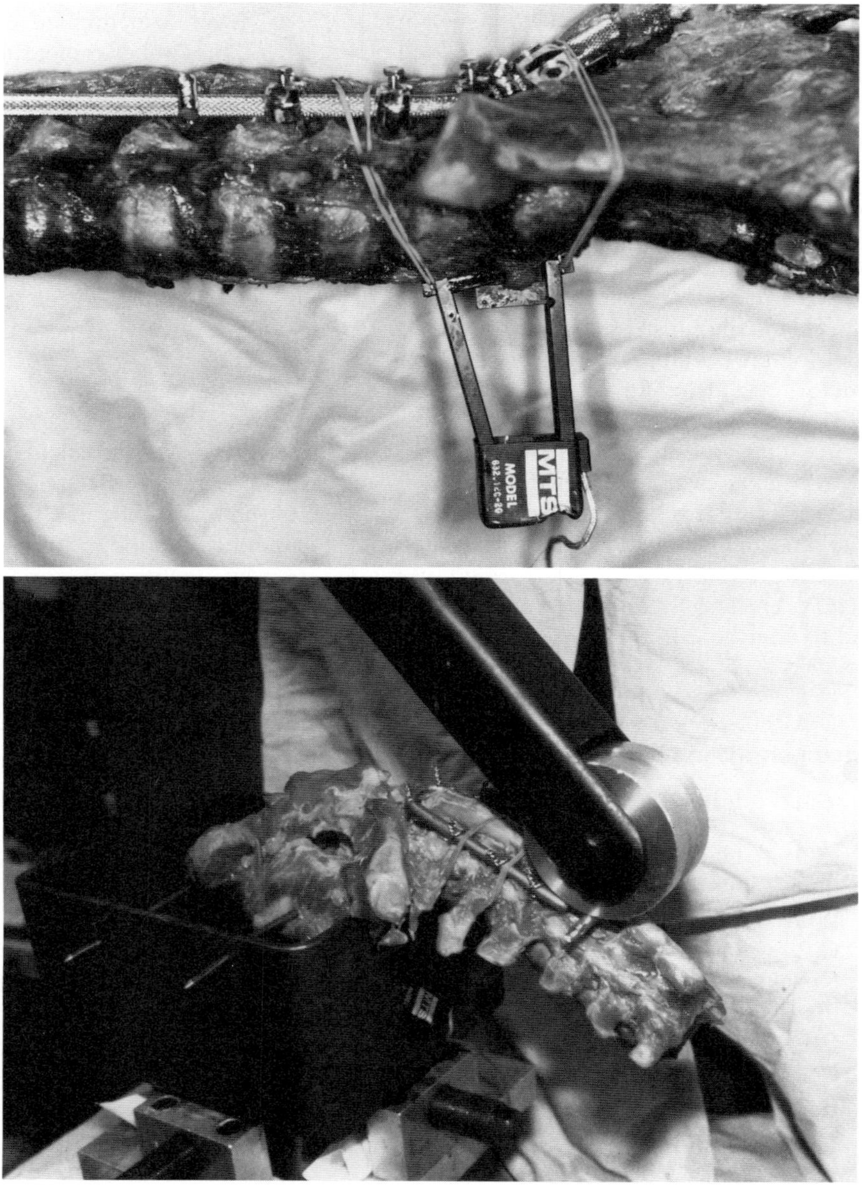

a

b

Fig. 1. **a** A mounted spine ready for testing. The extensometer is placed anteriorly across the lowermost disk spaces to measure anterior strain across the lumbosacral joint as the spinal segment is flexed. **b** A mounted specimen being flexed forward via a 22-cm level arm. Note the anteriorly placed extensometer with the metal tubing cut out in order to not interfere with the strain readings. **c** A schematic diagram depicting an instrumented spine loaded with a 22-cm lever arm originating over the S1–S2 spinous processes at 4.4 Nm/s. Strain is measured anteriorly

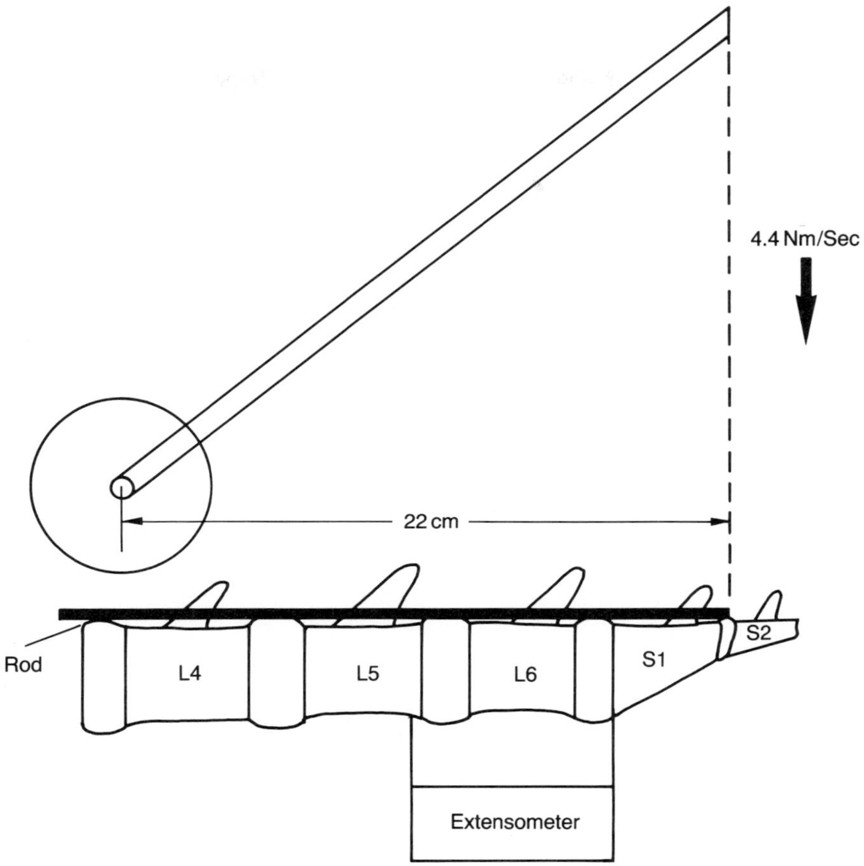

Fig. 1. c

Table 1. Design components.

Systems	Group	S1	S2	Iliac
Isola Galveston	1	screw		rod
Isola iliac screw	1	screw		screw
C-D iliosacral screw	1	screw		screw
Kirschner sacral plate	1	screw	screw	screw
C-D Chopin block	2	screw	screw	
C-D butterfly plate	2	screw	screw	
Isola sacral hook	2	screw	hook	
Harrington rods	3	hook		
Luque	3	wire		
Steffee plate	3	screw		
Control	4			

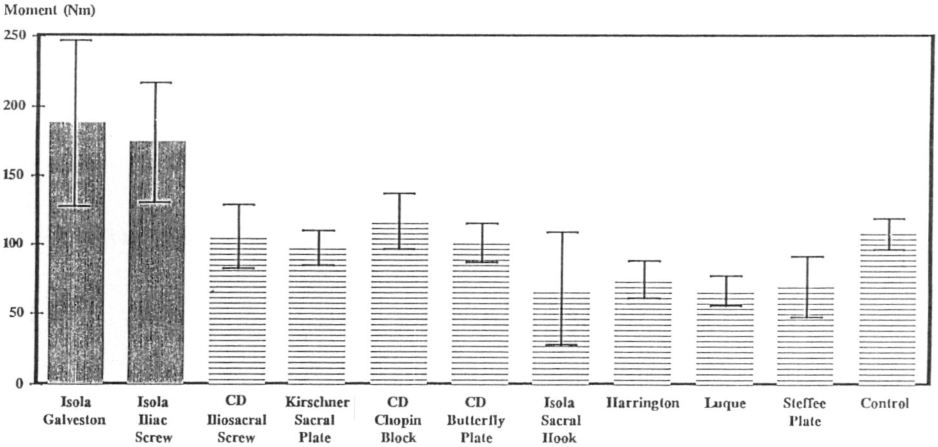

Fig. 2. Maximum moment at failure. Different subsets of moment are designated by different cross hatching. groups 1 and 2 (grey) were different ($P < 0.05$) from groups 3–11 (*horizontal lines*). Moreover there was no statistical difference between groups 3–11

Harrington and Luque systems by Union Memorial and St. Joseph Hospital (Baltimore, Md.).

It is important to note that although the longitudinal member of each system extended superiorly to the L1 spinous process, fixation to the lumbar vertebral column went to L4. In doing this, the applied rate of the flexion moment (4.4 Nm/s) was evenly distributed to the longitudinal rods. The lever arm was fixed while the specimen flexed under load control. The systems under evaluation can be divided into four principal groups based on sacroiliac purchase: group 1, Iliac; group 2, S2; group 3, S1 only; group 4, no instrumentation (Table 1).

Results

Statistical Analysis

Figure 2 is a bar graph of the 11 constructs showing the mean maximum moment at failure in Nm grouped by similarities in lumbosacral fixation. One standard deviation above and below the mean are also shown for each device. The first four constructs include iliac purchase, the next three have S2 fixation, and the next three S1 fixation only. A one-way analysis of variance demonstrated $F = 12.2$, $P < 0.001$, and $10\,df$. A Student-Newman-Keuls comparison of means between the 11 constructs was significant ($P < 0.05$) between devices 1 and 2, and the remaining 9 constructs. Construct one and two (gray bar) were

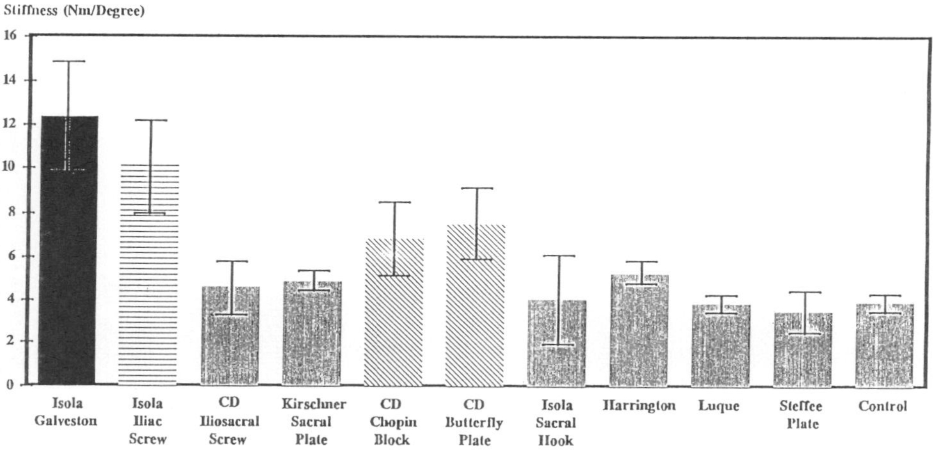

Fig. 3. Maximum stiffness at failure. Different subsets of stiffness are represented by different hatching

different ($P < 0.05$) from groups 3–11 (horizontal lines); moreover, there was no statistical significance between groups 3–11.

Figure 3 shows stiffness at failure in Nm/°. Again, the graph is arranged by similarities in lumbosacral fixation. A one-way analysis of variance demonstrated $F = 23.7$, $P < 0.001$, and 10 *df*. A Student-Newman-Keuls comparison of means was significant ($P < 0.05$) between devices 1 and 2. There was a significant difference ($P < 0.05$) between four subsets. Construct 1 (solid bar) was stiffer than construct 2 (left diagonal) versus constructs 5 and 6 (vertical line) versus the remaining seven constructs 3–11 (right diagonal lines).

An analysis was also derived from the maximum strain at ultimate failure for the 11 constructs (Fig. 4). This was determined by dividing the difference between the extensometer readings at the beginning and at failure by the original reading. A one-way analysis of variance revealed $F = 14.0$, $P < 0.001$, and 10 *df*. A Student-Newman-Keuls comparison of means between the 11 constructs was significant ($P < 0.05$) in 3 subsets: the first subset with the highest strain was comprised by constructs 2 and 11, the second subset included constructs 1, 4, 5, 6, 8, 9, and the third subset with the least strain across the lumbosacral junction was comprised by group 3, 7, and 10.

A comparison was also done showing maximum angulation at failure in degrees for all 11 constructs (Fig. 5). This theoretical angle was determined by obtaining the arctangent of the lever arm divided by maximal displacement at failure and was used in calculating stiffness. A one-way analysis of variance revealed $F = 12.8$, $P < 0.001$, and 10 *df*. A Student-Newman-Keuls comparison of means between 11 constructs was significant ($P < 0.05$) in the following three subgroups: construct 11 (control), which, as expected, angulated

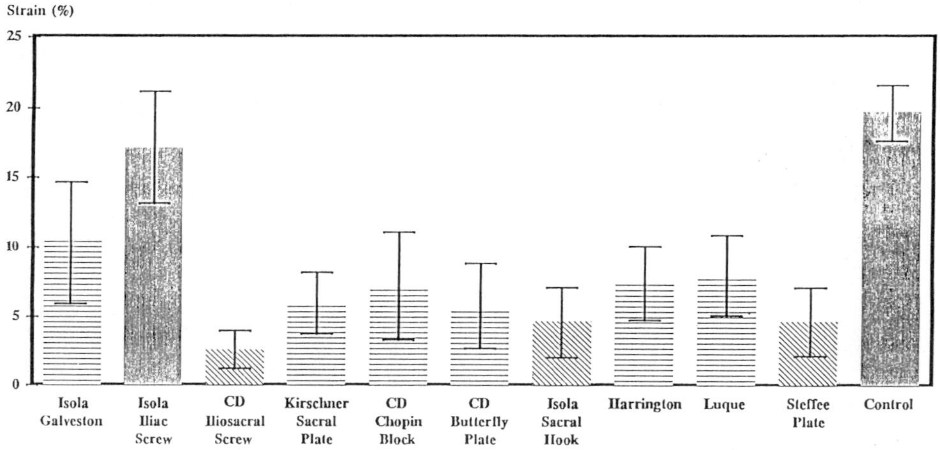

Fig. 4. Maximum strain at failure. Different subsets of strain are represented by different hatching

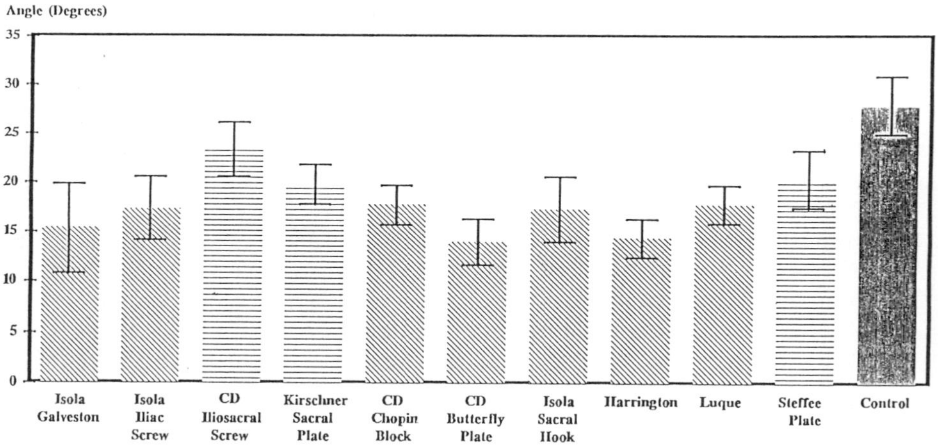

Fig. 5. Maximum angulation at failure. Different subsets of angulation are represented by different hatching

the most, followed by constructs 3, 4, and 10, followed by the remaining constructs (which angulated the least) 1, 2, 5, 6, 7, 8, and 9.

Figure 6 shows the percent strain per angulation at failure comparing all 11 constructs grouped by similarities in lumbosacral fixation. This was calculated from the data already obtained for both percent strain and angulation. A one-way analysis of variance revealed $F = 8.2$, $P < 0.001$, and $10\,df$. A Student-Newman-Keuls comparison of means between 11 constructs was significant (P

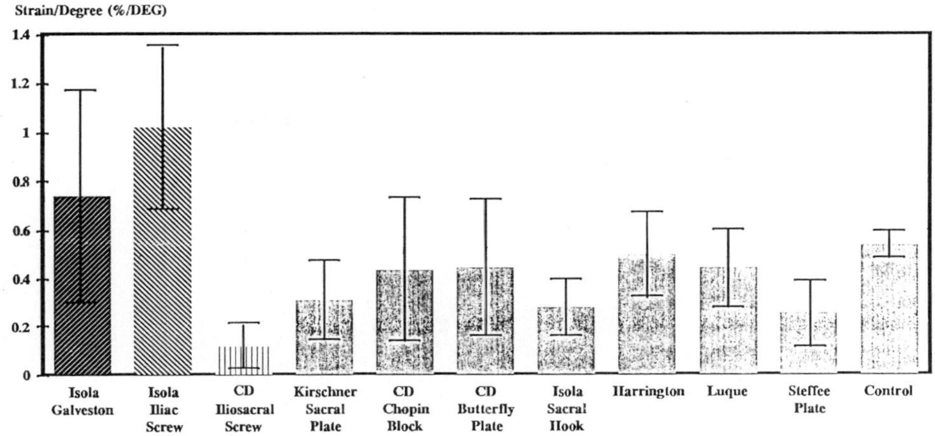

Fig. 6. Percent strain/angulation at failure. Different subsets of strain are represented by different cross hatching

< 0.05) for four subgroups: construct 2 (*solid bar*) versus construct (*horizontal lines*) versus the remaining constructs (*diagonal cross hatches*) except for construct 3 (*vertical lines*), which demonstrated the significantly ($P < 0.05$) lowest value.

Mechanism of Failure

Noting the mechanism of failure not only gives insight into the ultimate limitation of a device (whether or not the loads required are greater than clinically encountered), but may yield insight for improving a construct. For instance, single-level triangulated screws with a transverse plate fail at the bone-bone rather than bone-metal interface in straight pull out, indicating an ideal design. Finally, only by noting the failure mechanism was the low strain reading of the C-D iliosacral screw understood.

Each construct, other than the control, failed at the caudal bone-metal interface (the instrumented spines failed at the L6–S1 facet capsule). The Isola Galveston and Isola iliac screw specimens initially failed with delamination of the inner and outer tables of the iliac crest followed ultimately by fracture propagating to the S1 screw (Fig. 7). The Kirschner sacral plate began in the same location but propagated in a linear fashion across the S2 screws (Fig. 8). Once the ilium failed, the fracture extended to the caudal sacral screws rapidly, indicating that the major contributor to stability is the ilium.

The Cotrel-Dubousset (C-D) butterfly plate and Chopin block failed at the S2 screw with a fracture extending superiorly to the S1 screw. The posterior cortical bone within the rectangle formed by the bilateral S1 and S2 screws remained intact as the screws pulled out of the anterior cortex (Fig. 9).

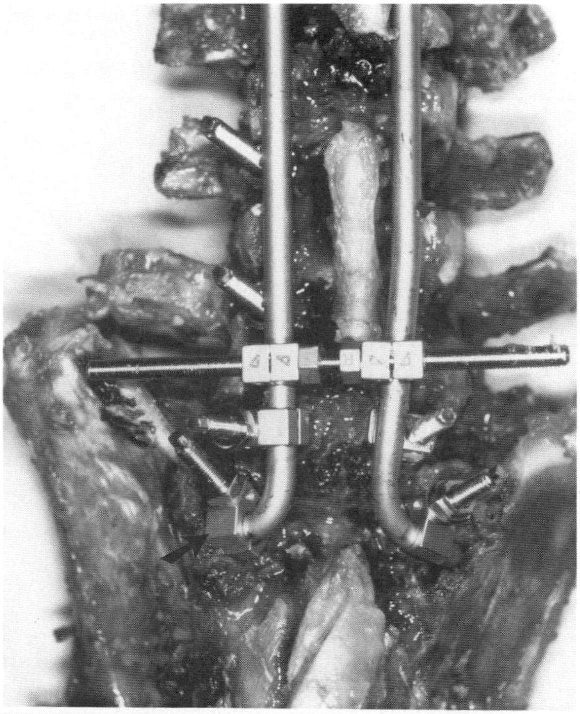

a

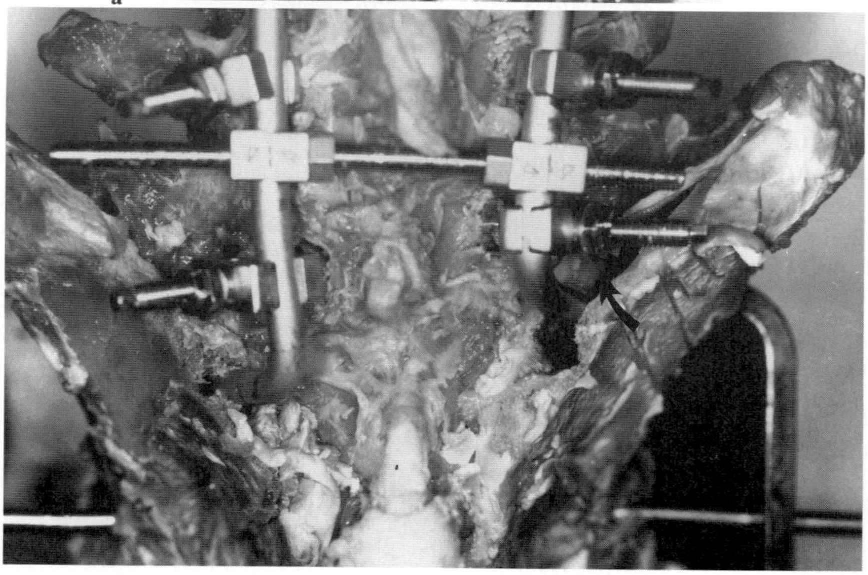

b

Fig. 7. **a** The Isola Galveston configuration (partially assembled) with 1/4-inch stainless steel rods imbedded between the iliac cortices and held by split connectors (*arrow*). **b** Iliac delamination (*arrow*) was noted with both Isola- and Galveston-type constructs. This resulted in early increased strain during failure and contributed to the increased percent strain per degree of angulation

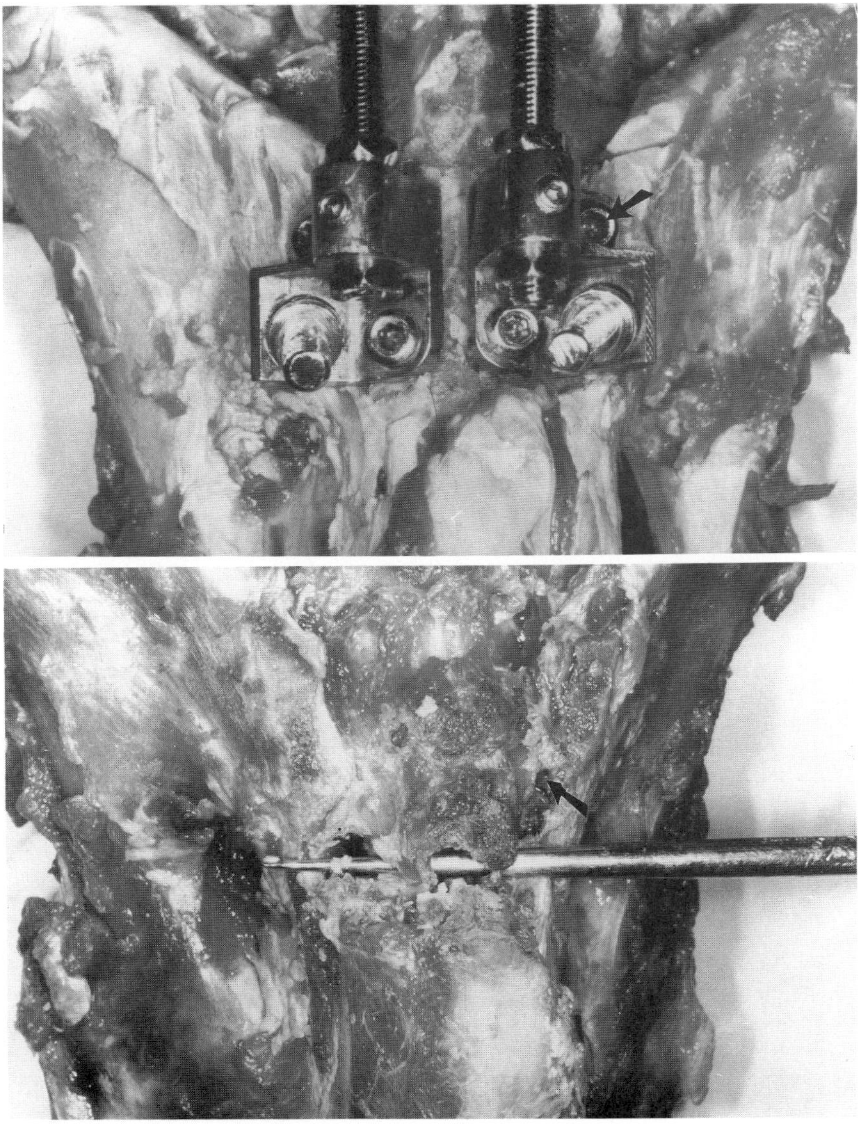

a

b

Fig. 8. **a** The Kirschner sacral plate construct demonstrates that the four caudal screws are placed in a linear fashion (iliac and S2). The iliac screw (6.5 mm × 40 mm) is laterally diverging as is the S2 screw. The S1 screw (*arrow*) is medially converging. **b** This shows the failed specimen following testing and hardware removal. A probe is inserted through a fracture site horizontally along the four iliac and S2 screw sites. Iliac delamination (*arrow*) also occurred at a relatively small load compared to the Isola Galveston and Isola iliac screw constructs which went more anterior to the middle osteoligamentous column

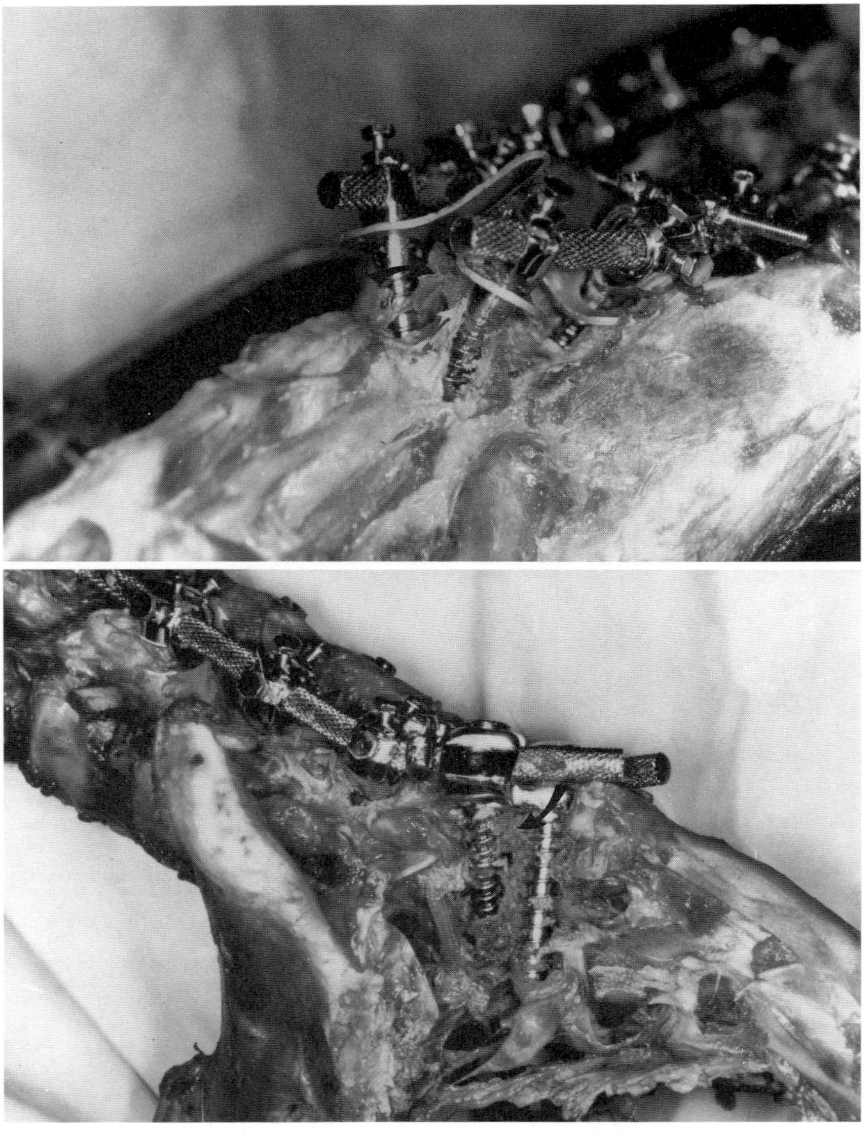

a

b

Fig. 9. **a** Failure of the C-D butterfly plate via fracture through the posterior bony arch (*arrow*) of S2 which propagated superiorly to the S1 screw. There is failure through the anterior cortex by screw pull out. **b** Failure of the C-D Chopin block, again, with fracture through the posterior aspect of the sacrum (*arrow*) from the S2 to the S1 screw and pull out from the anterior cortex.

Consequently, the increased area required for ultimate failure resulted in increased stiffnesss when compared to other non-iliac purchase constructs. The Isola S2 hook failed in five out of six constructs by simply pulling out of the S2 foramina with failure further noted at the S1 VSP screw. However, one construct obtained purchase and failed by fracture of the S2 lamina. As the dense cortical S2 lamina was the limiting point, this one construct tested much stiffer than the other five specimens. Indeed the remaining five specimens behaved almost identically to the Steffee plate which failed via S1 screw cut out in all modes tested.

The Harrington distraction rodded specimens demonstrated failure via sacral hook pull out while the Luque rectangular block failed by wire cut out through the S1 lamina.

The C-D iliosacral screw failed by fracturing superiorly through the ilium and distal to the iliosacral screw. Thus, the bone between this screw and the L6 pedicle screws remained intact (bypassing the area crossed by the extensometer) yielding a deceptively low strain reading.

Discussion

An optimal lumbosacral construct should be able to accept large loads before ultimately failing while maintaining strain within an optimum window between 2% and 10% [28,29,30]. Strain below 2% invokes device-related osteoporosis whereas strain above 10% leads to excessive instability. The two constructs which withstood the greatest load before ultimate failure were both constructs with iliac purchase. However, simple iliac purchase alone does not ensure enhanced stiffness over S2 purchase. Indeed, crossing the S1 joint with fixation is only biomechanically justified if the device obtains purchase of the iliac crest anterior to the middle osteoligamentous column (Fig. 10). This was supported by the statistically significant ($P < 0.05$) difference between groups 1 and 2 verses 4, 5, and 6 on both the maximum stiffness at failure and maximum moment at failure testing. The Kirschner sacral plate has outward iliac crest purchase also but the screw (Kirschner 40 mm versus 80 mm for the Isola iliac screw construct) did not cross far enough anterior to the middle column. The C-D Chopin block and C-D butterfly plate have S2 and S1 fixation, but lack iliac purchase.

Triangulation has been shown to significantly enhance load to pull out [31,32]. All pedicle and S1 screws were medially directed to ensure the maximum amount of triangulation which increases stability at the bone-metal interface. The iliac wing constructs included three outwardly divergent screw/rod constructs, the principal difference in purchase being anterior to the middle osteoligamentous column [33] for the Isola Galveston and Isola iliac screw constructs and shorter for the Kirschner sacral plate. The fourth construct which had iliac purchase was the C-D iliosacral screw. This screw is medially directed and purchase of the ilium and S1 is in linear fashion via a single screw as opposed

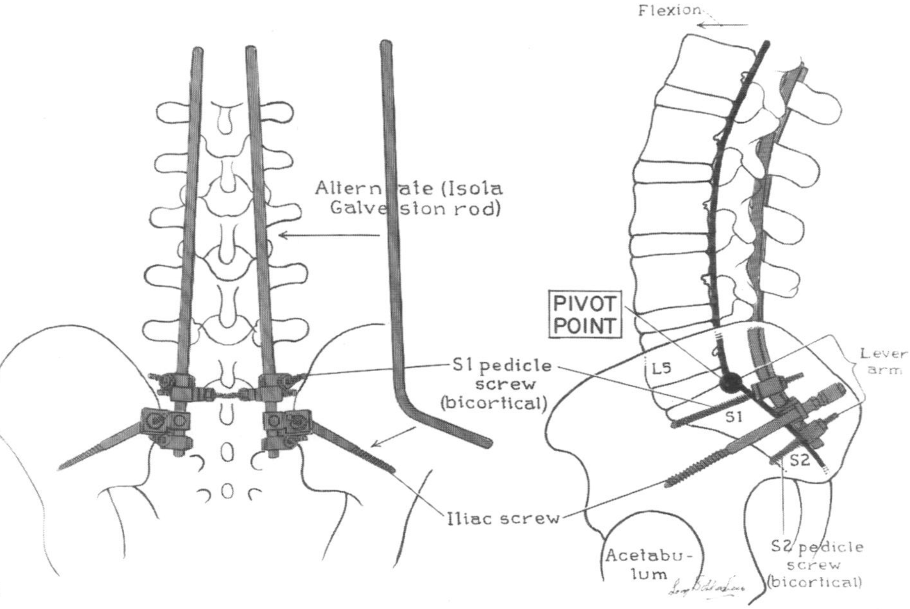
Flexion
Altern ate (Isola
Galve ston rod)
PIVOT POINT
S1 pedicle screw (bicortical)
Lever arm
L5
S1
S2
Iliac screw
Acetabu-lum
S2 pedicle screw (bicortical)

a

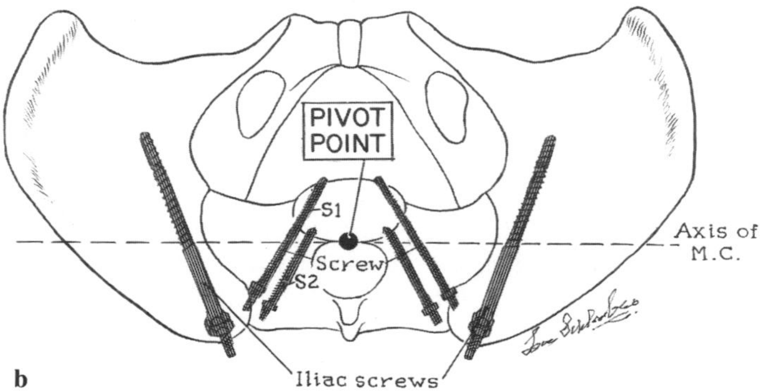
PIVOT POINT
S1
Screw
S2
Axis of M.C.
Iliac screws

b

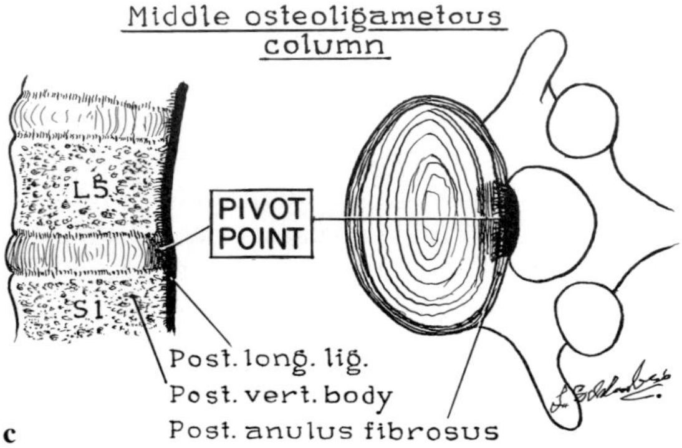
Middle osteoligametous column
L5
S1
PIVOT POINT
Post. long. lig.
Post. vert. body
Post. anulus fibrosus

c

to the Isola and Kirschner constructs which have outwardly deviated purchase of the ilium and medially deviated purchase of S1 (bilaterally triangulated). Consequently, the construct is triangulated only via medially convergent iliosacral screws. It lacks the separate triangulation on each side of the Galveston constructs and fails to cross anterior to the middle osteoligamentous column, thereby testing with less load to failure and stiffness.

Purchase of an S2 screw is more consistent than purchase of an S2 hook which is dependant on preload. Five of the six S2 hooks slipped out, leaving the only significant purchase point of this construct being a VSP S1 screw. Consequently, this tested essentially the same as the Steffee plate construct in all parameters measured. One construct, however, engaged and ultimately fractured the posterior sacral lamina. The maximum load at failure was 156.6 Nm with a stiffness of 8.4 Nm/° and a strain of 7.3%. This is comparable to the constructs comprising iliac purchase anterior to the middle column, thus demonstrating the strength of cortical S2 laminar purchase by a broad smooth hook when compared to the purchase of sacral screws. This may have some promise in future design as the constructs were designed and scaled for a human model and (as in this case) were sometimes prototypical.

There is a trend towards the idea that purchase of S2 with a screw increases stability as compared to an S1 screw alone. This is demonstrated by the statistically significant ($P < 0.05$) difference between groups 6 and 10 on the maximum stiffness at failure bar graph (Fig. 3). Purchase with an S2 screw greatly increases the area required for failure and consequently increases stiffness. The S2 hook construct, which engaged and ultimately fractured the S2 lamina, was even an order of magnitude stiffer and tolerated much greater loads to failure, suggesting that the cortical lamina in contact with a broad hook adds a certain desirable biomechanical depth when compared to screws alone.

Fig. 10. a Crossing the S1 joint is only biomechanically justified when fixation extends anterior to the projected image of the middle osteoligamentous column on the lateral radiograph. On the *left* is a coronal view of the Isola Galveston and Isola iliac screw constructs. Note the diverging iliac rods and screws between the inner and outer iliac cortices. The S1 screws converge medially in a triangular fashion. On the *right*, this sagittal view demonstrates the middle osteoligamentous column (*heavy black line*) and introduces the concept of a pivot point. The iliac screw goes a significant degree farther anteriorly towards the superior acetabular bone than bicortical S1 or S2 screws. (Note, this schematic depicts the human, not the calf, lumbosacral junction.) **b** A view of the pelvis looking distally. Note the iliac screws/rods are significantly farther anterior to the middle osteoligamentous column (*Axis of M.C.*). For illustrative purposes, the S2 screws are medially converging; however, they were placed laterally diverging for actual testing. **c** This illustration defines the biomechanical concept of the lumbosacral pivot point concerning lumbosacral instrumentation. It is the intersection point of the middle osteoligamentous column and the L5–S1 intervertebral disk

Strain was greatest for the two iliac purchase constructs which crossed the middle osteoligamentous column. However, these constructs showed early delamination, while accepting such a proportionally larger amount of load before failure, that ultimately they were the stiffest of all the constructs tested.

Comparing the percent strain per angulation at failure of each construct, gave good insight into the biomechanical properties of the lumbosacral fixation. The percent strain and angulation are not identical and, in fact, sometimes have little apparent correlation. The strain is determined across the caudal-most disk spaces while angulation is determined by the distal displacement (at 22 cm) required for failure, thereby calculating a theoretical angle at the lumbosacral junction. For any given flexural load, there will be stress, particularly at the caudal bone-metal interface. A construct with rigid fixation will have less strain and angulation for a given load. As the load increases significantly, however, the strain and angulation will likewise continue to increase. As the load increases, both the strain and angulation increase in similar fashion unless other factors occur which affect one or the other parameters. The Isola Galveston constructs demonstrate significantly ($P < 0.05$) higher percent strain per angulation in Fig. 6 which is explained by the early iliac delamination resulting in increased strain (Fig. 7). This was further enhanced by the slow increase in strain as the proportionately large load to failure was accepted. The Kirschner sacral plate, which also demonstrated iliac delamination, might have also shown increased strain and consequently higher percent strain per angulation, but it failed at a lower load across the linearly arranged caudal four screws. The C-D iliosacral screw demonstrated significantly ($P < 0.05$) low strain but relatively large angulation with a significantly ($P < 0.05$) small percent strain per angulation. This discrepancy is accounted for by the mode of failure, where the position of the screw fracture resulted in the bone between this screw and the L6 pedicle screws, remaining intact, thereby bypassing the extensometer (resulting in a deceptively low strain). The relative stiffness, however, is easily calculated by a load-displacement graph giving a more realistic picture of low stiffness.

As the remaining groups have no significant ($P < 0.05$) differences in percent strain per angulation, they are differentiated most strikingly by their respective load to failure (and further calculated stiffness) with the C-D Chopin block and C-D butterfly plate (group 2) being stiffer than ($P < 0.05$) the S1 fixation groups (group 3).

It remains for future clinical studies to determine the appropriate stiffness and flexion moments delineating between inadequacy and overkill. Furthermore, the ideal construct would balance fusion success and device-related osteoporosis. Nagel et al. [30] reported a strain of 10% led to solid fusion, whereas a 36% strain resulted in a pseudarthrosis in 87% of cases. At the moment, stiffer implants may be more appropriate in situations reducing and maintaining a significant correction, such as with neuromuscular scoliosis or reduction of a high grade spondylolisthesis.

Limitations of the Study

As with any in vitro study, there are certain limitations when extrapolating to a clinical situation. The most obvious perhaps is this analysis concerns only biomechanical properties immediately after surgery. The stiffness and strains will understandably be affected in the first 6 postoperative months as the fusion consolidates.

The second limitation of the study was that only one mode of biomechanical loading, flexion, was tested. This was felt to be the most clinically relevant parameter. The lumbosacral joint has more sagittal (flexion-extension) motion than any other segment in the lumbar spine. In addition, it has the least amount of lateral bending or axial rotation. Extension is limited due to facet joint orientation, leaving forward flexion as the most clinically relevant test mode [20].

Thirdly, the calf spine model was chosen due to interspecimen uniformity and adequate size. However, certain differences between this and the human model are obvious. The bovine spine has smaller vertebral width, six lumbar vertebrae, less pronounced lordosis, and relatively large transverse processes [21–23]. Due to these anatomical considerations, the transverse approximators were placed at L6–S1 instead of their location clinically which would be inferior to the S1 pedicle. All specimens were thawed and tested within 2 h after removal from the deep freezer. Moreover, biomechanical properties have been shown not to be significantly altered by this process [20].

Finally, each specimen was tested in a horizontal rather than vertical (weight bearing) position due to technical considerations. Each specimen was instrumented with pedicle screws for three levels (L4–L6) above the sacrum, except for the Harrington distraction rod, Luque rectangular block, and control. It is doubtful that upright weight bearing would have significantly affected the results.

Conclusion

The calf spine model is a good model for studying biomechanics of the lumbosacral junction. Flexion-extension strain and actual measurements are similar to the human model. Crossing the S1 joint is warranted only if the instrumentation crosses anterior to the middle osteoligamentous column. There is a pivot point near the junction of the middle osteoligamentous column and the L6–S1 disk space. Stiffness in flexion improves the further from this point the instrumentation extends. The importance of triangulation of pedicle screws in the sacrum cannot be overemphasized. The increased stiffness of a triangulated system bilaterally was also demonstrated when comparing the two Isola Galveston constructs and the C-D iliosacral screw.

The inherent difficulties in using an S2 hook were also demonstrated biomechanically. The stability is extremely variable and dependant on the distraction preload. Finally, two traditional methods of instrumentation, the Harrington distraction and Luque rectangular constructs, offer little resistance to strain, casting some doubt as to their clinical usefulness.

Acknowledgment. Supported in part by N.I.H. Grant AR38489 and an OREF Career Development Award

References

1. Boucher HH (1959) A method of spinal fusion. J Bone Joint Surg [Br] 41:248
2. Cleveland M, Bosworth DM, Thompson FR (1948) Pseudarthrosis in the lumbosacral spine. J Bone Joint Surg [Am] 30:302
3. Jacobs RR, Saunders EA, Sabatelle PE (1974) Posterolateral spine fusion with and without nerve root decompression: A primary procedure for low back pain. South Med J 67:177
4. King D (1944) Internal fixation for lumbosacral fusion. Am J Surg 66:357
5. King D (1948) Internal fixation for lumbosacral spine fusions. J Bone Joint Surg [Am] 30:560
6. Kornblatt MD, Casey MP, Jacobs RR (1986) Internal fixation of the lumbosacral spine fusion. A biomechanical and clinical study. Clin Orthop 293:141–150
7. Louis R (1986) Fusion of the lumbar and sacral spine by internal fixation with screw plates. Clin Orthop 203:18
8. MacNab I, Dall D (1971) The blood supply of the lumbar spine and its application to the technique of intertransverse lumbar fusion. J Bone Joint Surg [Br] 53:628
9. Shaw EG, Taylor JG (1956) Results of lumbosacral fusion for low back pain. J Bone Joint Surg [Br] 38:485
10. Stauffer RN, Coventry MB (1972) Posterolateral lumbar spine fusion; Analysis of Mayo Clinic series. J Bone Joint Surg [Am] 54:1195
11. Watkins MB (1959) Posterolateral bone grafting for fusion of the lumbar and lumbosacral spine. J Bone Joint Surg [Am] 41:388
12. Shirato O, Zdeblick TA, McAfee PC, Warden KE (1991) Biomechanical evaluation of methods of posterior stabilization of the spine and posterior lumbar interbody arthrodesis for lumbosacral isthmic spondylolisthesis. A calf-spine model. J Bone Joint Surg [Am] 73:518–526
13. Hibbs RA (1924) A report of 59 cases of scoliosis treated by a fusion operation. J Bone Joint Surg 6:3–37N
14. Albee FH (1911) Transplantation of a portion of the tibia into the spine for Pott's disease. A preliminary report. J Am Med Assoc 57:885–886
15. Brunski JB, Hill DC, Meskowitz A (1983) Stresses in a Harrington distraction rod: Their origin and relationship to fatigue fractures in vivo. J Biomech Eng 105: 101–107
16. McAfee PC (1985) Biomechanical approach to instrumentation of thoracolumbar spine: A review article. Adv Orthop Surg 8:313–327
17. Ogilvie JW, Bradford DS (1984) Lumbar and lumbosacral fusion with segmental fixation. Annual Meeting of the Scoliosis Research Society, Orlando, Florida, September

18. Panjabi MM, Goel VR, Takita K (1982) Physiologic strains in the lumbar spinal ligaments. An in vitro biomechanical study. Spine 7:192–203
19. Puno RM, Beechtold JE, Byrd JA, Winter RB, Ogilvie JW, Bradford DS (1987) Biomechanical analysis of five techniques of fixation for the lumbosacral joint. Orthopaedic Research Society, San Francisco, California, January
20. White AA, Panjabi MM (1990) Clinical biomechanics of the spine, 2nd edn. Lippincott, Philadelphia
21. Cotterill PC, Kostuik JP, D'Angelo G, Fernie GR, Maki BE (1986) An anatomical comparison of the human and bovine thoracolumbar spine. J Orthop Res 4: 298–303
22. Gurr KR, McAfee PC, Shih CM (1988) Biomechanical analysis of anterior and posterior instrumentation systems following corpectomy. A calf spine model. J Bone Joint Surg [Am] 70:1182–1191
23. Gurr KR, McAfee PC, Shih CM (1988) Biomechanical analysis of posterior instrumentation systems following decompressive laminectomy. An unstable calf spine model. J Bone Joint Surg [Am] 70:680–691
24. Lachin JM (1981) Introduction to sample size determination and power analysis for clinical trials. Controlled Clin Trials 2:93–113
25. Steel RGD, Tobble JH (1980) Principles and procedures of statistics. A biomechanical approach, 2nd edn. McGraw-Hill, New York
26. Allen B, Ferguson R (1984) The Galveston technique of pelvic fixation Luque rod instrumentation of spine. Spine 9:388
27. Luque ER (1982) The anatomic basis and development of segmental spinal instrumentation. Spine 7:256
28. Edwards WT (1990) Spine Stabilization – How Much is Enough PhD thesis, NASS Monterey, CA
29. McAfee PC, Farey ID, Sutterlin CE, Gurr KR, Warden KE, Cunningham BW (1989) Device-related osteoporosis with spinal instrumentation. 1989 VOLVO AWARD in Basic Science. Spine 14:919–926
30. Nagel DA, Kramers PC, Rahn BA, Cordey J, Perren SM (1991) A paradigm of delayed union and nonunion in the lumbosacral joint. Spine 16:553–559
31. Coe JD, Warden KE, Herzig MA, McAfee PC (1989) Load to failure strength of spinal implants in osteoporotic spines. A comparison study of pedicle screws, laminar hooks, and spinous process wires. Orthopaedic Transactions (from ORS 1989)
32. Ruland CM, McAfee PC (in press) Triangulation of pedicular instrumentation–Biomechanical analysis. Spine
33. Denis F (1984) Spinal instability as defined by the three column spine concept in acute spinal traumas. Clin Orthop 189:65–76

4.2 Comparative Study of Three Pedicle Screw Devices

Reinhard Steffen[1], Lutz-Peter Nolte[2], and Jürgen Krämer[1]

Introduction

There are a wide variety of indications for lumbar fusion in orthopedic and traumatic surgery. Lehmann et al. reported that the incidence of lower lumbar fusions for orthopedic diseases in the United States doubled between 1979 and 1983 [1]. In the field of trauma surgery of the spine, various authors have described the advantages of operative treatmet of compression and burst fractures over conservative non-operative treatment [2–4]. Considerations as to whether internal fixation devices are necessary differ depending on the trauma or orthopedic indications. Operative treatment of thoracolumbar fractures requires internal stabilization to maintain position and reduce the load on the anterior and middle column of the spine until the fracture has healed, irrespective of the necessity of simultaneous posterolateral fusion [4]. Lower lumbar or lumbosacral fusions in orthopedic cases are generally performed as *in situ* fusions except in cases of spondylolisthesis where some authors recommend reposition so only stability is required to support the bone fusion. The main problem of lumbar fusion is the considerably high rate of pseudarthrosis, that ranges between 18% and 49% depending on the number of fused segments and the kind of fusion (posterolateral or interbody) [5]. Various authors support the assumption that the rate of pseudarthrosis can be reduced by the use of an internal fixation device [5]. This could be explained by the relatively effective stabilization provided by an internal fixation as against the insufficient effect of external bracing. Animal studies have shown that the stability of bony fusion could be improved by the use of an implant [6,7]. Thus the main reason for the use of an internal fixation device in orthopedic cases is the internal stability provided. In addition the implant allows compression of the anterior bone graft

[1] Department of Orthopaedic Surgery, St. Josef Hospital, Ruhr University Bochum, Gudrunstr. 56, D-W-4630 Bochum, Germany
[2] Bioengineering Center, Wayne State University, 818 W. Hancock, Detroit, MI 48202, USA

in combined anterior and posterior fusions [8]. These requirements are met by the so-called fixateur interne first described by Dick [3]. The easy handling of this system led to the development of a number of devices along the same lines that differ in pedicle screw design, type of distraction rod, and connection of the two. In view of this Panjabi has suggested for the evaluation of spinal fixation devices that they should first be evaluated biomechanically in a standardized procedure to compare their effectiveness [9,10]. He distinguished strength, fatigue, and stability tests. Assuming that the strength and fatigue characteristics had been sufficiently evaluated and that these had been declared by the manufacturers, we performed a comparative in vitro stability study of three different fixateur interne devices. Although several internal fixation devices have been tested by various authors [3,11–19], there are considerable difficulties in comparing the results of these studies: different testing machines were used, different loads were applied, and different kinds of spine models and injury models were used in combination with or without simulated fusions.

This study follows Panjabi's proposals [9] and considerations by Wittenberg et al. [20] concerning the influence of bone mineral density. In a three-dimensional in vitro model the stability provided by the various devices was determined.

Material and Methods

Besides the two fixateur interne systems established on the European market (AO-Synthes, Bochum; Kluger-Endotec, Leverkusen), the new SOCON fixateur (Aesculap, Tuttlingen) was investigated. All the systems are described as constrained and fulfill the demands of Wörsdörfer for the treatment of thoracolumbar fractures [19]. Each system consists of two pedicle screws and an adjusted distraction rod which can be fastened to one another at different angles. In clinical practice the devices are applied dorsally on both sides of a two- or multi-segmental part of the thoracolumbar spine. The screws are placed transpedicularly in the vertebral body as first described by Roy-Camille [21]. The AO fixateur consists of 5-mm Schanz screws with a short, flat thread, ribbed distraction rods, and clamps which can be adjusted and freely moved. The SOCON fixateur uses a 6-mm pedicle screw with an increasing cone diameter, a deep thread, and a similar distraction rod and clamp system. In contrast the Kluger fixateur has a 6-mm pedicle screw with a shallow thread and a specially developed telescopic distraction system which can be directly fixed to the pedicle screw (Fig. 1).

Eighteen fresh human cadaveric spines from the level L3–L5 were harvested from donors with a mean age of 43 years and stored at −24°C. The day before testing the specimen was thawed at room temperature and all the soft tissue was carefully dissected leaving the ligamentous and osseous structures intact. Bone mineral density was quantified using dual photon absorptiometry (HOLOGIC QDR-100, lumbar spine version 4.20) and X ray control (anteroposterior

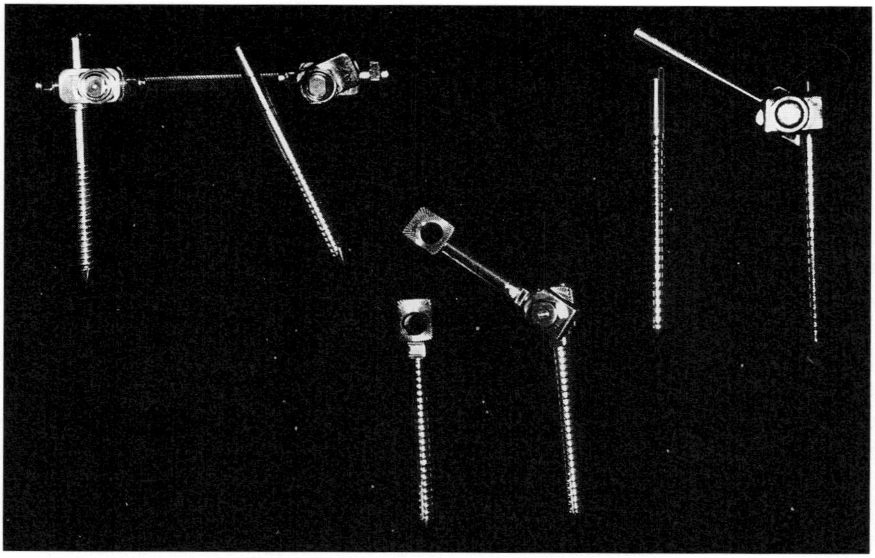

Fig. 1. The applied internal fixateurs. From left to right: Dick Fixateur (AO), Kluger Fixateur (Endotec), SOCON Fixateur (Aesculap)

and lateral) was performed for all the specimens. Both upper (L3) and lower (L5) vertebra were embedded in an epoxy block to provide fixation to the test table and the loading/measuring unit. The specimens were aligned with the help of an electronic correction device to set up a clinical coordinate system with an XZ plane perpendicular to the Y direction, formed as the intersection of the centres of L3 and L5.

The specimens were divided into three comparable groups after standardized preparation, determination of the bone mineral density, and biomechanical testing of the intact specimens. The specimens of each group were provided with one of the fixateur interne systems. The following conservative loads were applied incrementally in combination with a small stabilizing preload of 40 N: (a) axial compression ($-FY = 0 - 1{,}000\,N$), (b) flexion/extension ($\pm MX = 0 - 7.5\,Nm$), (c) lateral bending ($\pm MZ = 0 - 7.5\,Nm$), and (d) axial torsion ($\pm MY = 0 - 10\,Nm$). Special care was taken to minimize viscoelastic effects during the experiment. The resulting three-dimensional motion of the upper (L3) vertebra was measured using electronic displacement transducers and computer data acquisition equipment. From the resulting discrete load displacement paths the following clinically related parameters were studied: (a) range of motion (ROM), (b) neutral zone (NZ), both (a) and (b) according to the definition by Panjabi et al. [22], (c) strain energy, and (d) the center of rotation.

Table 1. Stabilizing capacity of an implant.

$$\frac{M\ (\mathrm{Sumrom}\ I)_i - M\ (\mathrm{Sumrom}\ F)_i}{M\ (\mathrm{Sumrom}\ I)_a}$$

M, mean value; I, intact without instrumentation; F, intact with instrumentation; i, individual subgroup, i.e., AO, Kluger, SOCON; a, total.

The specimens were investigated in the following groups: (1) intact, (2) intact with one of the internal fixateurs applied, and (3) after corpectomy (only in the SOCON group). In addition, the influence of transverse connectors was analyzed in selected cases of the SOCON group. For quantitative comparison of the various devices independent of the basic characteristics of the specimen, a new relative stabilizing capacity was defined (Table 1).

Results

The average bone mineral density of all specimens was 0.849 as measured against a 20-year-old control group. There was no difference between the three sub-groups. There was no occurence of osteoporosis.

Typical load displacement curves of a single specimen are shown in Fig. 2. The loads are marked on the horizontal axis and the resulting dominant deformations are marked on the vertical axis. Thus the shape of the path demonstrates clearly the stabilizing effect of the chosen internal fixation device. In all three dimensions of movement the intact specimens demonstrated a non-linear shaped path with decreasing deformation under increasing load. In contrast to this, after application of the internal fixateur, the path became linear, i.e., the deformation showed a constant correlation to the applied load. Under smaller loads the intersegmental stiffness of the specimens with applied devices was between 15 and 50 times higher than that of the non-instrumented specimens. Under maximum loading there was no great divergence in the degree of stiffness. Assuming a non-linear behaviour of the enclosed intervertebral disks and the ligamentous structures, the results suggested that the deformation after instrumentation was due to a certain deformation in the interface pedicle screw bone and in the implant itself.

Another parameter of clinical relevance is the deformation energy, i.e., the energy that is necessary to produce an equal deformation with and without instrumentation. The increase of the deformation energy after application of an internal fixateur was at most 13 times higher in flexion/extension and lateral bending and 3 times higher under axial torsion. The flexibility of the intact non-instrumented specimens is shown in Fig. 3. The values are given as the mean of the sum range of motion (SUMROM) for the three dimensions of movement. With the exception of some deviations under axial torsion, all the

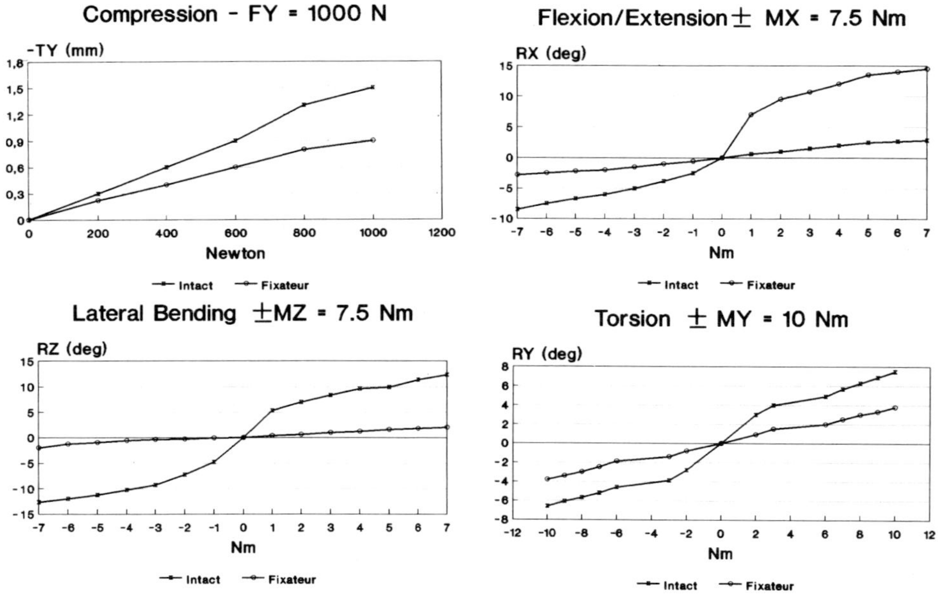

Fig. 2. Load displacement curves of a single specimen L3–L5 with and without instrumentation (SOCON). Applied loads: *FY*, force on y axis; *MX*, moment on x axis; *MY*, moment on y axis; *MZ*, moment on z axis. Resulting deformation: *TY*, axial compression; *RX*, flexion/extension; *RZ*, lateral bending; *RY*, axial rotation

sub-groups of specimens demonstrated similar behaviour of load-dependent deformation.

After application of the various internal fixateurs, a similar reduction of flexibility expressed as SUMROM for the different dimensions of movement was recorded (Fig. 4). The results demonstrated for the investigated fixation devices nearly the same decrease of SUMROM flexion/extension and lateral bending from 20° to 4°. The effectivity of instrumentation was considerably lower under axial torsion with a decrease from 10° to 5°. Further analysis of the data demonstrated that the stability provided by the fixation device depends on the original degree of flexibility of the specimen. To enable a reliable comparison of the three investigated devices we had to eliminate the above mentioned discrepancy as far as possible. Therefore we developed the normalization process described in Table 1. In contrast to the formula described by Panjabi et al. [10], we took into consideration the possible discrepancies in the basic characteristics of the sub-groups and introduced the mean values of all investigated specimens. The newly defined stabilizing capacity for the three investigated internal fixateurs is demonstrated in Fig. 5 for the various dimensions of movement. Once again a distinct decrease in stabilizing effectivity for axial torsion was established.

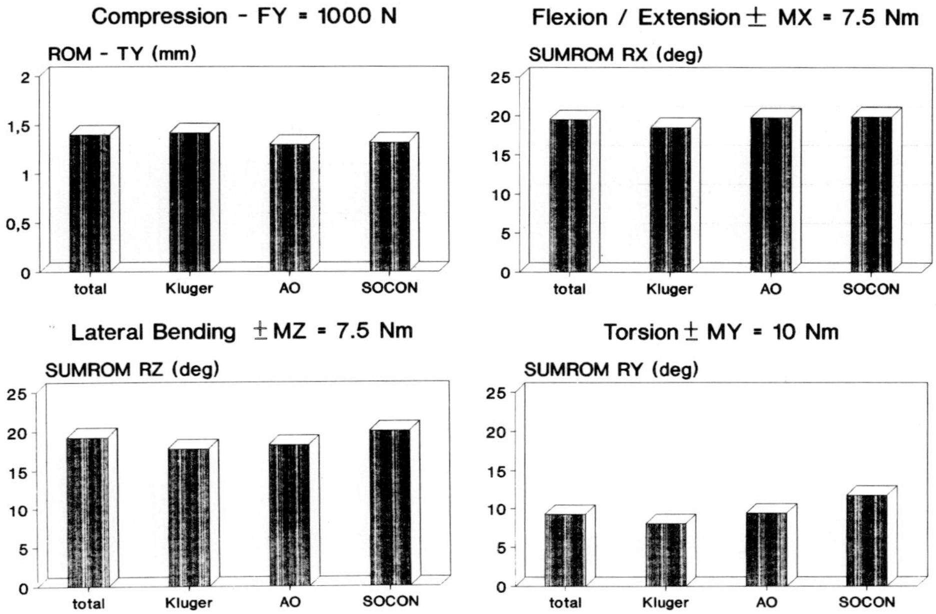

Fig. 3. Biomechanical characteristics of the specimens intact without internal fixateur. *ROM*, ranger of motion

Further investigation for the clinical effectivity of the internal fixation devices in the treatment of thoracolumbar fractures was carried out on a corpectomy model. This was carried out on three specimens with the SOCON internal fixateur. The corpectomy simulated a severe instability in the anterior and middle column of the spine. The following test procedure demonstrated a considerable decrease in instability compared with the specimen with instrumentation but without injury. Nevertheless the resulting flexibility expressed in SUMROM did not exceed the values of the intact non-instrumented segments.

The additional application of a transverse connector after corpectomy provided only a minimal increase in stability for lateral bending and axial torsion of less than 5%. In contrast, the increase in stability due to the transverse connector was about 15% for torsion before the corpectomy was performed. In a case of a single artificial screw loosening in combination with a corpectomy, a severe decrease of stability was seen which could not be reduced by the additional use of the transverse connector.

Discussion

The described in vitro investigation of three different internal fixateurs is based on 18 bisegmental lumbar specimens from the level L3–L5. All specimens with

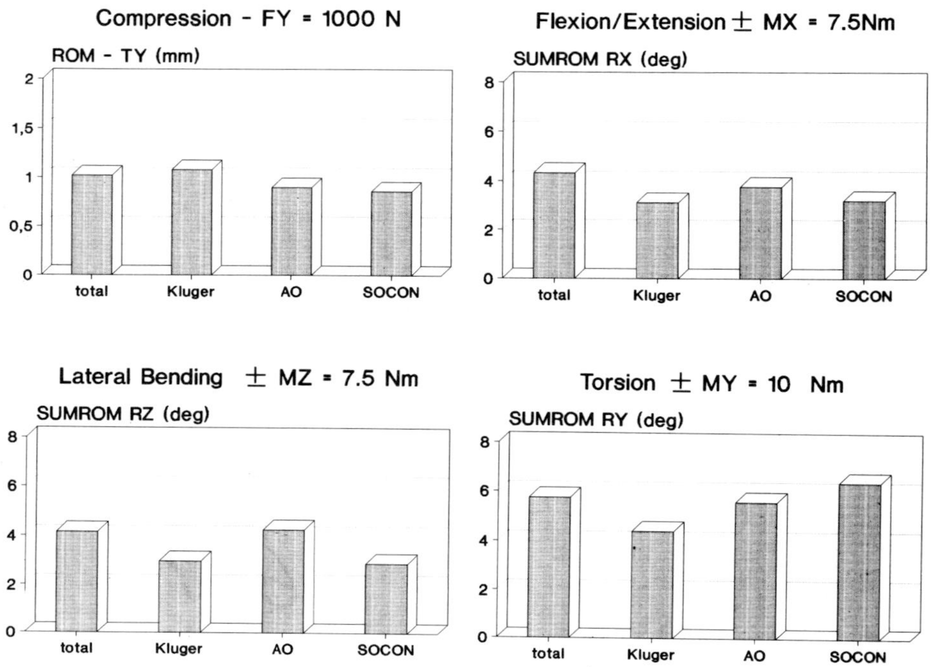

Fig. 4. Biomechanical characteristics of the specimens intact with different internal fixateurs

a mean age of 43 years showed regular bone mineral density and no osteoporosis. Thus the results are comparable with no detectable influence of differing bone quality [20]. In addition, the basic biomechanical parameters of the chosen sub-groups demonstrated a comparable picture. After the application of the various devices the specimens were investigated without additional injury to establish the expected in vivo effects in orthopedic cases, i.e., without severe degrees of instability. All the investigated systems provided almost the same degree of stabilization with a distinct weakness under axial torsion. The newly defined stabilizing capacity made it possible to minimize different basic characteristics of the individual specimen. The so-called physiological loads applied are comparable to the loads measured in an in vivo experimental set-up by Wörsdörfer [19]. It should therefore be possible to apply measured parameters to the expected effects in clinical use. The determined linear deformation behaviour of the specimens after instrumentation was comparable to results by Panjabi et al. [10]. They established a linear or slightly non-linear behaviour in the load displacement graph. In addition, the results correspond to the investigations of Mann et al. [23] who described a bisegmental deformation of 8° under a load of Mx = 10 Nm for the intact specimen. After bisegmental

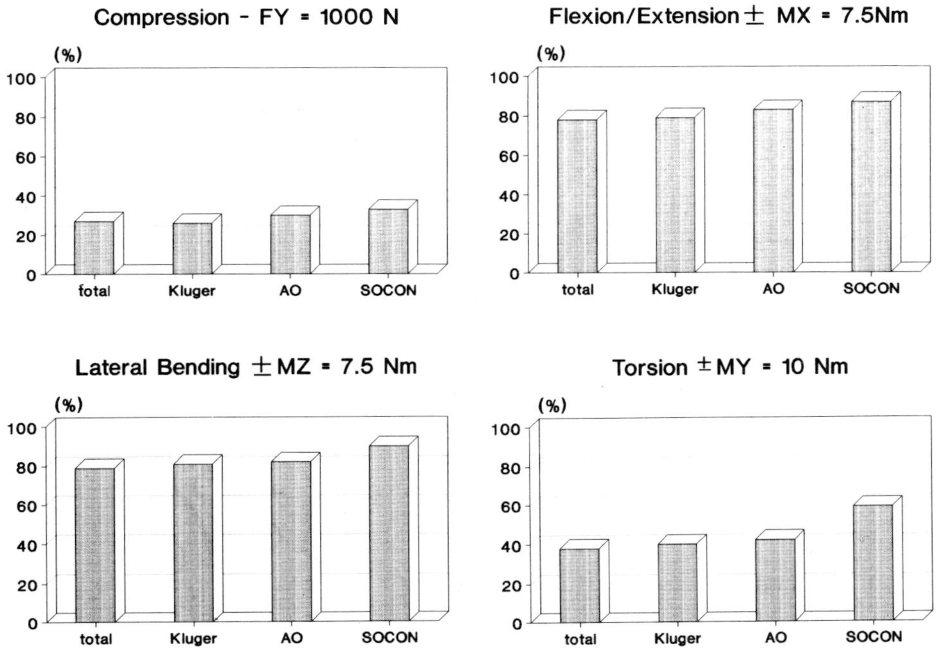

Fig. 5. Stabilizing capacity of the various internal fixateurs under different loads

application of the AO fixateur and additional injury performed as a transsection of the vertebral body, the deformation inflexion was reduced to 2.5°.

The in vitro flexibility for flexion and extension measured at L3–L5 with a bisegmentally adjusted AO fixateur was 3.8° (SUMROM) under a maximum load of MX = 7.5 Nm in contrast to the findings of Dick [3] who described a flexion of 0.9° for a bisegmentally adjusted AO fixateur under a load of 10 Nm. This discrepancy can be accounted for by the different test machines used and the various methods of load application and deformation measurement. The injury model of corpectomy confirms the capacity of the investigated internal fixation devices in the treatment of thoracolumbar fractures. However, the results of testing procedures under cyclic loads [18] have demonstrated a certain failure rate of the implant by screw or rod breakage between 60,000 and 90,000 load cycles. Another failure mode is described by Goel et al. [24], who, in a finite element model, established a stress shielding along the pedicle screw in the vertebral body and deduced the risk of screw loosening. These investigations suggest implant failure after a certain period of time and lead to the conclusion that we have to protect the internal fixation device in in vivo use from uncontrolled strain and movement during the period of fracture healing or consolidation of spinal fusion. Under particular consideration of our findings, it becomes clear that extensive loads for compression and axial torsion conceal the highest risk of implant failure. For further clinical use of an internal fixateur we recognized that it is necessary to apply a brace for the first 4 months after operation.

References

1. Lehmann TR, Spratt KF, Tozzi JE, Weinstein JN, Reinarz SJ, El-Khoury GY, Colby H (1987) Long-term follow-up of lower lumbar fusion patients. Spine 12: 97–104
2. Denis F (1983) The three column spine and its significance in the classification of acute thoracolumbar spinal injuries. Spine 8:817–831
3. Dick W (1984) Innere Fixation von Brust- und Lendenwirbelfrakturen. Aktuelle Probleme in Chirurgie und Orthopädie Bd. 28. Huber, Bern
4. Jacobs RR, Casey MP (1984) Surgical management of thoracolumbar spinal injuries. Clin Orthop 189:22–35
5. Kozak JA, O'Brien JP (1990) Simultaneous combined anterior and posterior interbody fusion. Spine 15:322–328
6. Johnston II CE, Asham RB, Corin JD, Welch RD (1989) Effect of spinal construct stiffness on early fusion mass incorporation. Trans Ann Meet Orthop Res Soc 14:364
7. McAffee PC, Farey ID, Sutterlin CE, Gurr KR, Warden KE, Cunningham BW (1991) The effect of spinal implant rigidity on vertebral bone density: A canine model. Spine 16:190–197
8. Krödel A, Refior H, Plitz W (1991) Biomechanical basis of compressive ventral interbody fusion. Abstracts of the 18th Annual Meeting ISSLS, Heidelberg, 12–16 May, p 29
9. Panjabi MM (1988) Biomechanical evaluation of spinal fixation devices. I. A conceptual framework. Spine 13:1129–1134
10. Panjabi MM, Abumi K, Duranceau J, Crisco JJ (1988) Biomechanical evaluation of spinal fixation devices. II. Stability provided by eight internal fixation devices. Spine 13:1135–1140
11. Abumi K, Panjabi MM, Duranceau J (1989) Biomechanical evaluation of spinal fixation devices. III. Stability provided by six spinal fixation devices and interbody bone graft. Spine 14:1249–1255
12. Ashman RB, Birch JG, Bone LB, et al. (1988) Mechanical testing of spinal instrumentation. Clin Orthop 227:113–125
13. Ferguson RL, Tencer AF, Woodard P, Allen BL (1988) Biomechanical comparisons of spinal fracture models and stabilizing effects of posterior instrumentations. Spine 13:453–460
14. Goel VK, Nye TA, Clark CR, Nishiyama K, Weinstein JN (1987) A technique to evaluate an internal device by use of the selspot system. Spine 12:150–159
15. Gurr KR, McAffee PC, Shih CM (1988) Biomechanical analysis of posterior instrumentation systems after decompressive laminectomy: An unstable calf spine model. J Bone Joint Surg [Am] 70:680–691
16. Gurr KR, McAffee PC, Shih CM (1988) Biomechanical analysis of anterior and posterior instrumentation systems after corpectomy: A calf spine model. J Bone Joint Surg [Am] 70:1182–1191

17. Krag MH, Beynnon BD, Pope MH, et al. (1986) An internal fixateur for posterior application to short segments of thoracic, lumbar, or lumbosacral spine: Design and testing. Clin Orthop 203:75–98
18. Wittenberg RH, Coffee MS, Edwards WT, White AA (1990) Zyklische Belastungstests verschiedener Wirbelsäulenimplantate. Hefte zur Unfallheilkunde 212: 528–529
19. Wörsdörfer O (1981) Operative Stabilisierung der thorakolumbalen und lumbalen Wirbelsäule: Vergleichende biomechanische Untersuchungen zur Stabilität und Steifigkeit verschiedener dorsaler Fixationssysteme. Thesis, Klinisch-Medizinische Fakultät, Ulm
20. Wittenberg RH, Shea M, Swartz DE, Lee KS, White AA, Hayes WC (1991) Importance of bone mineral density in instrumented spine fusions. Spine 16: 647–652
21. Roy-Camille R, Saillant G, Berteaux D, Salgado V (1976) Osteosynthesis of thoracolumbar spine fractures with metal plates screwed through the vertebral pedicles. Reconstr Surg Traumatol 15:2–16
22. Panjabi MM, Goel VK, Takata K (1982) Physiological strains in lumbar spinal ligaments. Spine 7:192–201
23. Mann KA, McGowan DP, Fredrickson BE, Falahee M, Yuan HA (1990) A biomechanical investigation of short segment spinal fixation for burst fractures with varying degrees of posterior disruption. Spine 15:470–478
24. Goel VK, Kim YE, Lim TH, Weinstein JN (1989) Mechanics of load transfer across a spinal fixation device. Trans Ann Meet Orthop Res Soc 14:363

4.3 Biomechanical Study of Pedicle Screw Fixation Systems for the Lumbar Spine

Masatsune Yamagata, Hiroshi Kitahara, Shohei Minami, Kazuhisa Takahashi, Hideshige Moriya[1], and Tamotsu Tamaki[2]

Introduction

Since the pedicle screw system has a strong reduction force and a stabilization effect on unstable conditions of the spine, it is used not only in cases of spinal injury [1–5] but also for spondylolisthesis, spinal canal stenosis, total vertebral replacement, and other segmental instabilities [6–12]. At present, various types of pedicle screws which have different mechanical properties have been developed and applied in many cases [10,12–20]. However, complications of pedicle screw fixation have been reported in a variety of different applications [2,4,12,21–24]. These complications include the spinal implant failures whose incidence is higher than that of other orthopedic implants [22].

In general, pedicle screw fixation of the spine serves two main purposes: correction and stabilization. The component factors determining the biomechanical strength of a pedicle screw fixation technique include the strength of the screw itself, the strength of the screw system, the strength of the bone and the binding strength between the screw and bone.

The purpose of this study was to compare the mechanical strengths of these different kinds of pedicle screw systems, and also to determine the ideal indication of pedicle screw systems from the biomechanical viewpoint. To evaluate each factor independently, four mechanical tests were performed: a fatigue test to evaluate the screw, a three-points bending test for rods and plates, a bending test for the connection between the rods and screws, and a compression and torsional test for the pedicle screw system.

[1] Department of Orthopaedic Surgery, School of Medicine, Chiba University, 1-8-1 Inohana, Chuo-ku, Chiba, 260 Japan
[2] Department of Mechanical Engineering, Nippon Institute of Technology, 4-1 Gakuendai, Miyashiro, Saitama, Japan

Table 1. Dimensions of pedicle screws for fatigue tests.

Screw	Minor diameter (mm)	Major diameter (mm)	Thread pitch (mm)
AO cortex screw	3.2	4.5	1.78
AO cancellous screw	3.2	6.5	2.78
Zielke screw	3.6	6.0	3.04
Tapered screw	3.9–5.0	6.0	2.03
Schanz screw	3.9	5.0	1.76
Diapason L	3.0–5.0	4.9–6.6	1.80
Diapason S	3.5–6.6	5.1–7.9	1.80

Materials and Methods

The fatigue strengths of different screw designs were investigated to evaluate the fatigue strengths of the screws themselves. The screws tested were the AO-cortex screw (OR-214-55), the Schanz screw, and the AO-cancellous screw (AO-218-55) (Robert Mathys, Bettlach, Switzerland), the Zielke screw (Heinrich C. Ulrich, Ulmdonau, Germany), the Diapason screw (L, S) (Dimso, Cestas, France), and the Tapered screw (Tanaka Medical Instrument Manufacturing, Tokyo) which was developed by ourselves and which has been used clinically since 1986. The design of each screw is shown in Table 1. The minor diameter of the Schanz and the Tapered screw is 3.9 mm, which is the maximum of the screws tested. The minor diameter of the Tapered screw tapers from 3.9 to 5.0 mm. The Diapason screws are made of titanium-6Al-4V and both minor and major diameters taper. The minor diameter of the Diapason S screw tapers from 3.5 to 6.6 mm.

The testing machine used was a universal fatigue testing machine (Shimadzu-UF-15 Shimadzu, Kyoto) which could apply pure bending moment at the center point of the test specimens using supports at two points and a two-point loading system. The loading span was 30 mm and each screw was loaded cyclically at 1,000 times/min until failure or until 5 million cycles (infinite life) were reached. Eight different sinusoidal loads of 0, 40, 60, 80, 100, 150, 500, 1,000 and 2,000 N were applied to each screw and the pure bending moment was calculated. The number of loading cycles required to cause a failure was recorded. Using different bending moment levels, the resulting data was plotted as a stress cycle diagram (SN curve).

The three-points bending test of the rods and plates was performed to measure the stiffness and the yield strength of these screw systems. The rods tested were the Diapason rod (Dimso, Cestas, France), the AO-ISSF rod, the Modified Zielke rod (Tanaka Medical Instrument Manufacturing, Tokyo), and the CD rod. The plates tested were the VSP plate (AcroMed, Cleveland, Ohio), the Luque II plate (Danek Medical, Memphis, Tenn), and the Chiba-type plate (Tanaka Medical Instrument Manufacturing, Tokyo). The dimensions of each rod and plate are shown in Table 2. Three sizes of SUS316L

Table 2. Dimensions of rods and plates for bending strength tests. All units are mm.

Rods	Diameter	Outer diameter	Thickness of cut surface
1. Luque rod	5.00		
2. Chiba solid rod	6.00		
3. Chiba solid rod L	7.00		
4. Diapason (titanium)	6.00		
5. AO-ISSF rod	6.00	6.80	5.00
6. Modified Zielke rod	4.00	4.90	
7. CD rod	6.80		
Plates	**Thickness**	**Width**	**Width of slit**
1. Steffee VSP plate	4.70	12.60	5.10
2. Luque II plate	4.90	12.70	6.70
3. Plate-screw (Chiba)	2.90	10.40	5.00

stainless steel were also tested as controls. The rods were placed on the universal testing machine (Shimadzu DCS2000) and a load was applied to the center of the rods and plates at 3 mm/min with a 30-mm loading span. The load deformation curves were recorded on an X-Y plotter and the stiffness and the yield strength were determined.

The bending strength test was performed to measure the strength of the screw connection. A longitudinal load was applied to the screws. The moment arm between the point of application of the load and the axis of the rod was 30 mm.

For the mechanical test of the pedicle screw systems, six different pedicle screw systems were selected. The systems were the AO Fixator Interne system (Robert Mathys, Bettlach Switzerland), the VSP Steffee plate system, the Luque II system, the modified Zielke system, the Diapason system and the Chiba-type plate screw system (experimental device). Each type of pedicle screw system was applied to lumbar models made from the polyester resin rigolac (Showa Highpolymer, Tokyo) with one motion segment from L4 to L5. The models were embedded in loading fixtures of a universal testing machine and compression loads were applied. The compression load was applied at the anterior edge of the vertebral body (eccentric compressive load) at a load rate of 3 mm/min. The torsional load was applied at a load rate of 10.8°/min. The compressive and torsional stiffness were obtained from the load-deformation curves of each pedicle screw system.

Results

Fatigue Test for Screws

The fatigue data for the screws tested is presented in Fig. 1. Calculation of the pure bending moment showed that the endurance limits of the AO cortex

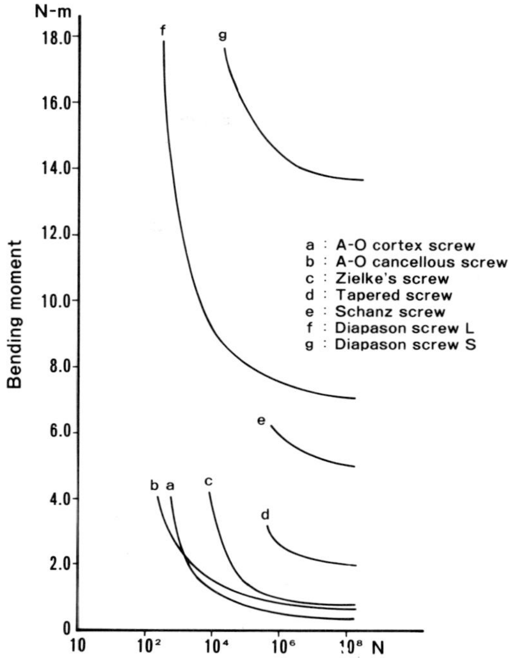

Fig. 1. Results of fatigue tests of pedicle screws

screw, the cancellous screw, and the Zielke screw were less than 1.0 Nm. The endurance limits of the Tapered screw, the Schanz screw, and the Diapason screw L were respectively 2.0 Nm, 5.5 Nm, and 7.2 Nm. The Diapason screw S showed the highest endurance limit in bending moment at 15.3 Nm. However, if the load at the anterior part of the vertebral body in the upright position was one half of the body weight, 70 kgf, and the distance between the loading point and the shank of the pedicle screw was 5 cm, the moment at the shank of the pedicle screw was 17.5 Nm which was beyond the endurance limit of all seven types of pedicle screws.

Bending Test for Rods and Plates

The bending stiffness for each design is shown in Fig. 2a. The AO-ISSF rod, the VSP plate, and the Luque II plate were stiffer than the others. The Diapason rod was less stiff than a SUS316L steel rod with the same diameter.

The yield strengths of the AO-ISSF rod, VSP plate, and Luque II plate were also greater than the others (Fig. 2b). The yield strength of the Diapason rod was greater than that of a 316L steel with a 7-mm diameter.

Bending Test for the Screw Connection

Each yield strength is shown in Fig. 3. The yield strength of the Diapason screw was 0.7 Nm, and loosening of the connection was found. On the other

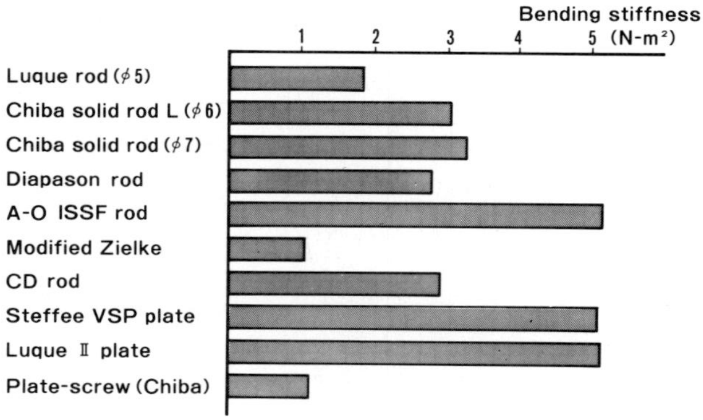

a

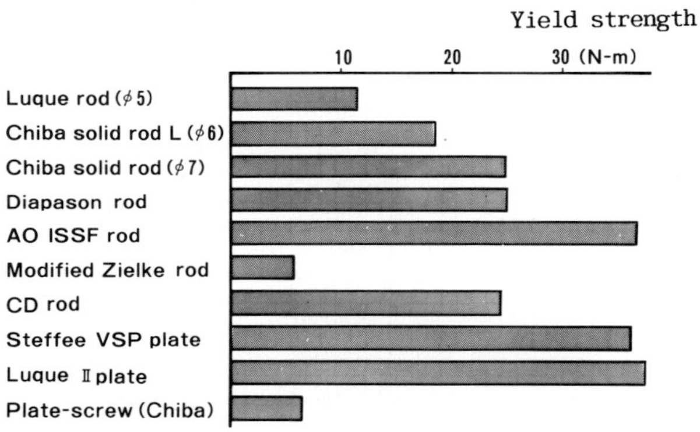

b

Fig. 2a,b. Three point bending tests of rods and plates. **a** Bending stiffness. **b** Yield strength

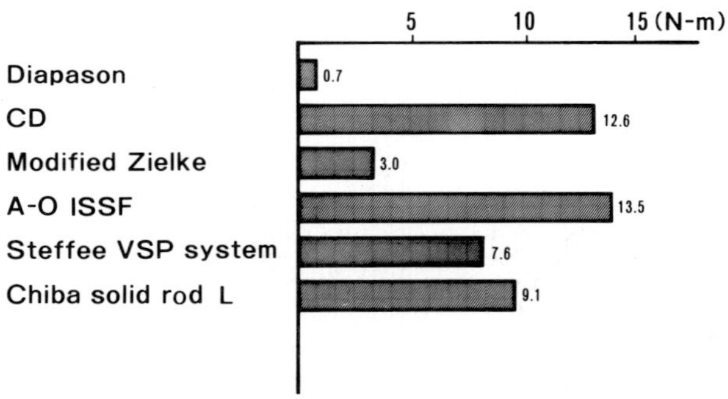

Fig. 3. Yield strength of the screw connection

Fig. 4a,b. Relative stiffness of 6 different pedicle screw systems. **a** Compressive stiffness. **b** Torsional stiffness

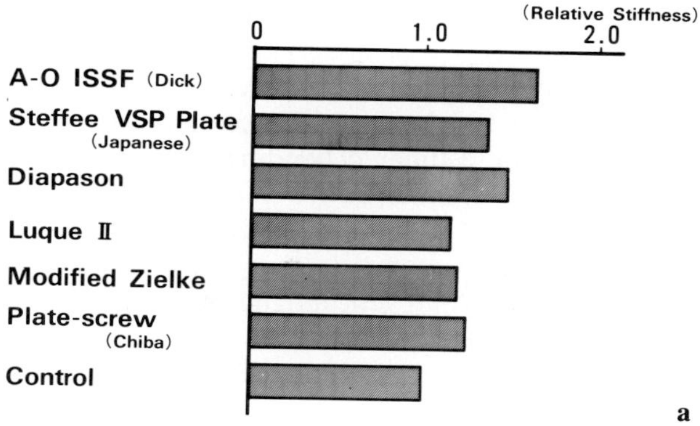

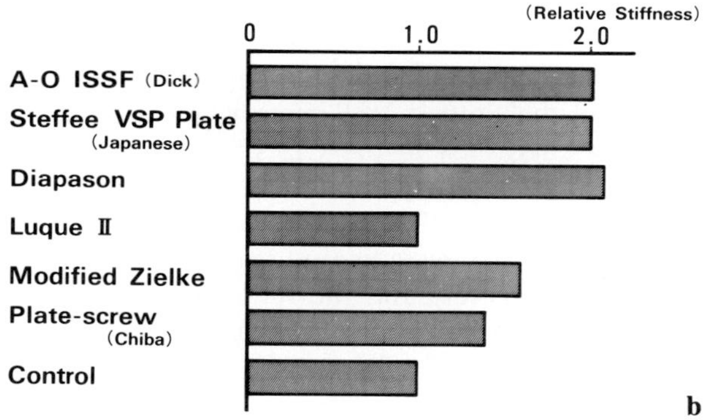

hand, the rods of the CD and the modified Zielke system were bent without any loosening of the connection, and the screw of the AO-ISSF and the VSP plate system were bent without any loosening.

Mechanical Tests for Pedicle Screw Systems

Compression Test (Fig. 4a)

The compressive stiffness of the AO-ISSF was 1.6 times higher than that of the uninstrumented control model and that of the Steffee VSP plate was 1.4 times higher. However, the stiffness of the Luque II, the modified Zielke, and the plate screw system (Chiba) were only 1.2 times higher than the control.

Torsional Test (Fig. 4b)

The stiffness of the AO-ISSF and the Steffee VSP plate was 2.0 times higher than that of the control. The stiffness of the Luque II, the modified Zielke, and the plate screw system (Chiba) was only 1.0–1.5 times higher.

Discussion

The fatigue tests of seven different pedicle screws showed that the Diapason screw had the highest endurance limit. However, its bending moment was lower than the estimated bending moment at the shank of the pedicle screw systems in the human body. If continuous stress was applied to the pedicle screws, they would certainly fracture. These pedicle screw systems should be thought of as temporary spinal instrumentation. Careful bone graftings are very important to prevent fatigue fractures.

The yield strength of the screw connection in the Diapason screw system was quite low compared to the other systems. However, this connection system does allow multidirectional screw insertions using the ball lock system. The system is also easy to handle, but there is still the problem of the connection sometimes becoming loose with usual daily activities. In cases of heavy activity, it may be better to fix the screw to the rod directly without a ball lock system.

Pedicle screw systems were divided into two groups from the results of these mechanical tests. One of the groups consisted of the rigid type such as the AO-ISSF and the Steffee VSP plate which have rigid link systems. The biomechanical strength test of the CD system was not completed, so this system may belong to the rigid type because of the result of the bending test of the rods and the strength of the screw connection. Since this type of pedicle screw system has a strong reduction force, severely slipped spondylolistheses can be reduced completely and the reduction can be held. However, Farey [25] and Goel [26] reported that device-related osteoporosis occured within vertebrae in response to rigid spinal instrumentation from their animal experimental studies. Instrumentation systems that are too rigid may produce loosening between the screws and the bone, or fatigue fractures. In this volume, Hsu reports the effects of rigid spinal instrumentation on the adjacent vertebral levels and insists that the use of internal fixation in lumbar spine fusions accelerates the rate of adjacent normal segment deterioration (Chap. 2.4).

The other group consists of semi-rigid types, such as the modified Zielke system, the plate-screw system (Chiba), and the Luque II. The Diapason pedicle screw system proved stiff in the compression and torsional tests on the models, but is included in this group because a loosening of the screw connection which was tightened at a torque of 2.0 Nm was observed during the bending strength test of the connection and the yield strength of the screw connection was lower than the others. This type corresponds to the semi-rigid plate of the AO plate for fractures which attempts to unite the fracture sites while allowing interfragmental micromotion. This produces less stress concentration in the screws, thereby decreasing the risk of fatigue failure. However, the forces of reduction or correction are less than those in the rigid type which is better indicated for reduction of fracture-dislocation and spondylolisthesis. On the other hand, the semi-rigid type is suitable for segmental unstable spines, and for spondylolisthesis which does not need the reduction but does need *in-situ* fusion. Postoperatively, it may also need external supports if a long fusion area was needed. These surgical indications are all from the standpoint of the mechanical stability of the implants. In practice it may be necessary to consider the level of the spine fusion before choosing the type of instrumentation. Spine surgeons should consider the constitution of the patient and estimate their postoperative physical activity. It is important to understand the mechanical characteristics of the pedicle screws to be used.

Conclusions

1. Even the Diapason screw, which showed the maximum endurance limit, may break under the continuous loading conditions within the body. It seems that the pedicle screw system should have a removable design because these spinal instrumentations cannot be used as endoprostheses but only as temporary implants.
2. Pedicle screw systems are divided into two groups. The rigid type may be applied to various unstable conditions. In particular, it has a good indication for diseases which require reduction, such as spinal fracture dislocation and severe spondylolisthesis. On the other hand, the semi-rigid type is indicated for degenerative diseases which require fixation *in-situ*. However, instrumentation should be properly selected with consideration to the original purpose for which they were developed.

References

1. Aebi M, Etter C, Kehl T, Thalgott J (1987) Stabilization of the lower thoracic and lumbar spine with the internal spine skeletal fixation system. Spine 12:544–551
2. Daniaux H, Seykora P, Genelin A, Lang T, Kathrein A (1991) Application of posterior plating and modifications in thoracolumbar spine injuries: Indication, techniques, and results. Spine 16:S125–S133
3. Dick W (1987) The "Fixatuer Interne" as a versatile implant for spine surgery. Spine 12:882–890
4. Esses SI, Botsford DJ, Wright T, Bednar D, Bailey S (1991) Operative treatment of spinal fractures with the AO internal fixator. Spine 16:S146–S150
5. Eysel P, Meinig G (1991) Comparative study of different dorsal stabilization techniques in recent thoracolumbar spine fractures. Acta Neurochir (Wien) 109:12–19
6. Honma G, Murota K, Shiba R, Kondo H, Satomura T, Funasaki H (1989) Pedicle screw fixation for lumbar spondylolisthesis (in Japanese). Seikei Saigai Geka 32: 637–642
7. Horowitch A, Peek RD, Thomas JC Jr et al. (1989) The Wiltse pedicle screw fixation system: Early clinical results. Spine 14:461–467
8. Miyashita H, Kumano K (1989) Internal fixation of the lumbar spine with Cotrel-Dubousset instrumentation (in Japanese). Rinsho Seikeigeka 24:1077–1083
9. Otani K, Izumi K, Kono T, et al. (1987) Transpedicular screw fixation for degenerative lumbar canal stenosis and degenerative lumbar spondylolisthesis (in Japanese). Seikeigeka 38:5–13

10. Steffee AD, Biscup RS, Sitkowski DJ (1986) Segmental spine plates with pedicle screw fixation. Clin Orthop 203:45–53
11. Thalgott JS, LaRocca H, Aebi M, Dwyer AP, Razza BE (1989) Reconstruction of the lumbar spine using AO DCP plate internal fixation. Spine 14:91–95
12. Tsunoda N, Kurose S, Sasaki K, Tanimura S, Harada H, Adachi H (1982) Transpedicular fixation for stabilization of the lumbar and thoracic spine Zielke instrument (in Japanese). Seikeigeka Saigaigeka (Orthopaedics and Traumatology) 31: 59–62
13. Cotrel Y, Dubousset J (1988) New universal instrumentation in spinal surgery. Clin Orthop 227:10–23
14. Dick W, Kluger P, Magerl F, Woersdorfer O, Zach G (1985) A new device for internal fixation of thoracolumbar and lumbar spine fractures: The Fixateur Interne. Paraplegia 23:225–232
15. Dove J (1986) Internal fixation of the lumbar spine: Hartshill rectangle. Clin Orthop 203:135–139
16. Guyer DW, Wiltse LL, Peek RD (1988) The Wiltse pedicle screw fixation system. Orthopedics 11:1455–1460
17. Krag MH, Beynnon BD, Pope MH, Frymoyer JW, Haugh LD, Weaver DL (1986) An internal fixator for posterior application to short segments of the thoracic, lumbar, or lumbosacral spine. Clin Orthop 203:75–98
18. Luque ER (1986) Interpeduncular segmental fixation. Clin Orthop 203:54–57
19. Puno RM, Bechtold JE, Byrd III JA, Winter RB, Ogilvie JW, Bradford DS (1991) Biomechanical analysis of transpedicular rod systems, a preliminary report. Spine 16:973–980
20. Roy-Camille R, Sailant G, Mazel G (1986) Internal fixation of the lumbar spine with pedicule screw plating. Clin Orthop 203:7–17
21. Esses SI, Sachs BL (1991) Complications of pedicle screw fixation. 25th Anniversary Meeting of Scoliosis Research Society, Minneapolis, Minn, September
22. McAfee PC, Weiland DJ, Carlow JJ (1991) Survivorship analysis of pedicle spinal instrumentation. Spine 16:S422–S427
23. Matsuzaki H, Hoshino M, Nagaoka T, Kiuchi T, Toriyama S (1989) Complications and techniques for pedicle screw plating instrumentation (in Japanese). J West Jpn Res Soc Spine 15:252–256
24. West JL III, Ogilvie JW, Bradford DS (1991) Complications of the variable screw plate pedicle screw fixation. Spine 16:576–579
25. Farey ID, McAfee PC, Gurr RK, Randolph MA (1989) Quantitative histologic study of the influence of spinal instrumentation on lumbar fusions: A canine model. J Orthop Res 7:709–722
26. Goel VK, Lim T, Gwon J, Chen J, et al. (1991) Effects of rigidity of an internal fixation device. A comprehensive biomechanical investigation. Spine 16:S155–S161

4.4 Lumbosacral Fusion with Pedicular Screw Plating Instrumentation: 10-Year Follow-up Results

Raymond Roy-Camille, Jean-Pierre Desauge, and Jean-Pierre Benazet[1]

Introduction

The use of pedicular screw plating (PSP) according to the procedure that we have proposed for lumbosacral fusion (LSF) permits the immediate stabilization of the vertebral segments while waiting for graft consolidation. Therefore, a high rate of fusion is obtained [1,2].

This work examines not only the outcome of fusion at long-term follow-up (more than 10 years), but also studies the spine above the fusion, the disks, and the articular processes [3,4].

Patients and Instrumentation

Of the 558 lumbosacral fusions performed between 1976 and 1990, 91 patients have had more than 10 years of follow-up. Of these 91 patients, 25 patients had undergone unusual procedures without plates, 9 patients were deceased, 10 patients were lost to follow-up, and 21 did not respond to our request for review; therefore 26 patients were examined for this study.

The patients' ages ranged from 31 to 67 years with an average age of 44 years. There were 13 males and 13 females. Their occupations before surgery were classified into 3 groups according to the physical labor required in their work and to the stresses placed on the spine. There were 13 patients who were heavy laborers and 13 who were active (office work, professional). No one was sedentary or retired.

The preoperative symptoms consisted of low back pain (LBP) only in 6 patients and LBP associated with radicular pain in 20 patients.

The most common underlying etiology was degenerative disk disease, and standard X ray examination was used to determine whether the pain came from

[1] Orthopedic Surgery Department, Pitié-Salpetriere Hospital, 83 Boulevard de l'Hôpital, 75651 Paris Cedex 13, France

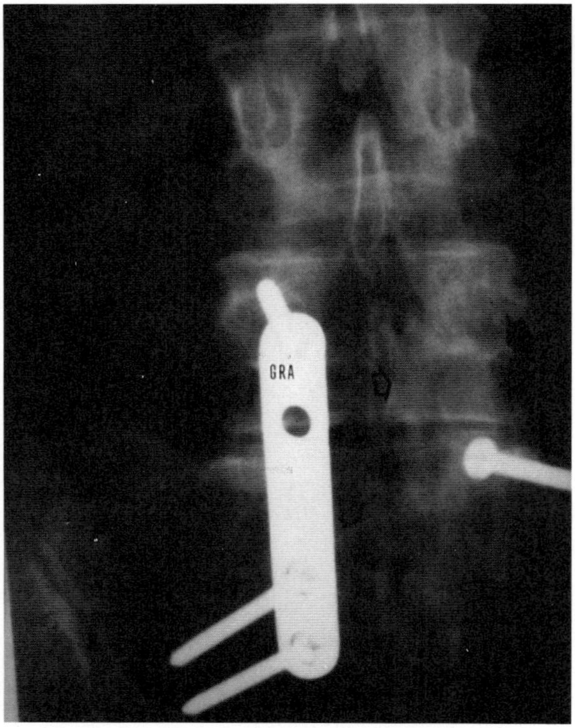

Fig. 1. Asymmetric technique with one plate on one side and pedicular screws on the other side, followed by a posterior graft. *Solid arrows* and *open arrows*, limits of graft

the disk or from the articular processes. We had nine cases of spondylolysthesis in our series, all of which were grade I or II, and four cases that had been treated by previous diskectomy. It was important however to know if the failure of the operation was secondary to fibrosis or arthritis; the indications for surgery depended on it. Finally, there was only one spinal stenosis. The indication for fusion was anytime when there was a risk of destabilization (large arthrectomy, disk excision, degenerative spondylolisthesis) or when there was a lumbar dislocation.

The instrumentation consisted of plates and screws. There were three types of plates (5, 7 or 9 hole) with 13-mm hole spacing. The plates were unique because they were reinforced except for the 2 last holes, which were oblique in a lateral direction (30°). The pedicular screws were 45 mm in length and 4.5 or 5 mm in diameter. The head diameter was 8 mm at lumbar level and 6 mm at sacral level.

Operative Technique

The patient was always placed in a supine prone on the operative table, as with disk surgery. The incision was a midline posterior.

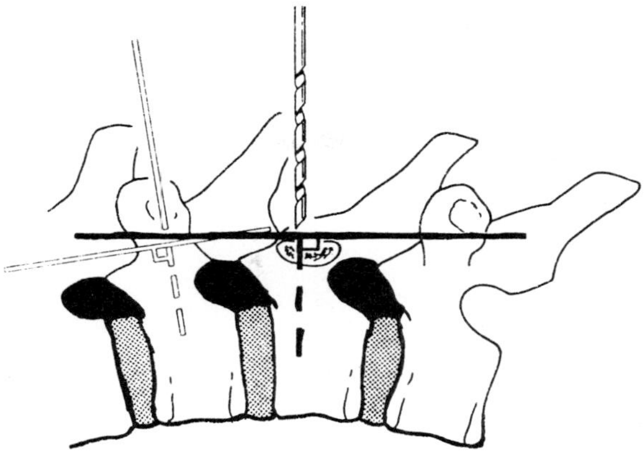

Fig. 2. Screw entrance point and direction of drilling. *Solid line*, perpendicular to the posterior arch; *dotted line*, direction of the pedicular; *black area,* foramen; *dotted area*, disk

Two procedures were used. In the first procedure, one plate was implanted on one side with pedicular screws and the facet joint screwed on the opposite side, followed by a posterior graft (Fig. 1). Lumbar pedicular screw aiming followed the usual rules of respecting the lateral vascularization of muscles. The entrance point was situated at the intersection of two lines, the horizontal line corresponding to the transverse process and the vertical line corresponding to the middle of the articular process. This point of insertion was 1 mm below the articular line, on the summit of a small crest. The direction was "right on", perpendicular to the posterior arch (Fig. 2). The S1 screw was unique because two directions were possible: either the same as the lumbar screw, or oblique upward and inward. The articular processes were prepared by excising the cartilage and placing bone graft. The screw was implanted exactly perpendicular to the orientation of the joint line (Fig. 3).

The second procedure was utilized when a large laminectomy was performed. In these cases, bilateral plating was followed by bilateral posterolateral grafting (Fig. 4). The bone graft extended from the lateral facet of the articular process to the summit of the transverse process. This was in contrast to the first procedure, where the bone grafting was posterior and laterally extended to the bases of the transverse processes including the lateral facet of the articular process.

Indications for Fusion

LSF was indicated in patients with recurrent LBP for more than 1 year. This permanent and incapacitating pain had to be associated with radiologic findings due to degenerative changes or spondylolysthesis. If radicular pain was associated with lumbar pain, canalar exploration with myelographic scan or MRI was necessary prior to surgical exploration.

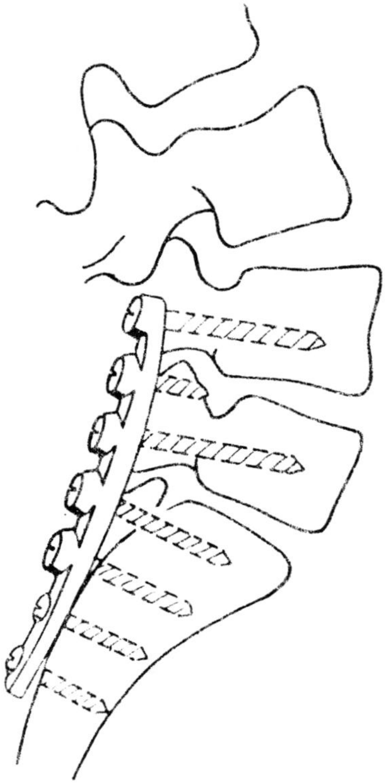

Fig. 3. Implantation of screws and plate

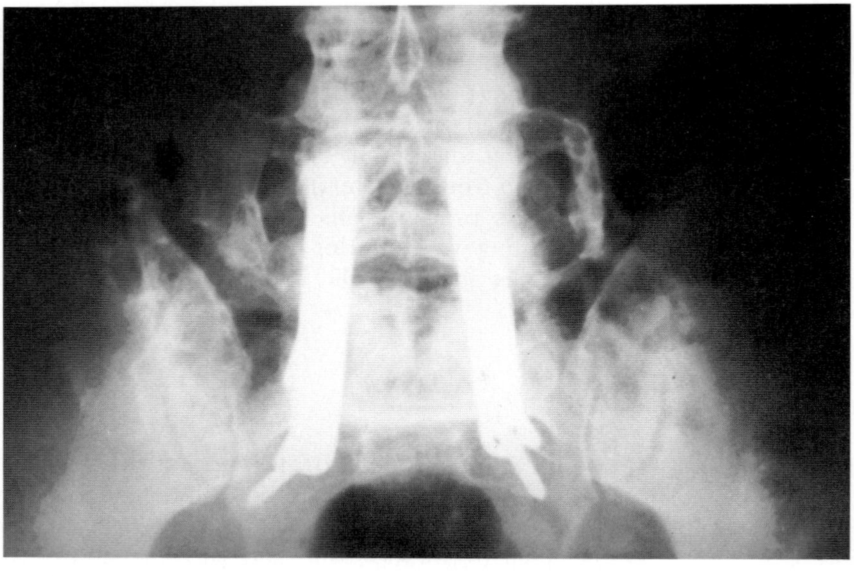

Fig. 4. Symmetric technique with two plates and bilateral posterolateral grafts.

Table 1. Stauffer and Coventry criteria [5] modified according to Friberg.

Result	Parameters
Excellent	No pain Able to do the same work Able to perform same daily activities No pain medication
Good	Attenuated pain Work sometimes interrupted Daily activities moderately diminished Occasional treatment
Fair	Frequent pain, but different to preoperative pain Frequent work interruptions Daily activities diminished Occasional treatment
Bad	Same pain as preoperative pain No work possible Daily activities difficult Permanent pain treatment

Diskography is important to many authors in determining the level of fusion. Here, we considered that standard X ray examination, or better yet MRI, was sufficient to appreciate the hinge or degeneration of the disk at the new lumbopelvic motion segment disk. When diskography was used, the injection pain was more important than disk appearance to locate the painful disk.

We studied the efficacy of the plaster cast and found that a positive test was a good indicator for determining the success of fusion, while a negative test was non-diagnostic. About 50% of patients with a negative test had successful fusion; the other 50% did not obtain good symptomatic results.

Results

All the patients were reviewed with an average follow-up of 11.4 years (10–19 years). We adopted the Stauffer and Coventry criteria [5] modified according to Friberg (Table 1). The parameters examined were pain, working capacity, daily activities, and treatment. We observed 10 patients with excellent results, 11 patients with good results, 3 patients with fair results, and 2 with bad results.

If we analyze our results with regards to pain, 7 patients had no pain at all, 15 were improved, and 4 were unchanged; no patients became worse. At the same time, medical treatment was not necessary, or only occasionally necessary, for 22 patients. However, it was frequent for four patients.

In terms of postoperative occupations, 14 patients are still in the same occupation, but 9 patients are now in less strenuous occupations. Of the 13 who were heavy labourers, 8 patients did not return to their original occupation. This is not surprising because the patients had decided this before surgery.

The results for fusion were difficult to analyze. There was often residual mobility in the dynamic roentgenograms and interference secondary to the plates in CT scans or MRI. More reliable was the quality of graft and stability of instrumentation from standard X ray examination. Graft fracture was possible and it was important to observe the osteosynthesis after 3 months. If there was loosening or breakage of a screw, a pseudarthrosis was possible and surgical intervention necessary to examine the continuity of the graft. According to these criteria, fusion was obtained in 96% of cases, with one patient (4%) needing surgical verification.

Disk changes that occurred above the fusion level increased from 17% to 53% at the new hinge between 5 and 10 years postoperatively. For the articular processes, degenerative changes increased only from 31% to 35%.

If we observe the evolution of the functional result, we see few changes: only two patients had a worse result. This can probably be correlated with the changes occuring at the articular processes. Furthermore, poor functional results remain stable over time and they do not depend on the fusion; two patients with a bad result were surgically explored and found to have good fusion.

In conclusion, LSF with PSP gives a high rate of fusion and this rate does not decrease with time. Furthermore changes may occur at the level above the fusion. The findings seen at the articular processes have more influence on the functional result than the new lumbopelvic hinge disk.

References

1. Roy-Camille R, Soulas P (1984) L'arthrodèse lombo-sacrée dans les lombalgies in Roy-Camille. IVèmes journées de la Pitie. Masson, Paris, p 16
2. Steffee AD, Sitkowski DJ (1988) Posterior lumbar interbody fusion and plates. Clin Orthop 227:99–102
3. Eveleigh MC, Perrot Y, Burdin P, Castaing J, Valat JP (1986) Les arthrodèses postéro-latérales dans le traitement du spondylolisthésis et de la discarthrose lombo-sacrée – Résultats à long terme. Rev Chir Orthop 72(II):92
4. Lerat JL et al. (1987) Arthrodèse lombaire inter-somatique postérieure (ALIP). Cahiers d'enseignement de la Sofcot 1987. Expansion scientifique, Paris, pp 275–322
5. Stauffer RN, Coventry MB (1972) Posterolateral lumbar spine fusion. J Bone Joint Surg [Am] 54:1195–1204

4.5 Simmons Plating System for Spinal Fusion Surgery

James W. Simmons[1]

Introduction

The purpose of this clinical study was to evaluate the safety and effectiveness of using the Simmons Plating System as an adjunct to posterior lumbar fusion. The System may be used to address a wide variety of indications which require spinal arthrodesis, including degenerative disk disease, pseudarthrosis, fractures, and unsuccessful spinal fusions. The System provides superior stability for maximum fusion augmentation without limiting surgical flexibility.

The System is simple in design but can be used to create a wide variety of spinal constructs. The system uses plates fixed to the pedicle. Two fixation methods are available (plate/bolt, plate/screw), and may be used exclusively or in combination (Fig. 1). The choice of fixation methods ensures that the surgeon can control the degree of rigidity present in the construct. "All-bolt" constructs provide maximum rigidity, whereas "all-screw" constructs provide minimum rigidity. Constructs made with bolts and screws allow a "customized" amount of rigidity.

A number of special features enhance stability and performance and facilitate application. These include closely spaced plate teeth for precise bolt or screw placement, cannulated bolts and screws for guide pin application, specially designed bolt and screw thread forms for enhanced pull out strength and increased stability, and pre-cut bolts for a shorter, simpler procedure.

Biomechanics and Design Rationale

The stabilization of the spine was first introduced by Hibbs and Albee in 1911 [1]. Cloward has been the prime proponent and propagator of posterior lumbar interbody fusion (PLIF) [2] and Crock indicated that the ideal operation for

[1] Alamo Bone and Joint Clinic, 8122 Datapoint Suite #1200, San Antonio, TX 78229, USA

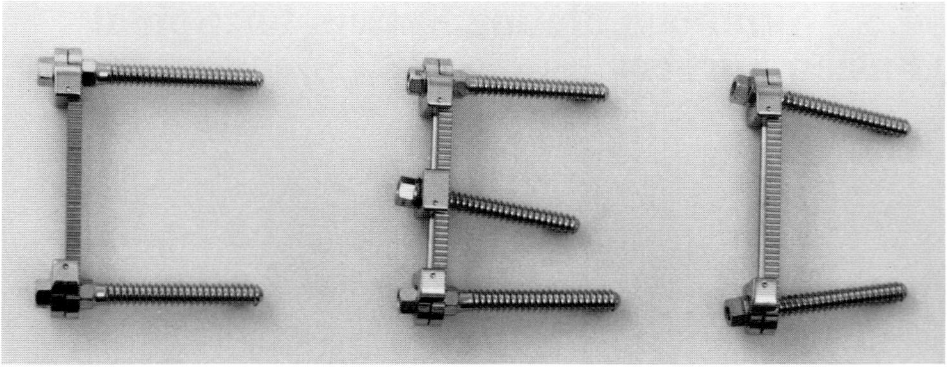

Fig. 1. All-bolt (*left*), combination bolt/screw (*center*), and all-screw (*right*) constructs

decompression and stabilization is the PLIF [3]. The use of metallic surgical implants provides the spine surgeon with a means of accurate bone fixation and helps generally in the management of fractures and reconstructive surgery. In 1970 Roy-Camille and Demeulenaere introduced the use of screws in the pedicle [4], and in 1987 Steffee et al., who popularized pedicle screw fixation in the United States, described the transpedicular fixation of spinal disorders with variable screw placement (VSP) [5]. The Simmons Plating System introduced in 1990 was developed to meet the spinal instrumentation need for an innovative fixation system that would offer a strong, versatile construct which is easy to use.

The design includes a variety of simple features. Bolts are precut to eliminate intraoperative trimming. Only one locking nut is necessary. Bolts and screws are cannulated for use with a blunt tip guide pin (Fig. 2). A stabilizing wrench allows for easy, controlled insertion of the bolts and screws. Removal and adjustment is a simple procedure.

The System's components were subjected to extensive testing, including strength, fatigue, and stability. All components are made of 316LVM stainless steel (ASTM 138), and bolts have a tapered minor diameter to eliminate the abrupt transition from major to minor diameter. Nuts, bolts, screws, and plate slots have large radii to eliminate sharp corners and provide built-in micromotion. Spiralock thread form is used on the nuts to reduce the chance of loosening due to vibration or fatigue (Fig. 3).

Technique and Components

The System includes plates, bolts, screws, washers, and locking nuts along with a complete array of surgical instruments. The following description illustrates the technique of instrumented lumbar spinal arthrodesis showing hardware

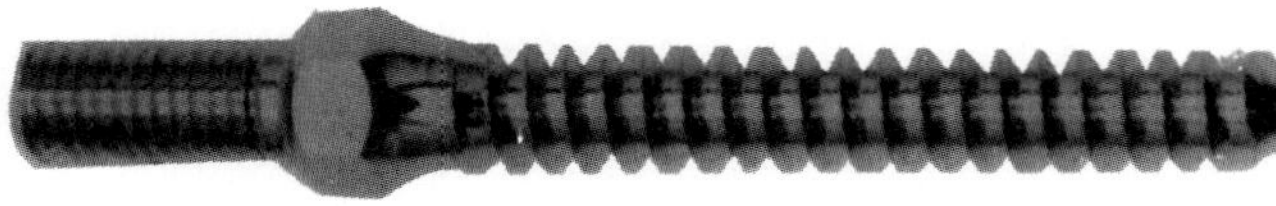

Fig. 2. Bolt

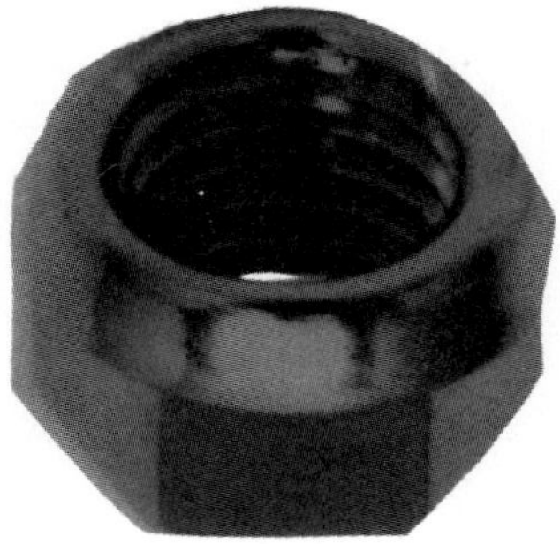

Fig. 3. Nut showing Spiralock thread

implantation. This technique is only one of many where the System may be used.

After the usual preparation and preliminary soft tissue dissection exposing the posterior elements, an osteotome is used to remove the inferior border of the superior lamina of the segment involved. The medial portion of the medial facets is removed along the exostosis causing spinal stenosis. The medial border of the lateral facet is exposed and removed as far as the pedicle to provide visualization of the segmental nerve root. By using spreaders, the superior portion of the lateral facet can be exposed for removal if it is causing narrowing of the foramina and/or nerve root impingement [6].

An osteotome is then used to take down the posterior annulus and the end-plates. Curettes are used to clean the intervertebral disk space. The disk is removed to the lateral and anterior edges of the annulus, including the cartilaginous end-plate. The remaining end-plate is punctured to obtain a bleeding surface for the bone plugs. Spanners are used to measure the width and depth of the intervertebral disk space with moderate distraction being placed with the lamina spreaders. An allograft bone plug is then fashioned to fit and is placed in the disk space with little resistance to impaction. Three to four tricortical or bicortical allografts blocks can usually be accomodated in the intervertebral disk space.

After sterile draping and positioning of the fluoroscopic C-arm (Fig. 4), the pedicles are identified above and below the disk involved. The entry sites into the pedicle are determined. Cortical bone is removed at each entry site using a rongeur or a high speed drill. A probe is used to verify its location with the aid of fluoroscopy (Fig. 5). For soft tissue protection each hole is tapped with the

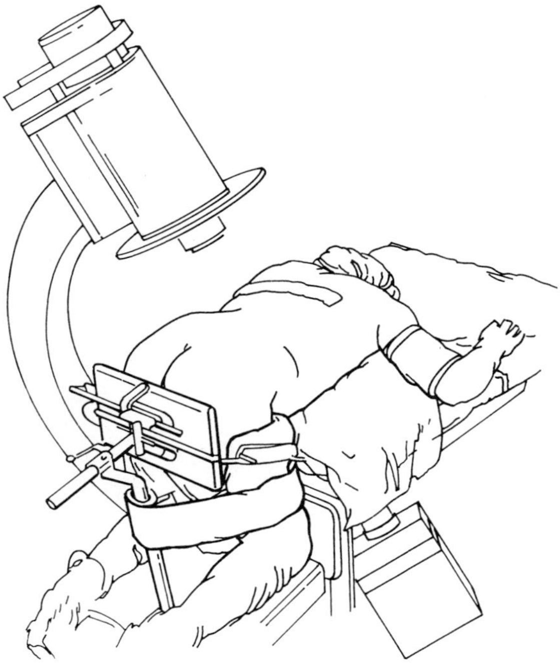

Fig. 4. Positioning of fluoroscopic C-arm

drill sleeve (Fig. 6). Both calibration of the tap and, periodically, fluoroscopy are used to check the tap depth. Using the wrench and stabilizing bar for bolts, appropriate size bolts are placed in each pedicle (Fig. 7).

A malleable aluminum template is used to gauge length and the lordotic curve (Fig. 8). An appropriate size plate is contoured for each side, and the plates are placed over the bolt heads (Fig. 9). A washer and a locking nut are placed over the bolt heads, using the contoured washers at the plate ends (Figs. 10,11), and a torque wrench to tighten the locking nut. A final check of the nerve roots should be carried out as well as a check to ensure that the foramina are not obstructed. Finally, a fat graft is obtained from the presacral fat and placed anterior to the dura, over the interbody grafts and dorsal to the dura.

The System is also versatile in that it provides an assortment of bolt and screw sizes, of different diameters and different lengths. Closely spaced teeth allow for 2 mm adjustment along the plate.

Materials and Methods

Between December 1990 and May 1992, 248 patients (149 males and 99 females) underwent lumbar spinal fusion with pedicle screw plate fixation at four institutions. Patient ages ranged from 21 to 80 years with a mean of 46 years. Of the 248 patients, 128 presented with degenerative disk disease, 118 with multiple operated back syndrome, and 2 with fracture. This was the first surgical intervention for the patients in the degenerative disk and fracture subgroups.

Pre- and postoperative back and leg pains were assessed and given numerical values ranging from no pain (0) to disabling pain (5). Determination of fusion was made radiographically using AP, lateral, and lateral flexion-extension views. Definite fusion was defined as the visible presence of bony trabeculae bridging the disk space of all motion segments undergoing fusion. Functional union was defined as the presence of a radiolucent line within or bordering the bone grafts, and no bony trabeculae visible across the disk space with no detectable movement on flexion-extension films. Non-union was defined as the presence of a radiolucent line or band within or bordering the graft and detectable movement on flexion-extension views.

Various bone graft placement techniques have been used including 201 posterolateral, 41 PLIF, 2 posterolateral and PLIF, and 4 posterolateral and ALIF. There were 91 one-level, 141 two-level, 14 three-level, 1 four-level, and 1 five-level fusions.

Clinical Results

Mean pain scores decreased from 3.7 (n = 128) preoperatively to 2.1 (n = 86) at 3 months postoperatively, 1.7 (n = 56) at 6 months postoperatively, and 1.9 (n = 14) at 12 months postoperatively. At 3 months postoperative, 48 (27.7%) patients were assessed as having definite unions, 28 (16.2%) functional union, and 1 (0.6%) definite non-union, with the remaining 96 (55.5%) cases being indeterminate as to fusion status. At 6 months, 105 (89.7%) patients were assessed as having definite unions, 1 (0.9%) as having functional union, and none as having definite non-union, with 11 (9.4%) cases being indeterminate. At 12 months postoperative, 28 (93.3%) patients were assessed as having definite unions, 2 (6.7%) functional union, and 1 (0.6%) definite non-union. No cases of definite non-union or indeterminate union have been reported thus far. This is an ongoing study. The numbers will have increased significance as data collection continues.

The mean operating time irrespective of graft placement for one-level fusion was 6.0 h (range: 2.0–7.0 h); for two-level fusion, 4.7 h (range: 2.7–12.3 h); three-level fusion, 6.5 h (range 3.6–8.0 h); four-level fusion, 4.0 h (range: 4.0–4.0 h); and five-level fusion, 6.5 h (range 6.5–6.5 h). Average blood loss was 778 ml for one-level, 1,174 ml for two-level, 1,711 ml for three-level, 700 ml for four-level, and 3,500 ml for the five-level fusion.

Interoperative complications included 4 pedicle fractures, 1 vertebral body fracture, 1 case of L5 nerve root damage during tapping, 17 cases of incidental durotomy (dural tears), 3 cases where we were unable to insert screw, and 5 other. Postoperative complications included 1 patient with a loss of bladder/

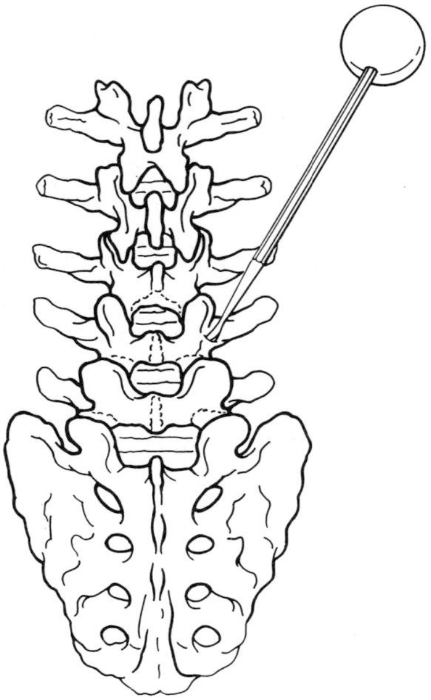

5

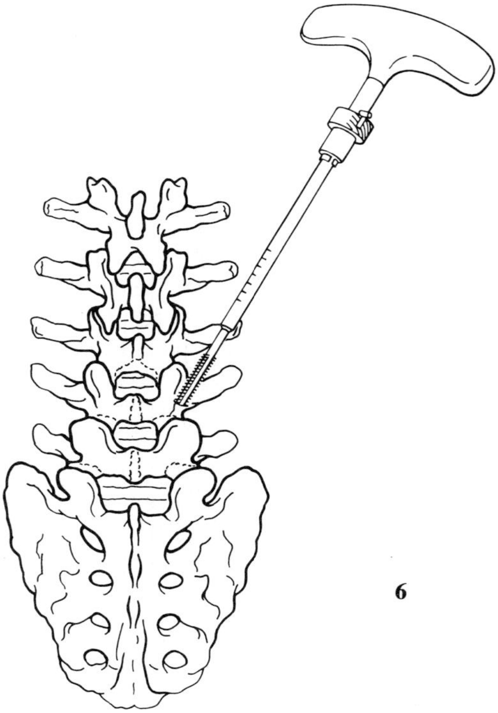

6

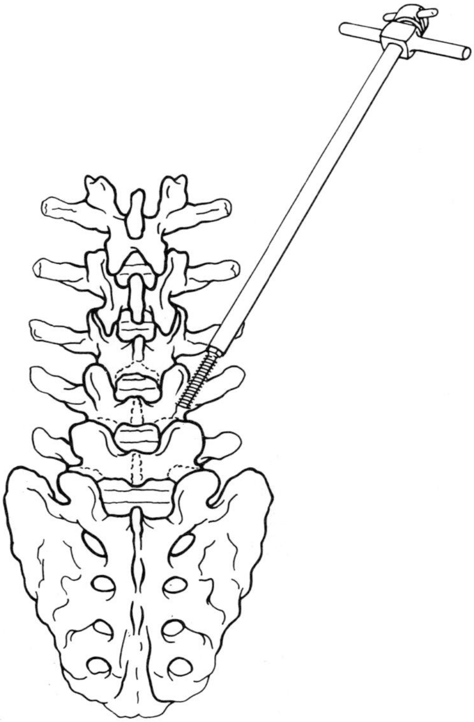

7

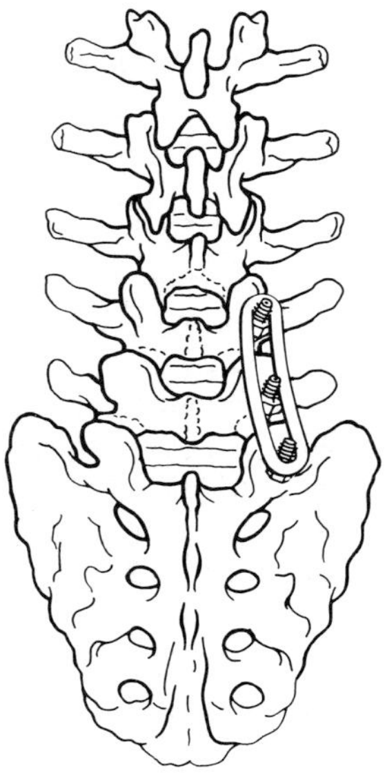

8

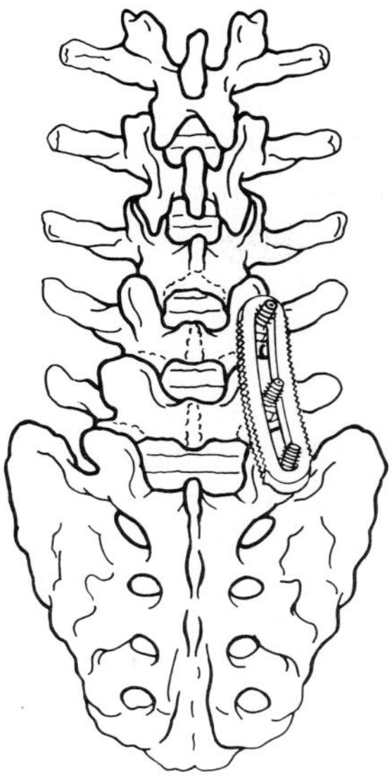

9

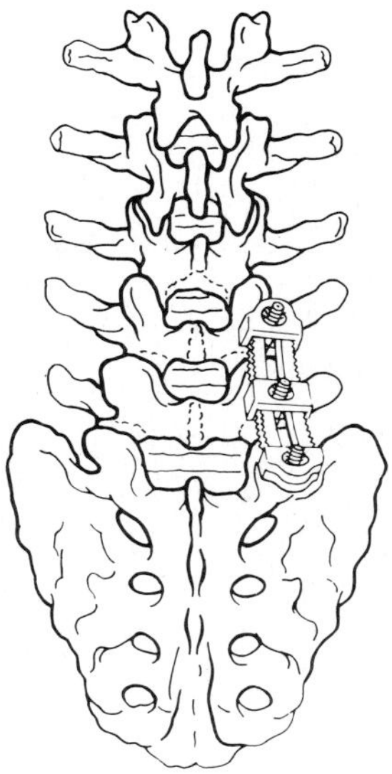

10

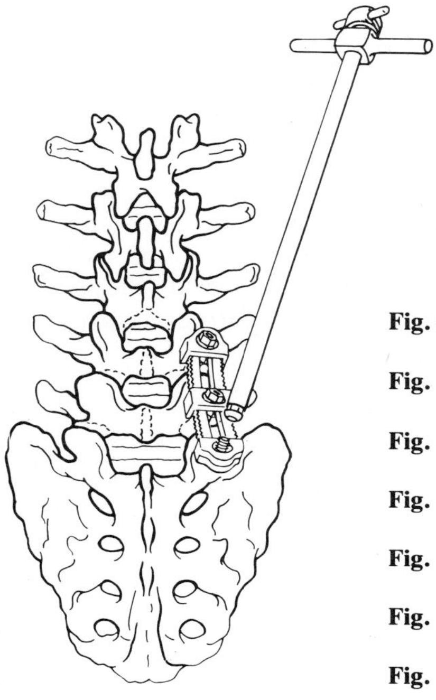

11

Fig. 5. Verifying location of the pedicle using a probe

Fig. 6. Tapping the hole

Fig. 7. Placing a bolt in the pedicle

Fig. 8. Determining plate size using a template

Fig. 9. Plate over the bolt heads

Fig. 10. Washer and over the bolt heads

Fig. 11. Locking nut over the bolt heads

bowel control, 5 with donor graft site pain, 1 with drainage without infection, and 4 with infection. Six patients underwent additional surgery. One patient required wound irrigation and debridement for persistent aseptic drainage. One required additional bony decompression along with the addition of a contoured washer at L5. One other patient required wound exploration and repair of a dural tear. No hardware failure has been observed.

Discussion

Complications in spinal surgery are known to occur and are inadvertent even in the best of hands. Complications relating directly to the pedicle could be avoided if the surgeon did not use interpedicular fixation. However, similar complications such as hook pull out and fracture of the posterior elements can occur with other types of fixation. Neurological complications can also occur with the hook and rod system, and in particular with sublaminar wiring. Although there is no perfect system available it is felt that the simplicity, versatility, and strength of this system allows for fewer complications and gives the surgeon a choice in the rigidity of the system.

In comparing the System to other systems available it was found that stresses in the System's components are significantly lower than those in others. Other systems reach a plastic deformation which reduces its expected fatigue life. The Simmons Plating System offers much longer fatigue life.

Conclusion

A system has been developed and designed to enhance spinal stabilization. The components and procedures described are for simplicity, versatility, as well as effectiveness. The safety of the system depends on the ability of the surgical technician. Safety features were a great consideration in its development, in particular the cannulation of the screws and bolts for the use of a guide wire. The guide wire can also be used with the taps thereby enhancing the safety of tapping the pedicle. The system is effective for spine stabilization and is safe when its technical application is appropriate.

References

1. Hibbs RA, Albee FH (1911) An operation for progressive spinal deformities. NY State J Med 93:1013
2. Cloward RB (1953) The treatment of ruptured lumbar intervertebral disks by vertebral body fusion: Indications, operative technique, after care. J Neurosurg 10: 154–168
3. Crock HV (1983) Practice of spinal surgery. Springer Verlag, New York
4. Roy-Camille R, Demeulenaere CL (1970) Osteosynthese du rachis dorsal, lombaire, et lombo sacre. La Presse Medicale 32:78

5. Steffee AD, Gainse RW, Henstorf JE (1987) Transpedicular fixation of spinal disorders with Steffee plates. Surgical Rounds for Orthopaedics 1:3
6. Simmons JW (1991) Posterior lumbar interbody fusion. In: Frymoyer JW (ed) The adult spine: Principles and practice. Raven, New York, pp 1961–1987

4.6 Stabilization of Spondylolisthesis: The Hartshill System

John Dove[1]

Our ideas about internal fixation of the spine were dramatically changed by Luque, who popularised sublaminar wiring [1]. There were, however, a number of problems with the original double rod Luque system, which we solved by joining the rods to form what we call the Hartshill rectangle [2]. The rectangles are called "Hartshill" because I work at the Hartshill Orthopaedic Hospital.

The rectangles are deliberately simple; they are made from a stainless steel rod which is welded. They have a roof at each end and they come in calibres of 5 and 6 mm. We implanted our first rectangle in January 1983 and we now have experience of more than 1,000 cases for a variety of spinal disorders [2–5].

This paper considers only our experience of the use of the Hartshill system for the internal fixation of spondylolisthesis. For the purposes of this publication the complex field of spondylolisthesis is split into two broad groups: a Grade 1 or 2 slip secondary to a spondylolysis and the more severe congenital slips Grade 3–5.

Spondylolysis Group

In the presence of a spondylolysis, if there is sufficient pain to require surgery and if an MRI shows that the neighbouring disc is normal, then a local anesthetic injection under X-ray control of the pars defect is carried out. If this gives good, temporary relief of the pain I would then simply repair the pars defect.

There are a number of different methods described for simple repair of the lysis but I normally use simple screw fixation, as described by Buck [6]. If a fit, young sportsman has a painful spondylolysis with normal adjacent discs then Buck's operation can get him back to sport at the highest level. If an MRI scan shows that the adjacent disc is abnormal then I would carry out a posterior

[1] Stoke-on-Trent Spinal Service, Hartshill Orthopaedic Hospital, Hartshill Road, Hartshill, Stoke-on-Trent, ST4 7NZ, UK

fusion in situ with internal fixation. The loose posterior arch is removed and stabilization is used with our Hartshill system. With the development of the new pedicle screw bridge to complement our Hartshill system it is possible to provide secure fixation at one level only [7].

Congenital Slips

Biomechanically a congenital slip is a different, more severe problem than a slip secondary to a spondylolysis. In biomechanical terms the patient presents with an acute lumbosacral kyphosis. The patient is often a growing child and in general terms an acute angular kyphosis in a growing child is best treated by combined anterior and posterior fusion.

In such cases I first perform an anterior transperitoneal L5/S1 disc excision and fusion, usually with the addition of two AO cancellous screws. Under the same anesthetic the patient is re-positioned and re-gowned and a posterior fusion with internal fixation with our Hartshill system and a pedicle screw bridge is performed, usually from L4 to S1.

Reduction

The question of the need for reduction in spondylolysis is highly controversial. In my practice, for a Grade 1 or 2 slip secondary to a spondylolysis, reduction is unnecessary. For a Grade 3 or 4 slip, to attempt a 100% reduction involves considerable surgery for the patient and significant risk. A perfectly satisfactory partial reduction can be obtained without the need for serial surgery. Once one has performed a transperitoneal discectomy with the patient lying supine on the operation table one finds that approximately a 30% reduction of the slip is thereby obtained. I stabilize the lumbosacral junction in that position and do not attempt to provide any greater reduction. Such a 30% reduction allows a very satisfactory correction of the lumbosacral deformity and the hamstring tightness gradually disappears.

Severe Congenital Slips

For the severe slips such as a Grade 5, if the symptoms demand it, then each case has to be tackled individually, but there is a case occasionally for performing L5 vertebrectomy from in front and then fixing L4 to the sacrum. I have experience of only two such cases.

Faced with unusually difficult cases, one has to be prepared to tailor one's surgery to the individual. If there is a pseudarthrosis from a previously attempted posterior fusion and a gross spondylolisthesis with early bladder symptoms then a wide, posterior decompression will be necessary and it may

Table 1. Spondylolisthesis: The Hartshill system.

	Spondylolysis	Congenital
No. of patients (*n*)	98	34
Results (*n*)		
Excellent	61	18
Good	26	4
Fair	5	3
Poor	6	9
Complications (*n*)		
Broken wires	7	9
Pseudarthrosis	2	3
Infection	0	1
Neurological	0	2

be necessary with the internal fixation to bypass the sacrum in order to link the lumbar spine above to the pelvis below. In such cases I cut off the bottom of a 6 mm rectangle. The upper part of the rectangle is wired to the lumbar spine in the normal way but the lower limbs of the rectangle are embedded in the pelvis on each side.

Results

The statistics are presented in Table 1. In the spondylolysis group the results in terms of relief of pain have been excellent. Although the results were very satisfactory in the congenital group they were not as good as in the spondylolysis group. One is dealing with a more severe slip and different pathology.

The complications are also presented in Table 1. It will be noted that the congenital group gave rise to more problems than the spondylolysis group. Despite not attempting a 100% reduction I have had two neurological problems in the congenital group: one patient had perineal loss of sensation which never fully recovered and one patient had a temporary, partial foot-drop which recovered completely in 3 months.

Pedicle Screw Bridge

The original Hartshill system with sublaminar wiring alone was simple and secure but was not entirely satisfactory for spondylolisthesis. Our new modification of the pedicle screw bridge answers these deficiencies [7]. The modification keeps the simplicity and adaptability of the Hartshill rectangle but allows one to link it securely to the pedicle. Fixation to the pedicle is obtained by a standard AO screw.

Conclusion

The Hartshill system is simple, secure, adaptable, and inexpensive. With the new pedicle screw bridge modification, secure fixation in spondylolisthesis can be obtained with fixation of the minimum number of levels. Although the system is in principle simple, attention to detail in technique is vital and surgeons thinking of using the system are encouraged to attend one of our regular hands-on instructional courses.

References

1. Luque ER (1984) Segmental spinal instrumentation. Slack, Thorofare
2. Dove J (1987) Luque segmental spinal instrumentation: the use of the Hartshill rectangle. Orthopedics 10:955–961
3. Dove J (1986) Internal fixation of the lumbar spine – the Hartshill rectangle. Clin Orthop 203:135–140
4. Dove J (1989a) Internal fixation of unstable spinal fractures: the Hartshill system. Injury 20:139–144
5. Dove J (1989b) Internal fixation of the cervical spine: the Hartshill system. In: Louis R, Weidner A (eds) Cervical Spine II. Springer Berlin, Heidelberg, pp 79–86
6. Buck JE (1970) Direct repair of the defects in spondylolisthesis. J Bone Joint Surg [Br] 52:432
7. Rahmatalla AT, Hastings GW (1991) A pedicle screw bridging device for posterior segmental fixation of the spine – preliminary mechanical testing results. J Biomed Eng 13:97–102

4.7 Lumbar Spinal Stabilization by the MOSS System

Myung-Sang Moon, Kyu-Sung Lee, Sung-Soo Kim, and Doo-Hoon Sun[1]

Introduction

Various internal fixation devices have been developed and used clinically to stabilize unstable spines [1–3], regardless of whether the cause is congenital or acquired. The more popular posterior fixation devices are pedicular fixation types, such as the Zielke, Cotrel-Dubousset (C-D), Puno-Winter, Rogozinski, modular segmental spinal instrumentation (MOSS), and Graf systems. All these devices have been known to provide secure fixation if they are properly applied, though each device has its disadvantages. Among the systems we have experience of, we will discuss here the use of the MOSS instrumentation system with a polyaxial adjustable screw head in the treatment of lumbar spinal disorders. The MOSS system (Biedermann MOTECH, Germany) (Fig. 1a–c) is a supporting, contouring, and stabilizing device for the spine that consists of:

1. Bone screws (neck dimensions, 4 mm) with either a mono- or polyaxial adjustable head
2. Hex nuts
3. Threaded rods (3-mm thick) that are slightly malleable (semirigid)
4. Washers
5. Transverse rod-stabilizers

One of the attractions of this system is that the instrumentation is simple. There are no specific indications. If for any reason the surgeon decides that stability of the lumbar spine is required, then the MOSS system is a straightforward way of providing that stability.

[1] Department of Orthopaedic Surgery, Catholic University Medical College, 505 Ban-po-Dong, Seo-Cho-Ku, Seoul, 137–040 Korea

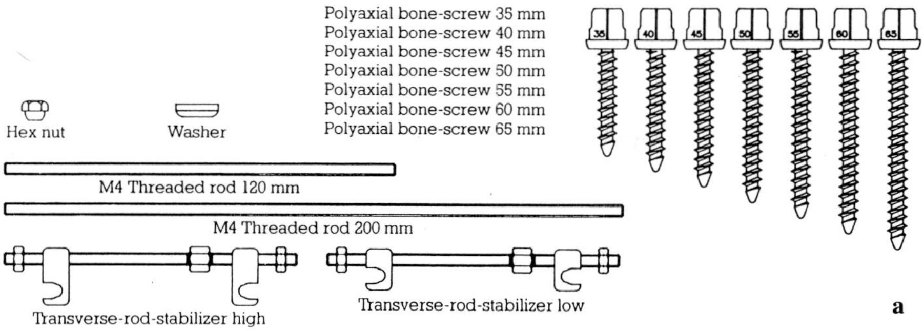

a

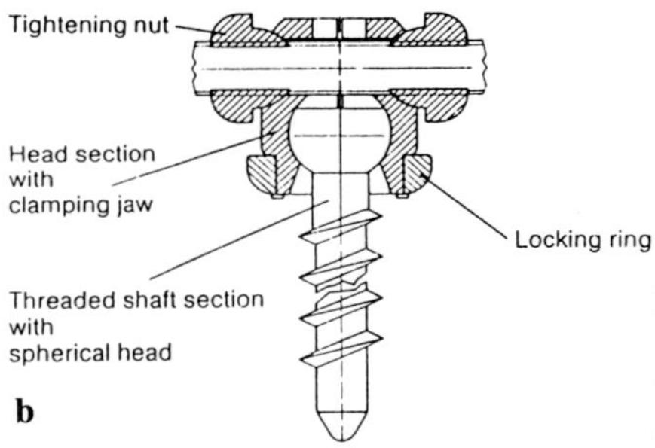

b

Fig. 1. a The components of the MOSS polyaxial bone screw, threaded rod and transverse rod stabilizer. **b** Names of screw parts. **c** Method of tightening the hex-nuts

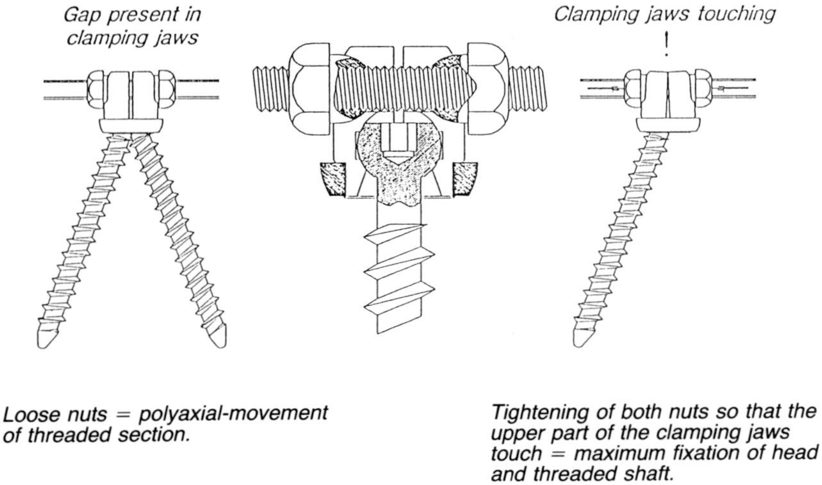

c

Table 1. Number of cases of two conditions.

Conditions	No. of cases (n)
Pure degenerative stenosis	20
Spondylolisthesis	25
Degenerative	13
Isthmic	12

n = 45; M:F = 13:32

Materials and Methods

Design and Application of MOSS System

The screw implant consists of a threaded shaft with a spherical head encompassed by two clamping jaws. The head section is connected to the threaded shaft section with a locking ring and cannot be dislocated. This permits movement of the head in all directions. The connection between the screw heads and the threaded rod is made so that the screw head is oriented in such a way that the rod can be inserted without bending (Fig. 1b,c). This can be done relatively simply and easily even in multisegmental situations. By manipulating the hex nuts on the rod, proper contouring can be accomplished. Tightening of the hex nuts beyond touching of upper part of the clamping jaws will not achieve more fixation of the rod, but can result in damage of the threaded rod (Fig. 1c).

Patients

We used the MOSS system in 20 patients with pure degenerative lumbar stenosis and 25 patients with symptomatic spondylolisthesis (13 degenerative, 12 isthmic types) to stabilize the lumbar spine after decompression surgery together with posterolateral fusion (PLF) (Table 1). In 5 cases of spondylolisthesis, anterior interbody fusion (AIF) was combined with PLF, and in 3 cases PLIF was combined. However, in this report, 5 cases who did not have posterolateral fusion were excluded because of a shorter follow-up and statistically insignificant numbers, and these cases will be presented later.

Of the total 45 patients, 13 were males and 32 were females. Olisthesis was graded from Myerding's I to II. The following complaints were seen: disabling low back pain in 41 patients (91.2%), sciatica in 38 patients (84.5%), and claudication in 29 patients (64%) (Table 2).

One-level fusion was carried out on 40 patients, and two-level fusion on 5 patients. Fusion at the L4–L5 level was performed on 25 patients, and L5–S1 fusion on 15 patients. Two-level fusion between L4–S1 was done on 5 patients (3 patients with pure stenosis, and 2 with spondylolisthesis) (Table 3).

Table 2. Complaints (symptoms and signs).

Complaints	No. of cases (n)
Low back pain	91.2% (41)
Sciatica	84.5% (38)
Claudication	64% (29)

Table 3. Levels of MOSS instrumentation and PLF.

Segment	Level	No. of cases (n)		Remarks
		Pure stenosis (n = 20)	Spondylolisthesis (n = 25)	
1 level (n = 40)	L4–L5	12	13[a]	AIF in 5 cases
	L5–S1	5	10[b]	PLIF in 2 cases
2 levels (n = 5)	L4–L5–S1	3	2[c]	PLIF in 1 case
Total (n = 45)		20	25	

[a] Includes 5 patients who underwent AIF
[b] Includes 2 patients who underwent PLIF
[c] Includes 1 patient who underwent PLIF

All patients were evaluated both clinically and radiologically at the time of the last follow-up, an average of 1.2 years (8 months to 2.2 years).

Assessment

All patients were evaluated both clinically and radiologically at the time of the last follow-up. In addition the patients were questioned as to how they rated their result from surgery using the following criteria:

1. Excellent: As good as before development of the disorder.
2. Good: Free from pain most of the time. Need occasional non-prescription pain medication for the back and to be careful when using the back.
3. Fair: Must be very careful when using the back.
4. Poor: Slightly better than before surgery.
5. Failure: No better or even worse than before surgery.

In all cases, the physical examination and the patients' subjective rating correlated well. All patients were given a rating 1 year after surgery, as well as a final rating at the follow-up examination.

Results

Symptomatic improvement was obtained in 42 patients (93.3%): 38 patients (84.4%) were rated excellent, and 4 patients (8.8%) as good. There was no

Table 4. Incidence of postoperative reduction and reslip in 25 spondylolisthesis cases.

	No. of cases (n)
Reduction	20 (80%)
Complete	12 (60%)
Partial	8 (40%)
Reslip	13 (52%)

Table 5. Clinical results.

Results	No. of cases (n = 45)	Remarks
Excellent	38 (84.5%)	Reslip (n = 11)
Good	4 (8.8%)	Reslip (n = 2)
Fair	0	
Poor	3 (6.7%)	
Failure	0	
Fusion rate	42 (93.3%)	Sum of excellent and good results

Table 6. Complications.

Reslip	13 (65%) out of 20 reduced cases
Loss of lordosis	3 (6.7%) out of 45 cases
Rod loosening	1 (2.3%)
Neurological injury[a]	1 (2.2%)[a]

[a] Drop: Transient palsy

improvement in 3 patients (6.6%). Reduction was obtained in 20 (80.0%) out of 25 patients with spondylolisthesis. However, reslip developed in 13 patients (52%), and occurred within 3 months postoperatively. The reslips did not influence the clinical end-results. Successful fusion was obtained in 42 patients (93.3%). Rod loosening and a mild drop foot developed in 1 patient as a complication. Loss of lumbar lordosis was found in 3 patients (6.7%) with spondylolisthesis (Table 4–6).

Discussion

Pedicular screw fixation is already an established technique available to spinal surgeons, and is known to improve fusion rates in cases of posterolateral fusion [4–8] and to allow earlier mobilization of patients after surgery [1,2,9,10]. Thus, the spinal stability provided by pedicle screw fixation is known to be better than that with any other fixation system [1,9,11].

The principal advantages of transpedicular fixation are: (1) direct control over all degrees of motion of the vertebral body and posterior elements, (2) a short fixation area limited to the pathological segment, and (3) increased stability of pedicular based fixation systems. In the MOSS system the rod can easily be inserted to the screw head without bending, because the screw design allows polyaxial motion at the screw neck. Thus, by interconnection of the screws via the threaded rod using nuts, a stable spondylodesis can be achieved. Also it was found that the incidence of complications associated with MOSS pedicular screw placement is low when performed properly [12]. We encountered no rod breakage, though rod loosening occurred in one case because of inadequate nut tightening. It is speculated that the MOSS polyaxial screw system could prevent screw breakage too, because the dimension of the rod is made to be smaller than that of the neck of the pedicular screw for safety reasons. Otherwise the screw neck inside the pedicle is likely to break in an overloading situation.

In comparison with other systems, this improved system could also effectively reduce slipped segments, and could initially provide rigid temporary fixation. However, in half the cases in our series the MOSS system could not maintain immediate postoperative reduction until the PLF consolidated, and also the system could not normalize the lumbar curve, particularly in those cases. We obtained successful fusion and satisfactory results in 93.3% of cases in our series, though this fusion rate was inferior to the 100% fusion rate achieved by Wiltse [11].

According to Lowe's survey report [13], the overall incidence of neurological complications in pedicular fixation surgery was 1.84%; 1.47% with the C-D hook system, 3.2% with the C-D pedicular screw device, 7% with the Roy-Camille pedicle screw plate, and 2.2% with the Louis screw plate. The figure of 2.2% for neurological complications in our series [14] was almost the same as that in Lowe's report. The high rate of forward reslip in the surgically reduced vertebral bodies in our series indicates that the polyaxial screw of the MOSS system cannot give optimal slip resistance for the bony architecture of the pedicle and cannot achieve rigid fixation through resistance of the lever action of the vertebral body because of the polyaxial motion. Therefore, it is thought that in conjunction with MOSS pedicular fixation, ventral fusion such as additional AIF or PLIF can be a solution to prevent reslip and to raise the fusion rate of PLF in the treatment of spondylolisthesis. Thus, it can be said that the polyaxial adjustable screw head of the MOSS system has merits, but it also has unexpected demerits.

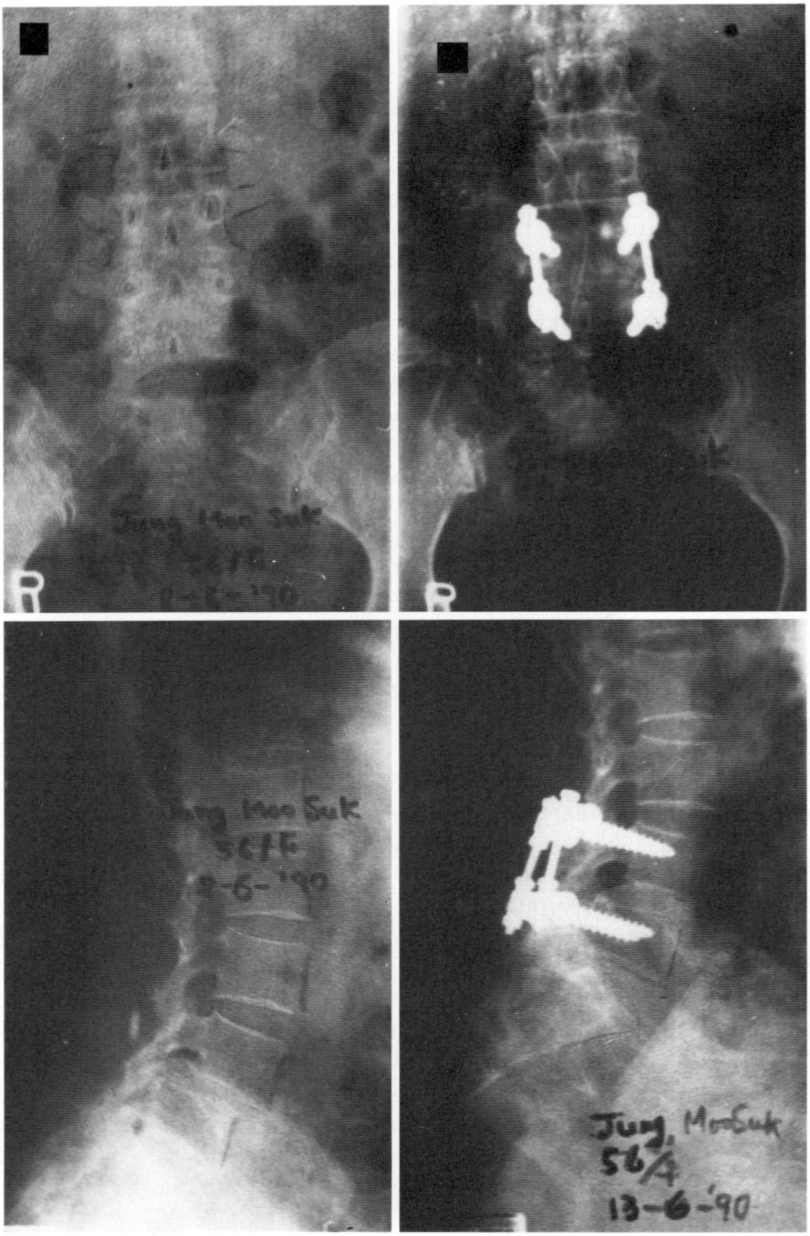

A C
B D

Case Studies

Case 1. This 56-year-old female suffered from low back pain and sciatica for several years. She said that the sciatica gradually worsened and became intolerable. Initial examination disclosed no neurological deficit except tension signs in the right leg (straight leg raising: 35°). X ray examination disclosed Grade 1 degenerative spondylolisthesis. Surgery was recommended, as 6

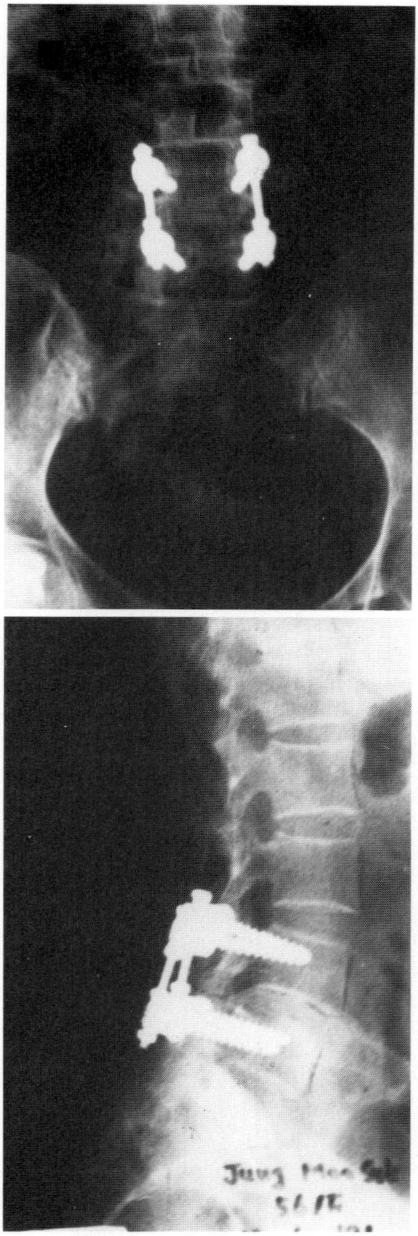

E

F

Fig. 2A–F. Case 1. Degenerative spondylolisthesis at L4–L5 (**A**,**B**). The patient was treated with decompression laminectomy, instrumented reduction, and PLF (**C**,**D**). There was no instrument failure or loosening. Good bony fusion between the transverse processes of L4–L5 was obtained without loss of reduction (**E**,**F**).

months of conservative treatment had failed. On June 13, 1990, posterior decompression surgery plus PLF and MOSS pedicular fixation was done (Fig. 2). Some reduction of L4 was obtained after surgery. She was kept in bed for 4 weeks postoperatively, and then gradually mobilized with a low back brace. In the postoperative 1-year X ray, we noticed good bony bridges between the transverse processes of L4–L5. The patient is faring well.

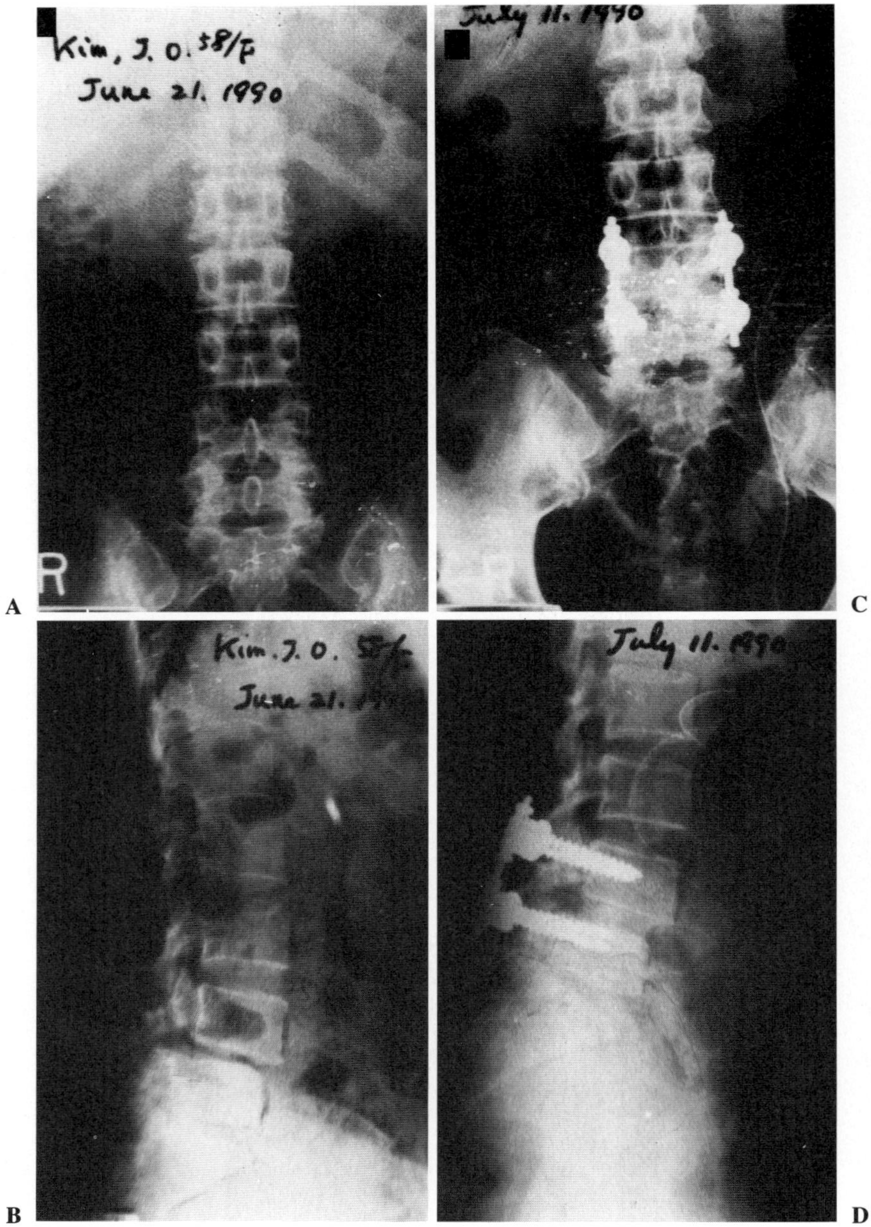

Case 2. This 58-year-old female suffered from disabling low back pain and intermittent claudication for which posterior decompression surgery, PLF and AIF, plus MOSS pedicular fixation was carried out on July 11, 1990 (Fig. 3).

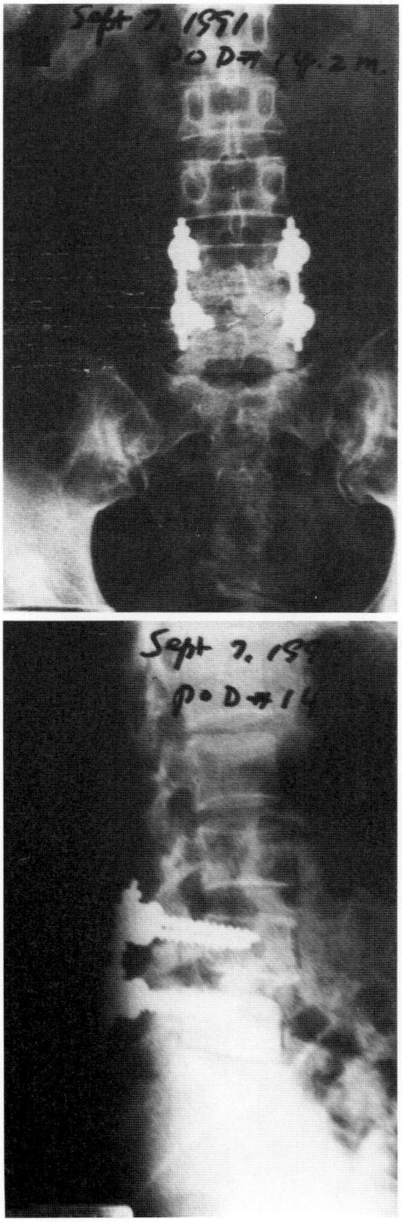

E

F

Fig. 3A–F. Case 2. Degenerative spondylolisthesis at L4–L5 (**A**,**B**). Decompressive laminectomy, instrumented reduction, PLF, and AIF were done. Some reduction of slip and restoration of disk height were obtained postoperatively (**C**,**D**). Segmental stabilization and the maintenance of slip reduction were obtained. Intercorporal fusion was obtained, though there was some reduction of disk height at the final follow-up (**E**,**F**)

Postoperatively there was some reduction of L4 over L5. During follow-up until September 7, 1991, 1 year and 2 months postoperatively, there was evidence of intercorporal fusion though some graft collapse was noticed. She was free from symptoms at the final follow-up.

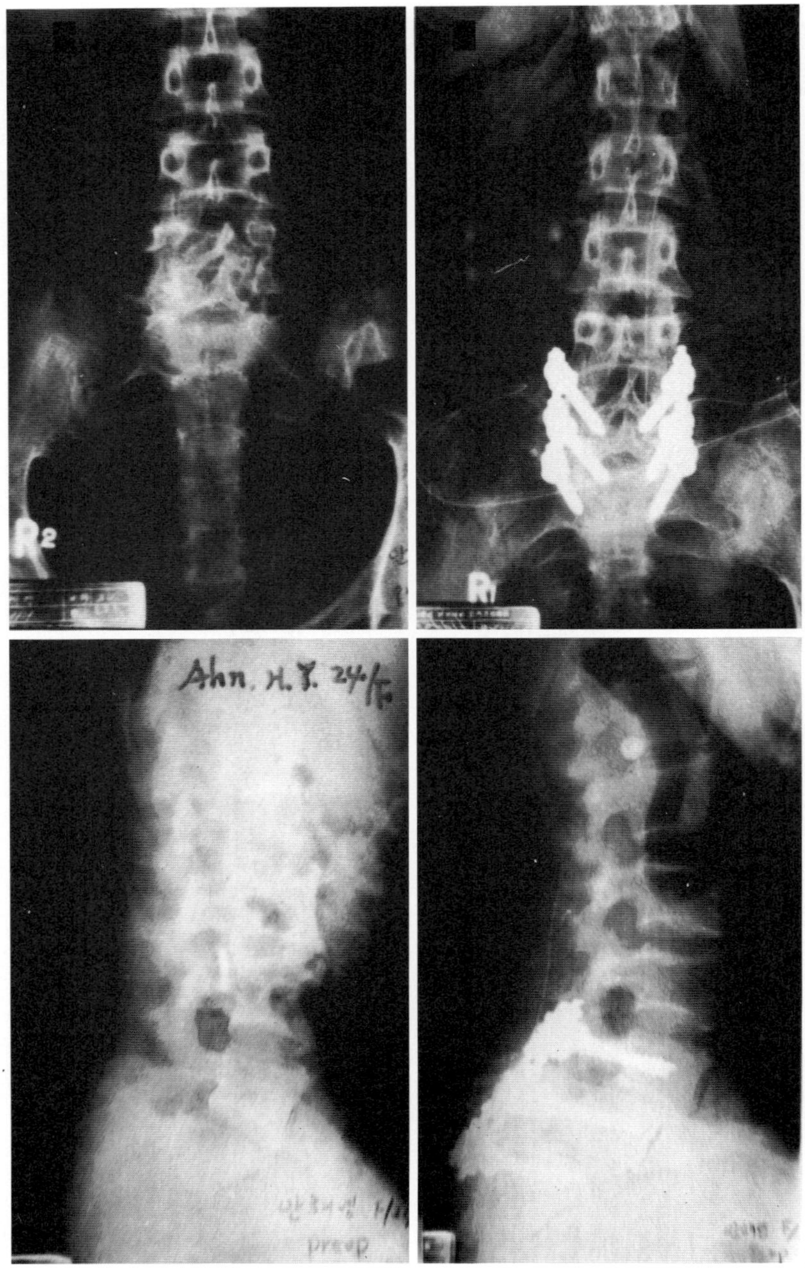

Case 3. This 24-year-old female had suffered from disabling low back pain for a few years and waddling gait since birth. X ray examination disclosed Grade 1 dysplastic spondylolisthesis at L4–L5 and L5–S1 (Fig. 4). For the two-level

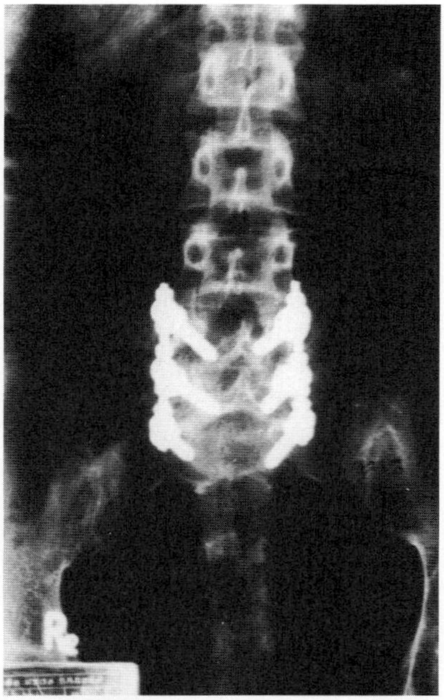

E

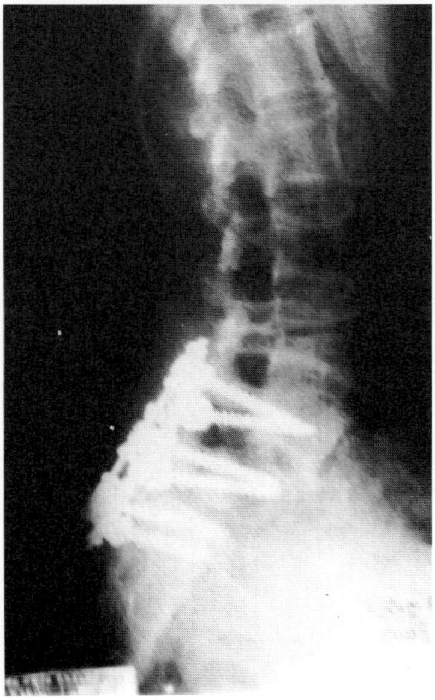

F

Fig. 4A–F. Case 3. Dysplastic spondylolisthesis at L4–L5 and L5–S1 (**A**,**B**). Immediate postoperative X rays (anteroposterior and lateral) following PLF and MOSS pedicular fixation (**C**,**D**) show the in-situ stabilization and fusion. At 9 months postoperatively good intertransverse fusion between L4–S1 was obtained without instrument failure (**E**,**F**)

slips, posterolateral fusion reinforced with MOSS pedicular fixation was carried out on January 15, 1991. At 9 months postoperatively there was good bony fusion between transverse processes of L4–S1, and no reslip and/or failure in the MOSS system. She is faring well.

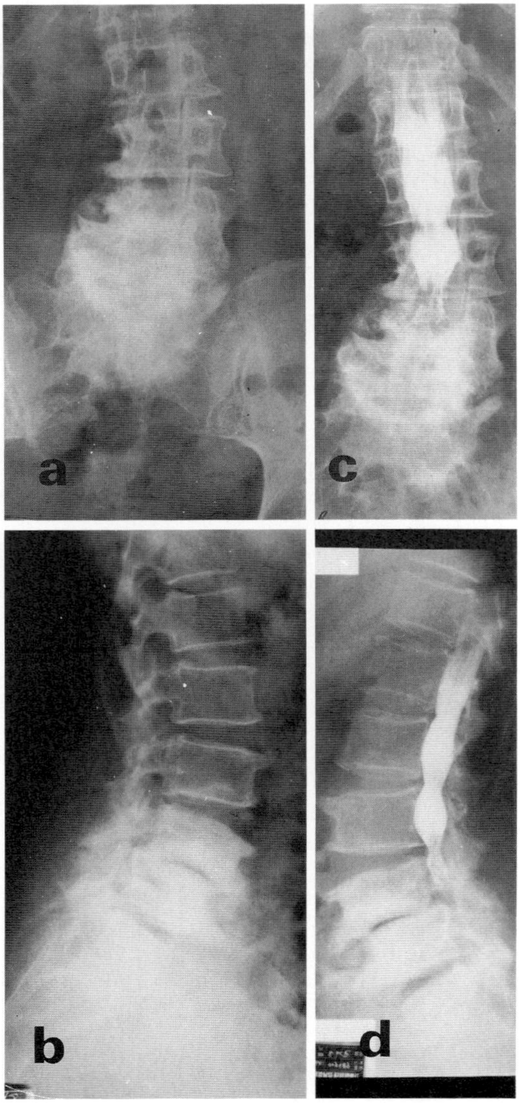

Fig. 5. Case 4. Preoperative X ray showing left degenerative lumbar scoliotic curve with severe subchondral sclerosis and forward slipping of L4 on L5 (**a**,**b**), and myelogram showing the complete block at level of posterior wall of L4 (**c**,**d**). MOSS instrumentation, and posterior lumbar interbody fusion between L4–L5 and L5–S1 (**e**,**f**), and posterolateral fusion between L4–S1 were carried out with successful final stabilization **g**,**h**)

Case 4. This 53 year-old female suffered from spinal stenosis at L4–L5 for several years. Preoperative X-rays show left degenerative lumbar scoliotic curve (Fig. 5a,b), and myelograms (Fig. 5c,d) show complete block at the level of the posterior wall of the L4 body. In this patient L4–S1 was immobilized with a MOSS device after decompression laminectomy, and PLF and PLIF of L4–L5 and L5–S1 were combined (Fig. 5e,f). In the 1-year postoperative

Fig. 5.
(*continued*)

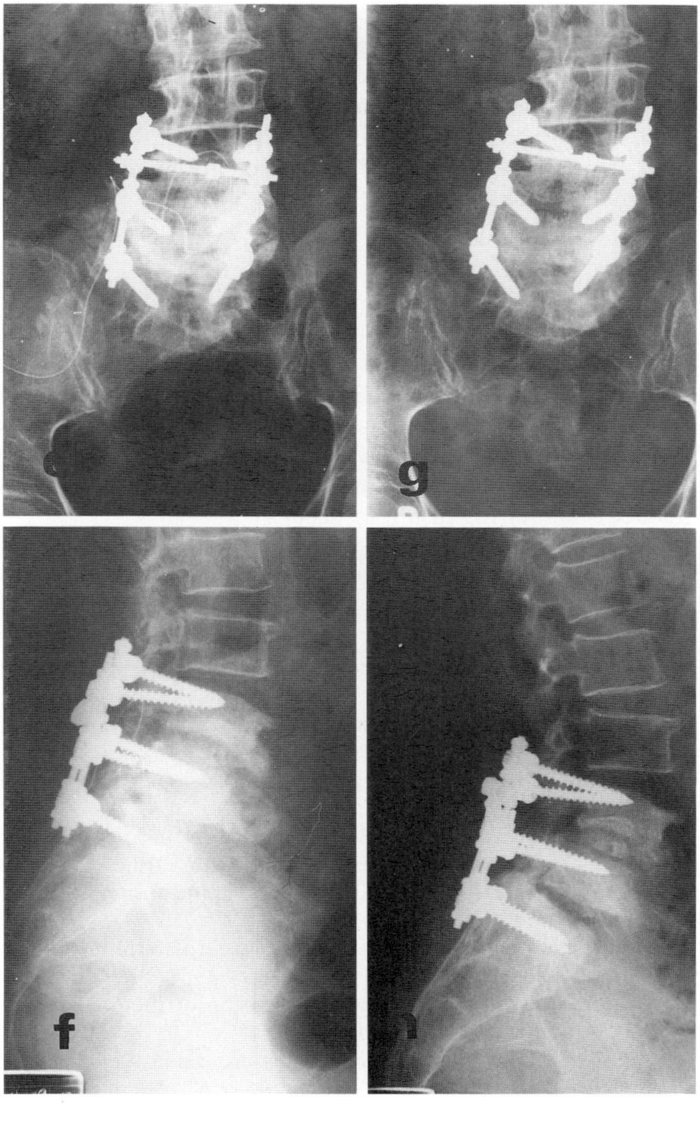

anteroposterior and lateral X-rays, no loosening of the fixative devices or metal failure were seen (Fig. 5g,h). During the follow-up period there was no forward vertebral reslip seen, though disk space became slightly narrowed between L4–L5 and L5–S1. Finally fusion between L4–S1 was obtained successfully (Fig. 5g,h), and she is now completely free from preoperative symptoms.

With increasing experience with transpedicular instrumentation, indications and techniques are becoming more clear and complications less frequent. If we can reduce the incidence of complications, this may be the best procedure. However, it is stressed that any pedicular fixation system for spinal stabilization is in no way a substitute for meticulous surgical techniques, adequate facet joint excision, and bone grafting, which are mandatorily required for long-term successful fusion.

Conclusions

This study has disclosed that the MOSS system can effectively raise fusion rates in cases of posterolateral fusion, though it cannot maintain instrumented reduction effectively in the spondylolisthetic vertebra. In our opinion, the MOSS system is a simple device which can easily be utilized even by non-specialist spine surgeons, and that internal fixation by the MOSS system can add the needed stability for fusion to occur.

References

1. Aebi M (1991) Transpedicular fixation. Indication, techniques and complications. Curr Orthop 5:109–116
2. Dick W (1987) The "Fixateur Interne" as a versatile implant for spine surgery. Spine 12:882–900
3. Harrington PR (1988) The history and development of Harrington Instrumentation. Clin Orthop 227:3–5
4. Tajima N, Kawano K (1989) Posterolateral fusion of the lumbar and lumbosacral spine – A review of long term results. J Jpn Orthop Assoc 63:262–268
5. Thompson WAL (1986) Lumbosacral spine fusion. J Bone Joint Surg [Am] 56: 1643–1647
6. Truchly G, Thompson WAL (1962) Posterolateral fusion of the lumbosacral spine. J Bone Joint Surg [Am] 44:505–512
7. Watkins MB (1953) Posterolateral fusion of the lumbar and lumbosacral spine. J Bone Joint Surg [Am] 35:1014–1018
8. Wilste LL (1968) The paraspinal sacrospinalis splitting approach to the lumbar spine. J Bone Joint Surg [Am] 50:919–926
9. Cotrel Y, Dubousset J, Guillaumat M (1988) New universal instrumentation in spinal surgery. Clin Orthop 227:10–23
10. Olerud S, Karlstrom G, Sjostrom L (1988) Transpedicular fixation of thoracolumbar vertebral fractures. Clin Orthop 227:44–51
11. Wiltse LL (1991) Treatment of degenerative spondylolisthesis. J Jpn Spine Res Soc 2(1):161
12. Moon MS (1991) Comparison of effectiveness of C-D, Zielke and MOSS transpedicular screw fixation systems in the lower lumbar spinal disorders. J Jpn Spine Res Soc 2(1):163

13. Lowe TG (1987) Morbidity and mortality report of scoliosis. Scoliosis Research Society Meeting, Vancouver, Canada, September 6–8
14. Moon MS, Ha KY, Jung DY (1990) Pitfalls, errors, and complications in the transpedicular screw fixation surgery. J Korean Orthop Assoc 25:169–176

4.8 Internal Fixation of the Lumbar Spine: Further Clinical Experience Using Computer Assisted Design and Manufacture of a Precise System

David C. Hemmy[1]

Introduction

Degenerative disorders of the lumbar spine cause loss of the normal disk space height, the formation of osteophytes, and facet joint osteoarthropathy, all of which singly or in combination cause encroachment upon the intraspinal and intraforaminal contents. This results in pain and neurologic dysfunction. The goals of therapy are restoration of normal function and prevention of further degenerative changes. Surgically, this is accomplished by enlargement of the spinal canal and intervertebral foramina (anatomical restoration) and prevention of further motion thus preventing further degenerative changes through fusion. Anatomic restoration of the caliber of the spinal canal and foramina may result in further instability of the spine also justifying fusion. For fusion to occur, a form of fixation or immobilization of the spine is necessary. The introduction of pedicle screw and dorsal plate fixation has provided us with a system permitting solid immobilization for patients undergoing fusion of the lumbar spine.

The technique is, however, not without drawbacks. Imprecise screw location can result in less than optimum stability. This lack of precision can also cause injury to the nerve roots and intrathecal contents or retro- or intraperitoneal structures. Furthermore, current techniques require time consuming X rays for screw location and are extremely dependent upon the skill and experience of the surgeon. Additionally, plates are often shaped and bent quite imprecisely. The system subsequently described obviates these problems and pitfalls.

Materials and Methods

The system to be described was used in 53 patients with degenerative disorders of the spine which resulted in pain and/or neurologic deficit. The system was

[1] St. Joseph Professional Bldg., 3070 North 51st St., Suite 406A, Milwaukee, WI 53210, USA

confined to patients with spondylolysis and spondylolisthesis when the pain was not of a radicular nature.

In addition to the clinical physical examination, conventional radiologic techniques including plain film X rays, contrast myelography, contrast enhanced computed tomography (CT), and magnetic resonance scanning were used singly or in various combinations to assess the disorder anatomically. Furthermore, all patients underwent CT performed in such a way to serve as both a substrate for design for the plating system and to provide precise anatomical information.

CT scans were obtained with the patient in the supine position. CT slices of 1.5 mm thickness, abutting one another are acquired from an anatomical landmark above the site of the proposed fixation to a landmark below the site of the proposed fixation. Scanning typically takes 1 h, with scan factors of 120 kV, 170 mA, and a 2-s scan time. No gantry tilt is used. All scans were acquired on a General Electric 9800 scanner (General Electric Medical Systems, New Berlin, WI). Several volunteers were scanned in both the supine and the prone positions to determine if position would alter the design of the fixation system. Scanning of the prone patient resulted in significant motion error or "artifact" due to the anteroposterior respiratory excursions and misregistration of adjacent CT slices. Although there was anteroposterior motion, little cephalocaudal motion was recorded. Therefore, supine and prone scanning procedures could be compared. Little or, in most cases, no difference was noted in studies suggesting no change in the osseous lumbar skeleton from the supine to the prone position. As a result, supine scanning was adopted to eliminate the respiratory artifact.

CT data thus obtained was reformatted in the three dimensional [1] format as well as in sagittal and axial projections for the diagnostic and planning use of the surgeon. The DMI (Dimensional Medicine, Inc., Minnetonka, MN) workstation was used in all cases. The information obtained from the reformatted three dimensional images was used by the surgeon to convey to the manufacturer (Artifex Ltd., Newport Beach, CA) the levels of the spinal column requiring fixation as well as the landmarks to be used in siting the guide for installation of the system.

A magnetic tape containing the CT scan data is sent to the manufacturer of the system. The scan image files are transferred to an imaging workstation equiped with ArtSys (Version 3.1) image analysis software (Artifex Ltd., Newport Beach, CA). In addition to typical grey scale formats, the system allows presentation of image data in a hued and colored format with colors corresponding to the threshold density levels above and below selected osseous values and a binary format depicting only those pixels which meet adjustable thresholding criteria. The system also allows evaluation of image data using an adjustable window which maps any range of the −1024 to 3072 Hounsfield unit CT scale to a 256 grey/color scale image. After review of the images, the appropriate CT threshold level is selected displaying only osseous structures.

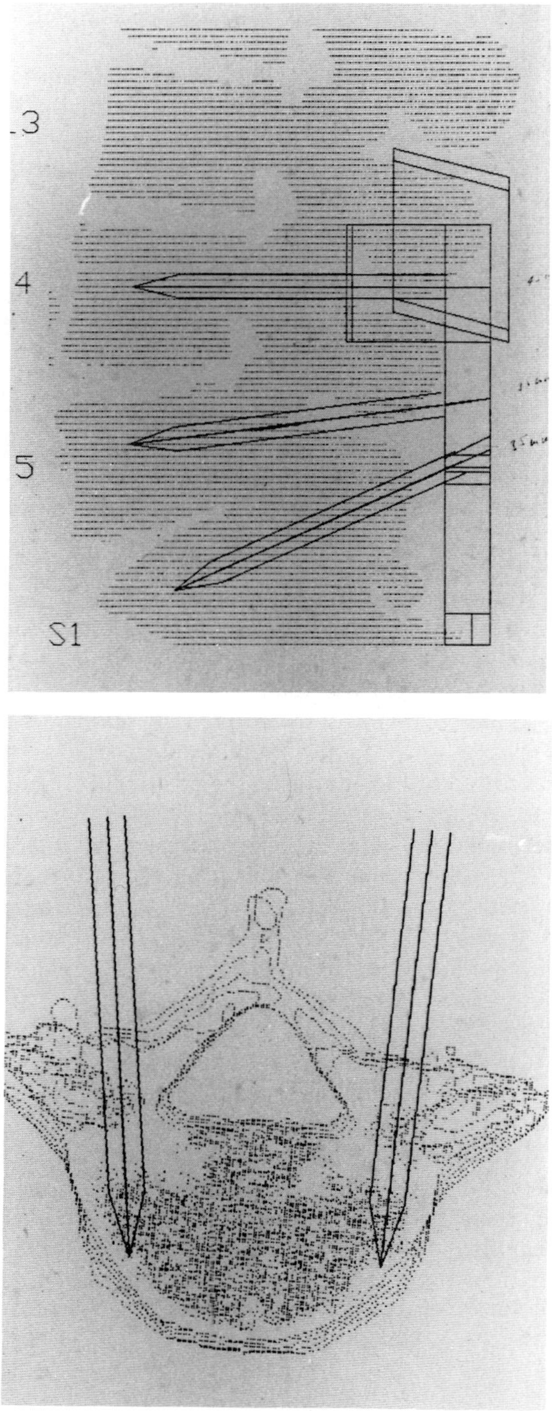

a

b

Fig. 1a,b. Lateral view (**a**) and axial view (**b**) of designed screw position

After selection of the threshold level, a database of geometric points is generated by applying an adjustable edging algorithm against all threshold qualifying pixels. The system makes a conversion of this qualifying point database to a format readable by a standard computer assisted design (CAD) system.

Once the data reside in the CAD system, the designer is responsible for collecting three sets of design information: (1) that which determines the appropriate screw locations, (2) that which determines the appropriate plate locations relative to the screws, and (3) the specific landmarks used for the design of the guide component (Fig. 1). In all cases the design is driven by both patient tissue geometry and the design preferences of the surgeon. Therefore, all components are specific to the patient and the surgeon.

When the design process is complete, the component geometry is transferred to a computer assisted manufacturing (CAM) system which generates the specific software to drive automated machinery in the production of all components. Within North America, the components can be generated within 4 days of receipt of the scan data.

The surgical procedure is carried out with the patient placed in the prone position with the chest supported by chest rolls. The table is not placed in flexion. The dorsal elements of the spine and transverse processes are denuded of all tissue and ligamentous attachements. Care is taken not to remove any bone as this serves as the substrate for the guide used for positioning of the screws.

The guide (Fig. 2) is positioned by resting on the dorsal elements of the spine as well as encircling selected spinous processes. When it is positioned so that no motion is permitted, transfixion pins are placed through the selected spinous processes to temporarily secure the guide.

Guide pins are next placed in the template. Their location is such that if correctly positioned, they will be immediately dorsal to the pedicles desired for fixation. A lateral X ray is obtained to confirm the location. This will be the only X ray which is necessary during the procedure. A gundrill is then used to provide pilot holes in the pedicles and vertebral bodies for the bone tap screw. The manufacturer provides the precise depth to place the tap holes. This is marked on the tap screw and it is driven to the necessary depth at each of the locations. Following this, the permanent screw is driven to the computed depth at each location. The guide is then removed.

If a laminectomy, facetectomy or foramenotomy is to be performed, it is accomplished immediately after the placement of the screws. Lastly, the plate (Fig. 3) is positioned between lock nuts and fastened permanently. Placement of the onlay bone graft on the tranverse processes follows.

Results

In most cases in the postoperative period, a "pedicle study" was performed by means of CT. In each case, the scan was performed so that the gantry was

2 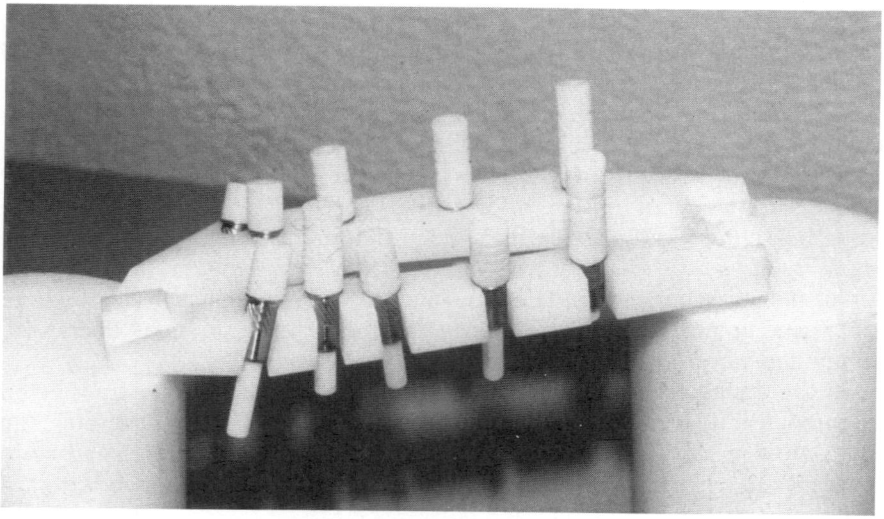

3 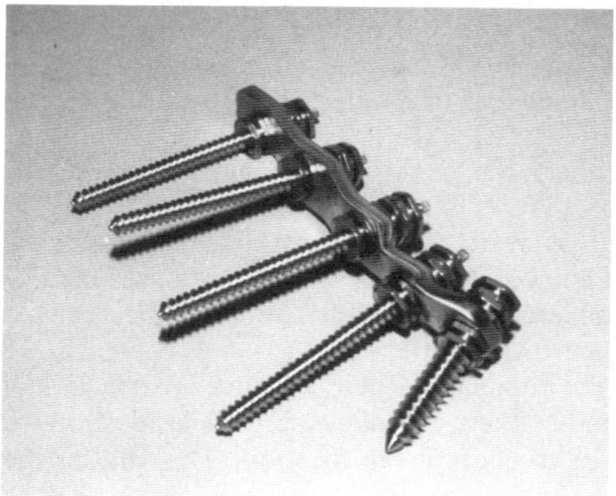

Fig. 2. Screw positioning guide

Fig. 3. Plate, screws, and nuts

positioned parallel to the screws. This view permitted the determination of the location of the screw and whether it was "in" or "out" of the pedicle. The geometric error that was noted was attributable to "sliding" or "skating" of the screw in that it entered the pedicle at the correct point but was misdirected from that point on. There were no definite instances of nerve root injury. One patient had radicular pain postoperatively which did not exist preoperatively. Radiographic studies did not confirm nerve root penetration or distortion, but removal of the screw at the suggested clinical location resulted in cessation of the patient's pain. In a second instance a patient continued to have postoperative pain resulting in removal of screws and plates. Post removal films showed extremely accurate location of screw holes. The patient's pain did not subside following removal of the plates and screws.

There was one instance of metal failure. A 54-year-old patient was placed in a work hardening program which necessitated conditioning by repeated flexion of the spine. Screw fracture was noted to occur 3 months postoperatively by means of serial X rays.

Conclusions

This is a spinal internal fixation system which is easy to install based on accurate fiducial coordinates obtained through CT scanning. The system obviates the "art" of screw placement, significantly reducing the length of the operation. To date only one neurologic and one structural failure have been noted. The cost of the system is only slightly more than off-the-shelf stocked systems but it avoids an expensive hospital inventory.

Reference

Hemmy DC, Tessier PL (1985) CT of dry skulls with craniofacial deformities: Accuracy of three dimensional reconstruction. Radiology 157:113–116

4.9 Complications of Lumbar Spinal Surgery with Transpedicular Fixation

Sanford H. Davne and Donald L. Myers[1]

Historical Perspective

Spinal fusion has been an important management technique for various degenerative and traumatic conditions of the lumbar spine. The addition of internal fixation during arthrodesis allows correction of deformity that might not otherwise be feasible. Instrumentation also will minimize motion during graft incorporation and there is substantial evidence this probably increases the rate of solid arthrodesis, especially over multiple anatomic motion segments [1–3]. The incidence of pseudarthrosis in posterolateral fusions without instrumentation has been reported to vary between 5% and 55% for one- and two-level fusions [1,3]. Unfortunately, most studies have not relied on re-exploration, but on radiological assessment which has been shown to have a significant margin of error [4]. Instrumentation in the lumbar spine has been difficult to apply because of the lumbar lordosis, surgical absence of laminae, and the problem of sacral fixation. Transpedicular instrumentation addresses these problems, is an excellent method of vertebral attachment in the lumbar spine [5], and allows specific levels to be fused with short segmental fixation. While use of the pedicle screw was first described by King [6] in 1944, considerable experience was subsequently developed by Roy-Camille et al. [7] and Louis [8]. Currently, a variety of transpedicular-screw-based devices are either in development or are being used clinically. These include the variable screw placement (VSP) system of Steffee et al. [9,10], the A-O fixateur interne [11], and systems developed by Luque [12], Wiltse [13], Edwards [14], Cotrel-Debousset [15], and others. The variable screw placement (VSP) instrumentation was used in all of our procedures. We began using this system shortly after its introduction because of our discouraging results with uninstrumented lumbar fusion. The system has undergone several design modifications during this series that will be discussed.

[1] Departments of Orthopaedic and Neurological Surgery, Thomas Jefferson University, 1015 Chestnut St., Philadelphia, PA 19107, USA

Materials and Methods

The series includes 533 consecutive procedures (including our first case) performed on 486 patients from April of 1986 to October of 1990 for diskal, degenerative, or spondylolytic pathology. Patients with fractures or tumors were excluded. Strong indicators for fusion were the presence of degenerative spondylolisthesis, symptomatic spondylolysis, and re-exploration at the same level. Relative indicators included facet degeneration, obesity, age, bulging central or degenerated disk, and predominance of back pain aggravated by activity. Diskectomy or decompression without fusion was used whenever appropriate and these patients were not included. All procedures were performed jointly by a neurological and orthopaedic surgeon.

Preoperatively, all patients were encouraged to donate blood autologously, and most did. We have used sequential compression boots on all patients for the last 3 years and patients with a history of thromboembolic problems received subcutaneous perioperative heparin. Prophylactic antibiotics were used in all patients with the initial dose given during the induction of anesthesia and every 3 h during the procedure. The antibiotics were continued for 2–3 days after the procedure, and longer if wound drainage persisted.

Operative technique consisted of initial dissection, exposure, exploration, decompression, and diskectomy when indicated. The lateral fusion site was then exposed and packed. The iliac crest bone graft was harvested through the same incision with subcutaneous dissection over the lumbodorsal fascia. Bone wax and Gelfoam were used for hemostasis of the graft donor site. When appropriate, posterior lumbar interbody fusion (PLIF) was performed either before or after screw placement. Lateral decortication was done before screw insertion, because the screws can obstruct access to the lateral fusion bed. The site of insertion was described by Steffee [16] and subsequently by Weinstein et al. [17] as the junction of the transverse process and the infero-lateral border of the superior articular facet. The accessory process and ridge of the transverse process were also helpful landmarks, when present. With a narrow rongeur, a small window was made in the cortex and then a bone awl was used to penetrate the first few millimeters. The pedicle probe or "gear shift" was used to establish the tract by guiding the tip of the probe along the lateral wall of the pedicle into the vertebral body. Early in the series, X ray markers in the pedicle were often used. Generally, the pedicle tract was tapped with a 7.0-mm tap, however if the pedicles were small on preoperative X ray evaluation, were unusually sclerotic, or probe placement was difficult, 5.5-mm and 6.25-mm taps were first used in sequence, which is effective because the thread is the same on all three taps. The pedicle feeler was then used to verify the presence of bone and threads circumferentially. The screw was then placed and should go in fairly easily and should not really be "steered" to avoid fracturing or breaking out of the pedicle. Intraoperative X rays were taken to help confirm proper screw placement before plate application to avoid having to remove the plate to adjust a screw. Spacing washers or wedges were placed and then the bone graft was packed laterally. In many of our first hundred patients, we used allograft mixed with local bone available from decompression and decortication. Subsequent to this, we have used allograft only when adequate autogenous iliac crest bone of good quality was not available. The plates were contoured, positioned and secured with nuts. To prevent impingement of the functional facet joint above, the plate was not allowed to project cephalad from the superior screw. The inferior portion of the foramen just above and the superior portion of the foramen below the decompressed interspace were carefully evaluated to insure that shifts of the vertebrae during application did not result in neural compression. The bolt ends were then cut as flush as possible.

Postoperatively, the patients were encouraged to ambulate the next day, and could usually be discharged by the 7th postoperative day. Bracing was not routinely employed, although many patients were given the opportunity to wear an elastic lumbar corset. A few patients with extensive fusions, "soft" bone, or with less than optimal fusion constructs were required to wear a brace. Activity was discouraged and active physical therapy was not employed during the first 3 months.

Demographics

The average age at surgery was 43 years. The average preop duration of symptoms was 45 months: 30 without prior surgery and 59 with prior surgery. The duration of follow-up ranged from 1 to 5 years, and was over 24 months for 392 procedures. 52% of the patients had had previous surgery, and 73% of the reoperations were at the same level. 96% of the patients had lumbar radiculopathy and all these had decompression and optional discectomy. 61% had a one level fusion, 34% had a two level fusion, and only 5% had three or more levels fused. There were 767 levels fused in 533 procedures; 49% were posterolateral fusions, 29% were PLIF, and 22% had combined or global fusions. We had at least 1-year follow-up in all patients, and have current data on 97%.

Complication Data

General complications included five (0.9%) patients requiring treatment for thromboembolic disorders with no serious sequellae. Two (0.4%) patients developed hepatitis, and both were early in the series. Perioperative death occurred once (0.2%) and was not directly related to surgery. The patient did very well initially but died 5 days postop from myocardial infarction.

Wound infection occurred in 14 (2.6%) patients. Three (0.6%) infections clearly tracked beneath the fascia and were classified as deep wound problems. Five (0.9%) tracked to the iliac crest graft site that had been harvested through the same incision. Six (1.1%) infections were superficial and did not track below any fascial plane. Culture results included eight staphylococcus areus, one beta hemolytic streptococcus, four different gram negative organisms, and one showed no growth. There was no significant difference in the infection rate between primary and reoperative patients. All infections were treated with appropriate intravenous antibiotics, debridement, irrigation with antibiotic solution, and most underwent delayed closure. Two of the iliac crest infections recurred and required re-exploration despite long courses of intravenous antibiotics consistent with treatment for osteomyelitis. These resolved with the second course of debridement and antibiotics. One deep wound infection recurred 11 months later and we opted to remove the device to help eliminate the infection.

Neural injury occurred in six (1.1%) patients in this series. Two (0.4%) involved screws partially outside the pedicle displacing the nerve. One of these patients had sensory impairment, which completely resolved with device removal. The other had sensory and motor symptoms and following screw removal has a mild sensory impairment with good motor function. Neural blunt injury occurred in two (0.4%) patients, one during probing the pedicle through an old lateral fusion mass, and one while cutting the PLIF channel. Both of these fully recovered. Two (0.4%) nerves were injured in retraction for performance of PLIF. One patient recovered, the other is the only patient in this series with a complete and persistent foot drop (0.2%). We feel this was related to retraction for PLIF in a patient with taut or non-mobile nerves. We experienced no exploration- or decompression-related neurologic problems in the series, which included 279 patients undergoing re-exploration. The nerve impingement problems tended to occur early in our experience as we had no device-related neural injuries in the last 330 procedures. Three (0.6%) neural injuries related to performance of PLIF, and three (0.6%) injuries related to the use of instrumentation.

Technical problems were seen with a higher frequency early in our series and included difficult screw placement, screw breakage, and nut loosening. In 43 (8.1%) of the procedures, screw placement was difficult or unsatisfactory because of variations in anatomic landmarks, bone density, pedicle size, or disk space penetration. Most of these occurrences were lateral pedicle breakouts that were corrected during the procedure. Screw fractures were more often the original design and occurred in 23 patients (4.3%), however the overall breakage rate was 28 of 2642 total screws placed (1.1%). The breakage usually became apparent early in the clinical course and 75% of these patients developed recurrent symptoms. Nut loosening occurred in about 20 of the first 100 patients (30 total or 5.6%) as seen on follow-up X rays or on re-exploration. We have only occasionally observed nut loosening after changing the nut application technique.

Discussion

We experienced the same spectrum of general complications one might expect in a surgical group of this size. Autologous blood donation, occasional use of the cell saver, and operative technique have dramatically curtailed our need for donor transfusion that in turn may have reduced our incidence of hepatitis over time. The incidence of phlebitis has probably been reduced by the compression boots now used. Dural tears occurred upon occasion and were repaired primarily; the patients were kept at bedrest for a few days and none required re-exploration. The wound infection rate of 2.6% is similar to that reported in other instrumented and uninstrumented series of spinal fusions, although our deep wound infection rate of 0.6% is somewhat lower than many other series [7,10,13,16,18–21]. Closed suction drainage was used in mainly the first half of our series and no difference in wound healing or infection rate was observed with or without drains. We have not seen closed suction drainage to protect against the persistent wound leakage that seems to occur with a higher frequency in lumbar spinal fusions than with other orthopedic procedures. If drainage persists, we continue the antibiotics to try to prevent secondary infection, although we have no evidence to support this practice. Several wound problems clearly related to suboptimal wound closure.

Technical Discussion

Difficult screw placement occurred in 8.1% of our procedures, although the rate of difficult placement per pedicle instrumented is only 1.6% (43 of 2624). This was usually related to variations in anatomy and increased bone density. Lateral pedicle breakout was the most common problem, and was recognized and generally corrected immediately without sequellae. If difficulty is encountered in establishing the tract with the probe, we recommend starting with the smallest tap and progressively enlarging the hole. In occasional situations, the bone is so dense that drilling is necessary to start the hole so as to place the pedicle probe. When prior lateral fusion had been attempted, or when landmarks are otherwise obscured, further decompression to access the pedicle more directly may be of benefit. Image intensification in not required and we do not use it routinely, although it may be very helpful for the first few cases [16,22]. The pedicle may be imaged obliquely, or with a lateral view carefully aligned to avoid parallax.

During our first year of VSP experience, we observed a relatively high incidence of nut loosening. When we began using the system, one nut was on the screw beneath the plate, and one or two nuts were placed above the plate (Fig. 1a). If any space existed at any point along the construct between the nuts and the plate, the possibility of loosening existed. In particular, the lower nut was more difficult to align properly and secure. If the lower nut was not secured to the bottom of the machine thread, the nut could loosen, especially with loss of mineral content in the adjacent bone. Locking two nuts beneath the plate (Fig. 1b) largely resolved these problems and further improvement was seen with the introduction of the integral-nut screw (Fig. 1c) now in use. The cannulated wrench is an important addition that allows the screw to be

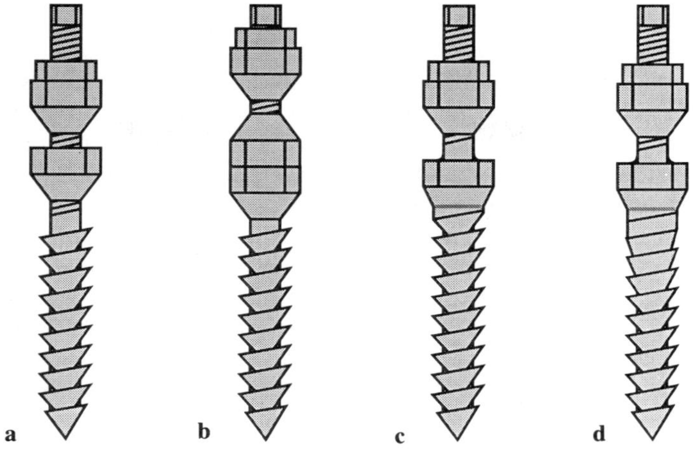

Fig. 1a–d. Design changes in the nuts used in VSP. **a** The original design. **b** Double nut design to reduce loosening. **c** Integral-nut screw currently in use. **d** Tapered root, the most recent modification

firmly held while tightening the nut. This wrench allows the upper nut to be tightened with much higher torque and prevents the screw from spinning or loosening in the bone. Lock nuts were not used initially and were later always used although their significance remains questionable [23]. It is important to contour the plate properly and use the appropriate washers and wedges to achieve optimal plate contact at all levels when the nuts are tightened. The use of spacing washers helps to protect the screw from failure, increases the bending stiffness of the device, prevents impingement on the normal facet joint above the fusion, and allows more room for bone graft beneath the plate. We strongly recommend their use. The facet joint above the fusion is very important and must be preserved. It is placed at some risk of compromise by the dissection, screw placement, and by plate impingement with postoperative motion.

Screw breakage is one manifestation of device failure and has been significantly reduced by device modifications. The original screw did not have an integral nut and breakage was seen at the junction of the machine and bone threads (Fig. 1a). The second modification made the nut integral to the screw and breakage was noted at the junction of the nut and the cancellous thread (Fig. 1c). The most recent modification tapered the root diameter (Fig. 1d) in this junctional area and if breakage occurs now, it is at the end of the taper. With the first screw design, we observed a significantly higher screw fracture rate especially when diskectomy was performed without PLIF. We feel this left the anterior column relatively unsupported and may have overstressed the device. If screw breakage occurred, it was usually early in follow-up and about 75% of our patients with screw fractures were symptomatic. Of the symptomatic patients who opted for re-exploration, several were found solidly fused, but most were not. We have observed that multilevel fusion is a predisposing factor, and that sacral screws are more likely to be involved. It is critical to avoid bending the screws at any point during the operative procedure as this weakens them structurally. If VSP screws have already been placed for a multilevel fusion and their alignment hinders plate positioning, these screws can now be incorporated into a rod system (ISOLA) that was not available during this series. This will prevent both bending of the screws and lateral pedicle breakouts, either of which may be induced by tightening the nuts.

Neurologic injury is a known complication of spinal surgery in general, and is of special concern with transpedicular instrumentation because of both the proximity of neural structures, and the relative inability to visualize directly most of the pedicle and screw path. In our series, three of six neural injuries were related to performance of instrumentation resulting in a device-related neural injury rate of 0.6%, which is somewhat lower than other reported occurrence rates [19,20,22]. Our neural screw impingements occurred fairly early in the series and to date (October 1991), we have not had any device-related injuries in the last 450 procedures and have performed more than 650 pedicular instrumentation cases. If significant unexpected radiculopathy is seen immediately postop, we recommend radiographic evaluation to verify screw position. Thin section CAT scanning is probably most helpful for this. If the screw is suspected of causing neural impingement, early re-exploration to reposition the screw should be recommended to the patient.

PLIF offers a more stable fusion construct, provides anterior column support, and can help significantly in restoring spinal alignment, particularly with spondylolisthesis. However, one must be judicious in the use of PLIF as in some patients the depth of the wound, size of the spinal canal, takeoff of the nerve roots, and "tautness" or difficulty retracting the dural sac are all factors that can make the technique considerably more difficult. Thorough wide decompression at the interspace that might even require complete facetectomy is essential for reliably safe performance of PLIF. We did not have experience with PLIF until the 2nd year of this VSP series. A very definite learning curve exists with PLIF as three of our neural injuries were associated with and occurred early in our experience with this technique. We feel that not all patients can safely have PLIF, and occasionally the best intraoperative decision might be to do just posterolateral fusion, or to add anterior fusion later if it is felt to be essential. Graft retropulsion has been a significant complication of PLIF [24] and as we have not observed this in 384 total levels of PLIF during our series, transpedicular instrumentation probably helps to prevent this problem.

Operative time is always a factor when considering an instrumentation system. After 2 years of experience with device application, we evaluated the operative time spent in activity directly related to device placement. We timed about 75 sequential procedures and observed that instrumentation at one level added about 20–30 min, and at two levels added 30–45 min to the procedure.

This included application of screws and plates, and obtaining a satisfactory intraoperative X ray. Our impression is that with experience, the intraoperative time is not unreasonably increased by instrumentation.

Although we used banked bone initially, and now use autograft whenever possible, we cannot prove that autograft is more effective. Some authors feel that allograft is satisfactory, have a good experience with it and feel the fusion rates are similar, while some feel that autograft is optimal and use it whenever possible [23,25]. In patients with ongoing or recurrent postoperative symptoms, pseudarthrosis must always be suspected, although radiological evaluation after instrumentation is exceedingly difficult. Visualization of the fusion mass is impeded by the plate, and flexion-extension views are not reliable as even minimal motion may be quite symptomatic and yet be difficult or impossible to detect without re-exploration. The true overall rate of fusion cannot be determined except by re-exploration [26], and in our patients with continued or recurrent symptoms (some associated with device failure), to date we have found fusion in 57% of 85 re-explorations.

The role of fusion in the lumbar spine remains controversial. The basic indications for spinal fusion are deformity and instability, although both the clinical significance of deformity and the diagnostic criteria for instability have yet to be satisfactorily defined. The term "mechanical insufficiency" of the motion segment may be a more accurate descriptive term to use in discussing the relative instabilities encountered in degenerative spinal conditions. Clearly, a learning curve is generally associated with the introduction of most new procedures or types of instrumentation. Our experience also influenced the technical evolution of the device and application system by the manufacturer. From a clinical standpoint, the first 6–12 months, or 50–100 cases, produced the most tangible improvements in operative time, blood loss, deformity reduction, and our ability to minimize technical problems. At this point, we have extensive experience in transpedicular screw fixation and we believe that with experience and proficiency, the device can be applied safely, without significantly increasing the complication rate.

References

1. Krag MH (1991) Spinal fusion: Overview of options and posterior internal fixation devices. In: Frymoyer JW (ed) The adult spine: Principles and practice. Raven, New York, pp 1919–1945
2. Schwaegler P, Lorenz M, Cram R, Zindrick M, Collatz MA, Behal R (1991) A comparison of singe level fusions with and without hardware. Annual Meeting of the Federation of Spine Associations, Anaheim, Ca, October 3
3. Zindrick MR (1991) The role of transpedicular fixation systems for stabilization of the lumbar spine. Orthop Clin North Am 22:333–343
4. Brodsky AE, Kovalsky ES, Khalil MA (1991) Correlation of radiologic assessment of lumbar spine fusions with surgical explorations. Spine 16:S261–265
5. Zindrick MR, Wiltse LL, Widel EH et al. (1986) A biomechanical study of intrapeduncular screw fixation in the lumbosacral spine. Clin Orthop 203:99–112

6. King D (1944) Internal fixation for lumbo-sacral fusion. Am J Surg 66:357
7. Roy-Camille R, Saillant G, Mazel C (1986) Internal fixation of the lumbar spine with pedicle screw plating. Clin Orthop 203:7–17
8. Louis R (1986) Fusion of the lumbar and sacral spine by internal fixation with screw plates. Clin Orthrop 203:18–33
9. Steffee A, Biscup R, Sitkowski D (1986) Segmental spine plates with pedicle screw fixation: A new internal fixation device for disorders of the lumbar and thoracic spine. Clin Orthop 203:45–54
10. Steffee AD, Sitkowski DJ (1988) Posterior lumbar interbody fusion and plates. Clin Orthop 227:99–102
11. Dick W (1987) The "fixateur interne" as a versatile implant for spine surgery. Spine 12:882–900
12. Luque E (1986) Interpeduncular segmental fixation. Clin Orthop 203:54–57
13. Horowitch A, Peek RD, Thomas JC, Widell EH, DiMartino PP, Spencer CW, Weinstein J, Wiltse LL (1989) The Wiltse pedicle screw fixation system: Early clinical results. Spine 14:461–467
14. Edwards CC (1987) Spinal screw fixation of the lumbar and sacral spine: Early results in treating the first fifty cases. Orthop Trans 11(1):99
15. Cotrel Y, Dubousset J, Guillaumat M (1988) New universal instrumentation in spinal surgery. Clin Orthop 227:10–23
16. Steffee AD (1989) The variable screw placement system with posterior lumbar interbody fusion. In: Lin PM, Gill K (eds) Lumbar interbody fusion: Principles and techniques in spine surgery. Aspen, Rockville, Md
17. Weinstien JN, Spratt KF, Spengler D, Brick C (1988) Spinal pedicle fixation: Reliability and validity of roentgenogram-based assessment and surgical factors on successful screw placement. Proceedings of the 23rd Annual Meeting of the Scoliosis Research Society. Baltimore, Maryland, September 29
18. Gepstein R, Eismont FI (1990) Postoperative spine infection. In: Weinstein JN, Wiesel S (eds) The lumbar spine. Saunders, Philadelphia
19. West JL, Ogilvie JW, Bradford DS (1991) Complications of the variable screw plate pedicle screw fixation. Spine 16:576–579
20. Whitecloud TS, Butler JC, Cohen JL, Candelora PD (1989) Complications with the variable spinal plating system. Spine 14:472–476
21. Zucherman J, Hsu K, White A, Wynne G (1988) Early results of spinal fusion using variable spine plating techniques. Spine 13:570–579
22. Matsuzaki H, Tokuhashi Y, Matsumoto F, Hoshino M, Kiuchi T, Toriyama S (1990) Problems and solutions of pedicle screw plate fixation of lumbar spine. Spine 15:1159–1165
23. Dalenberg D, Asher M, Jayaraman G, Robinson R (1991) The effect of a stiff spinal implant and its loosening on bone mineral content in canines. 6th Annual Meeting of the North American Spine Society, Keystone, Colorado, July 7–8
24. Lin PM (1989) Technique and complications of posterior lumbar interbody fusion. In: Lin PM, Gill K (eds) Lumbar interbody fusion: Principles and techniques in spine surgery. Aspen, Rockville, Md
25. Dodd CAF, Ferguson CM, Leedman GR, Houghton GR, Thomas D (1988) Allograft bone in scoliosis surgery. J Bone Joint Surg [Br] 70:431–434
26. Bosworth DM (1948) Techniques of spinal fusion: Pseudarthrosis and method of repair: AAOS Instructional Course Lecture V, pp 295–313

PART 5

Bank Bone and Bone Graft Substitutes

5.1 Recent Trends in the Use of Bank Bone in Spinal Surgery: Replies to Questionnaires from the United States

Masaaki Kakiuchi[1] and Keiro Ono[2]

Introduction

To understand the recent trends in the use of allograft in spinal surgery, we sent questionnaires to spine surgeons throughout the world. We present here the results from the questionnaires we sent to the United States, where allograft is easily obtained from qualified bone banks and there is more experience in its use.

Methods

The questionnaire was sent to 513 spine surgeons in the United States from 1989 to 1990. The surgeons were members in 1989 of the North American Spine Society or the International Society for the Study of the Lumbar Spine (ISSLS), or were participants in the 1989 meeting of the ISSLS in Kyoto.

An outline of the questionnaire is shown in Table 1.

Results

Of the 513 spine surgeons, 508 received the questionnaire and 153 responded to it. There were 134 orthopaedic surgeons, 7 neurosurgeons, 2 spine surgeons, and 10 who did not specify. Of the 153 respondents, 129 (84%) use allograft, while 24 (16%) never use allograft when doing spine fusion. Of the 129 respondents who do use allograft, 65 often use, 39 sometimes use, and 18 rarely use allograft.

[1] Department of Orthopaedic Surgery, Osaka Police Hospital, 10-31 Kitayama, Tennoji-ku, Osaka 543, Japan
[2] Department of Orthopaedic Surgery, Osaka University Medical School, 1-1-50 Fukushima, Fukushima-ku, Osaka 553, Japan

Table 1. Outline of the questionnaire.

1. What is your specialty? orthopaedic surgeon, neurosurgeon, other
2. Do you use allograft when doing spine fusion? yes (often, sometimes, rarely)/no
3. What kind of allograft do you use?
4. Where do you obtain the allograft?
5. Does the bone bank supply as much bone as you need?
6. How many days does it take to obtain the allograft after you have given an order to the bone bank?
7. How much does the allograft cost for one procedure for one-level spine fusions?
8. Have you experienced any complications with the allograft?
9. Do you usually use allograft or autograft? Please choose from "A. only autograft," "B. only allograft," "C. either autograft or allograft, depending on the case," or "D. both autograft and allograft at the same time" for the following procedures you have experienced.

Lumbar spine				
Anterior interbody fusion	A.	B.	C.	D.
Posterior interbody fusion	A.	B.	C.	D.
Posterolateral fusion	A.	B.	C.	D.
Posterior fusion	A.	B.	C.	D.
Cervical spine				
Anterior interbody fusion	A.	B.	C.	D.
Posterior fusion	A.	B.	C.	D.

10. Do you intend to continue using allograft when doing spine fusion?
11. What is your reason for not using allograft when doing spine fusion?

Of the 129 respondents who use allograft, 64 use fresh frozen bone, 52 use freeze-dried bone, 52 use ethylene-oxide-sterilized, freeze-dried bone, 20 use freeze-dried, irradiated bone, 12 use ethylene-oxide-sterilized, frozen bone, 12 use decalcified bone, and 12 use frozen, irradiated bone. Some respondents checked more than 1 item.

Of the 129 respondents who use allograft, 28 obtain all of their allograft from their own practices or from a bone bank operated by their own hospital, and 66 use only regional bone banks, which distribute allograft among hospitals. The other 35 secure allograft from both systems. Thus, 101 (78%) obtain it from regional bone banks. Respondents using their own sources chiefly use fresh frozen bone, while those making use of regional bone banks chiefly use freeze-dried bone or ethylene-oxide-sterilized, freeze-dried bone, which can be transported at room temperature and delivered easily to the hospitals (Fig. 1).

Of the 129 respondents who use allograft, 106 (82%) are supplied with as much bone as they need, while 23 (18%) are not able to receive an adequate supply. Most of them obtain allograft within 2 days after they place an order to the bone bank (Fig. 2). The usual cost of the allograft for a one-level lumbar interbody fusion is about $300 (Fig. 3).

According to the difference between the use of "autograft only" and "allograft only" in each procedure for lumbar fusion (Fig. 4a), allograft is preferred for posterior interbody fusion and anterior interbody fusion, but not for posterolateral fusion and posterior fusion. A combination of autograft and allo-

Fig. 1. Types of allograft used. *Black areas*, from regional bone banks; *white areas*, from own sources

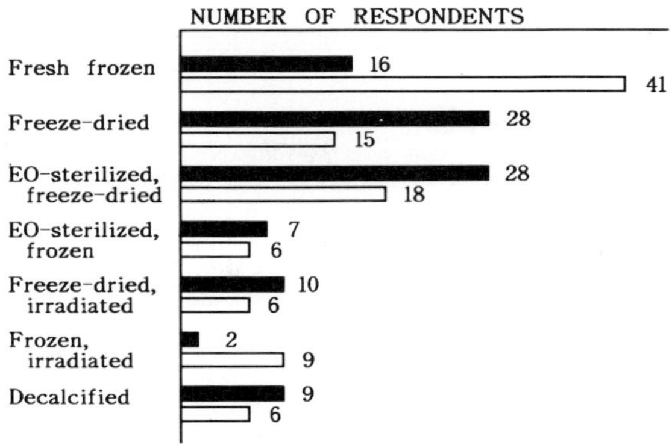

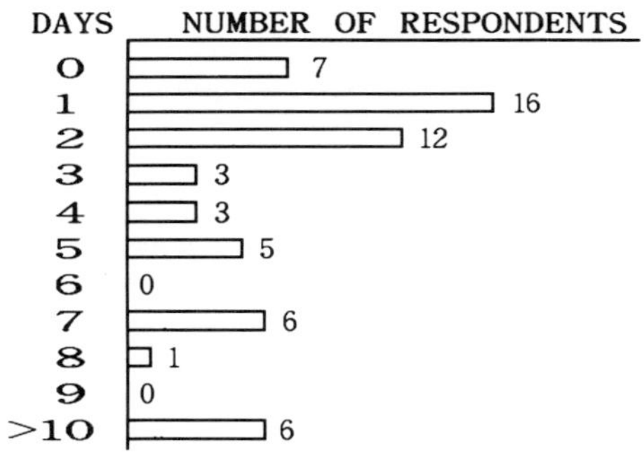

Fig. 2. Order to receipt: Waiting periods

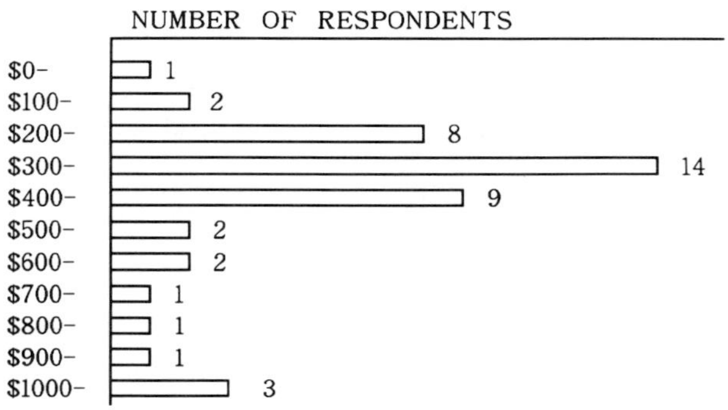

Fig. 3. Cost of allograft for a one-level lumbar interbody fusion

graft is preferred for each of the four procedures for lumbar fusion. For cervical spine fusions (Fig. 4b), in which the required volume of bone graft is small, autograft is preferred for both anterior interbody fusion and posterior fusion.

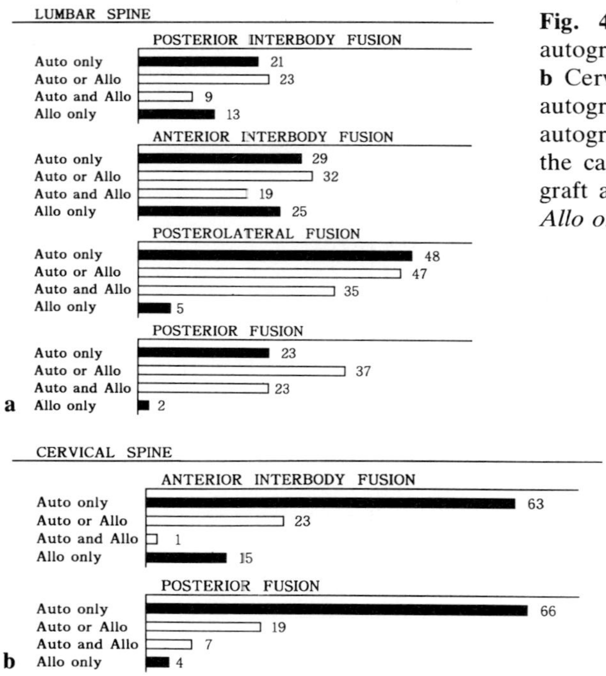

Fig. 4a,b. Use of allograft and/or autograft. **a** Lumbar spine fusions. **b** Cervical spine fusions. *Auto only*, autograft only; *Auto or Allo*, either autograft or allograft, depending on the case; *Auto and Allo*, both autograft and allograft at the same time; *Allo only*, allograft only

Of the 129 respondents who use allograft, 8 (6.2%) and 5 (3.9%) have experienced infection and rejection, respectively. Forty-two (33%) of the 129 who use allograft and 22 (92%) of the 24 who never use allograft gave their reasons for not using allograft when doing spine fusion. The reasons were:

1. Less effectiveness of allograft (52 respondents)
2. More complications with allograft than autograft (24)
3. Difficulty in obtaining allograft (8)
4. Expensiveness of allograft (5)
5. No need to use allograft (4)
6. The risk of transmission of HIV (4)

Of the 129 respondents who use allograft, 121 (94%) intended to continue using allograft, while 8 (6%) planned to discontinue using allograft because they thought it was less effective than autograft.

Discussion

More than 80% of the respondents use allograft. Of these, about 50% often use it and about 80% utilize regional bone banks. Most of them were promptly supplied with sufficient quantities of allograft. This may be due to (1) the activities and services of bone banks in almost all parts of the country, and (2) the increased use of freeze-dried bone and gas-sterilized, freeze-dried bone, which can be stored and transported at room temperature and delivered easily to hospitals.

As was expressed by some of the respondents, one problem with the present system of bone banking is that there is still a risk of transmission of bacteria or viruses in spite of strict donor screening. This is because (1) virus-infected donors sometimes test false negative in the early stages of infection, and (2) only small samples of the bone or attached blood can be used to culture for bacteria, which does not validate sterility of the whole area of the bone. Therefore, to increase the safety of allograft use for spinal surgery, effective and harmless sterilizaton methods should be established.

Another concern is the effectiveness of allograft. Allograft is as effective as autograft in some cases, and less effective in others. According to the increased use of allograft for lumbar interbody fusions (Fig. 4), allograft may be more effective and useful in lumbar interbody fusions than the other procedures. To eliminate inappropriate or ineffective use of allograft, guidelines on the use of allograft, based on scientific clinical studies, should be established.

Acknowledgment. We would like to express our thanks to the surgeons who kindly responded to this questionnaire.

5.2 Defatted, Gas-Sterilized Bone Allograft as Bank Bone: Preparation, Safety, and Utility for Lumbar Spine Surgery

Masaaki Kakiuchi[1], Keiro Ono[2], and Kazuo Shinka[3]

Introduction

Lumbar spine fusion usually requires a large volume of bone graft material, and therefore the use of allograft is sometimes of great value. However, using allograft runs the risk of transmitting bacteria or viruses. In addition, there are no adequate guidelines on the use of allograft. If allograft is used in the same way as autograft, complications often result. Therefore, we have introduced a new banking system, and based on our clinical results, have attempted to prepare guidelines on the use of allograft prepared by our system.

We present here the preparation, safety, and utility of our allograft for lumbar spine fusions.

Preparation of Defatted, Gas-Sterilized Allograft

Procurement of Bone

Donors must be free from systemic bacterial or viral infection. Bone was usually obtained from limbs amputated because of acute ischemic necrosis chiefly caused by arteriosclerosis obliterans, and cut into desired shapes and sizes with an electric cutting machine. The necrotic or infected portion of the bone was discarded, while bone contaminated with bacteria could still be utilized.

[1] Department of Orthopaedic Surgery, Osaka Police Hospital, 10-31 Kitayama, Tennoji-ku, Osaka, 543 Japan
[2] Department of Orthopaedic Surgery, Osaka University Medical School, 1-1-50 Fukushima, Fukushima-ku, Osaka, 553 Japan
[3] Medical Products Department, Industrial Equipment Division, Daido Sanso K.K., 1-20-16 Higashi-shinsaibashi, Chuo-ku, Osaka, 542 Japan

Procedures for Preparation of Allograft

The bone was treated sequentially under clean but not sterile conditions as follows: (1) the bone was washed with deionized water at 4°C, (2) it was defatted in a mixture of chloroform and methanol at room temperature [1], (3) the chloroform and methanol were allowed to evaporate in the open air in a well ventilated room at room temperature, (4) the bone was washed with distilled water at 4°C, (5) it was dehydrated by freeze-drying in a vacuum at −40°C, and (6) exposed to ethylene oxide gas in a doubly wrapped bag. The sterilized bone in the bag was stored at room temperature until it was ready to use.

Treatment with a mixture of chloroform and methanol and freeze-drying remove fat and water, which prevent diffusion of ethylene oxide gas into the bone during sterilization and diffusion from the bone after sterilization. These procedures do not have harmful effects on the osteogenetic properties of bone matrix [2].

Safety of the Allograft

Interstitial Sterilization vs Surface Sterilization

To evaluate the effectiveness of our method in destroying bacteria in the inner area of the bone, infected human bones from six patients with active chronic osteomyelitis were treated and sterilized by our method and cultured for bacteria. The six patients had suffered from the infection for 1–52 years, with an average of 21.4 years. Bacteria identified were *Pseudomonas aeruginosa*, *P. cepacia*, *P. maltophilia*, *Staphylococcus epidermidis*, *Streptococcus faecalis*, *S. pyogenes*, *Klebsiella pneumoniae*, *Enterobacter cloacae*, and *Escherichia coli*. After the sequential treatment and sterilization shown in the previous section, Procedures for Preparation of Allograft, all the bones tested negative for any bacteria.

Penetration of Ethylene Oxide Gas into Bone

To evaluate the effectiveness of prior defatting and freeze-drying in facilitating penetration of ethylene oxide gas into bone, distribution of ethylene oxide within bone during sterilization was examined as follows. Whole femoral heads were treated by three different procedures: (1) defatting and freeze-drying, a method introduced by us, (2) deep-freezing, or (3) freeze-drying. Each treated bone was exposed to ethylene oxide gas for 4 h and then quickly frozen to liquefy the gaseous ethylene oxide. The levels of ethylene oxide were measured using gas chromatography. As shown in Fig. 1, in the defatted, freeze-dried bone, ethylene oxide was distributed throughout the bone. In the freeze-dried bone or the frozen bone, the levels of ethylene oxide in the inner area were much lower than those in the surface area.

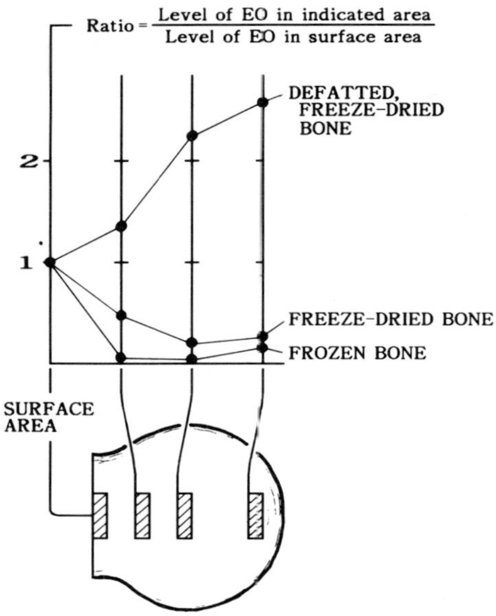

Fig. 1. Penetration of ethylene oxide gas into the whole femoral head excised for joint replacement. Values are the ratios of the levels of ethylene oxide measured at the indicated area to those measured on the surface area

Residual Ethylene Oxide and Its Toxic Byproduct

Ethylene oxide in bone is partially converted to a more toxic substance, ethylene chlorohydrin, through its reaction with chlorine ions and water contained in the bone. To evaluate the effectiveness of prior defatting and freeze-drying in reducing the residue levels of ethylene oxide and ethylene chlorohydrin after sterilization, the levels of the two substances were measured as follows. Cancellous bone of the femoral head was cut into 1 cm cubes and treated by: (1) defatting and freeze-drying, (2) deep-freezing, or (3) freeze-drying. Each treated bone specimen was exposed to ethylene oxide gas for 24 h in a polyethylene film bag (0.07 mm thick). The bone in the bag was aerated in the open air in a well-ventilated room. The residue levels of the two substances in defatted, freeze-dried bone were much lower than those in freeze-dried or frozen bone, and after 6 days' aeration, decreased to far below the FDA-proposed limits for a medium sized implantable devices (Fig. 2).

Discussion

These results validate the effect of prior defatting and freeze-drying on facilitating diffusion of ethylene oxide into the bone during sterilization and from the bone after sterilization. According to guidelines from the Welfare Ministry, ethylene oxide gas can destroy even viruses, such as HIV or HBV, as well as bacterial spores, when its humidity, temperature, and concentration are appropriate. Our method provides adequate conditions for ethylene oxide to destroy

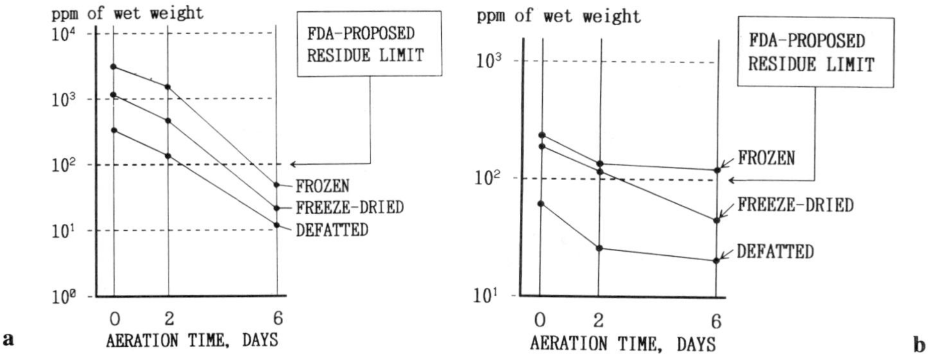

Fig. 2a,b. Residue levels of the toxic substances after sterilization and subsequent aeration. **a** Ethylene oxide. **b** Ethylene chlorohydrin. *FROZEN*, frozen bone; *FREEZE-DRIED*, freeze-dried bone; *DEFATTED*, defatted, freeze-dried bone

these microorganisms in bone. Therefore, sterile, non-toxic allograft can be prepared easily without aseptic handling.

Utility of the Allograft for Lumbar Spine Fusions

Methods

Bone graft for spine fusions, especially for interbody fusions, should have mechanical strength as well as osteogenetic properties. Cancellous bone autograft has excellent osteogenetic properties, and cortical bone, whether it is autograft or allograft, has sufficient mechanical strength. Therefore, we started using a combination of cortical bone allograft and cancellous bone autograft.

This study included cases of one-level lumbar spine fusions, using a combination of cortical bone allograft and a small amount of autograft, that were followed up for 1 year or more. The autograft was usually obtained from excised posterior elements. Cases with inadequate placement of graft or an internal fixator were excluded. There were 61 cases of posterior lumbar interbody fusion (PLIF), 14 cases of posterior fusion (PF), 7 cases of posterolateral fusion (PLF), and 4 cases of anterior lumbar interbody fusion (ALIF).

In PLF and PF, plates of cortical bone allograft were placed on the decorticated recipient beds, and chips of cancellous bone autograft obtained from excised posterior elements were packed into the gap between the recipient beds and the cortical bone allograft. In PF, the allograft was attached to the spinous processes by a stainless steel wire. The patients were recumbent for 3 weeks after operation.

In PLIF and ALIF, several pieces of cortical bone allograft were placed as struts, and cancellous bone autograft was usually packed anteriorly and laterally to the cortical bone allograft (Fig. 3a). The cancellous bone autograft in PLIF

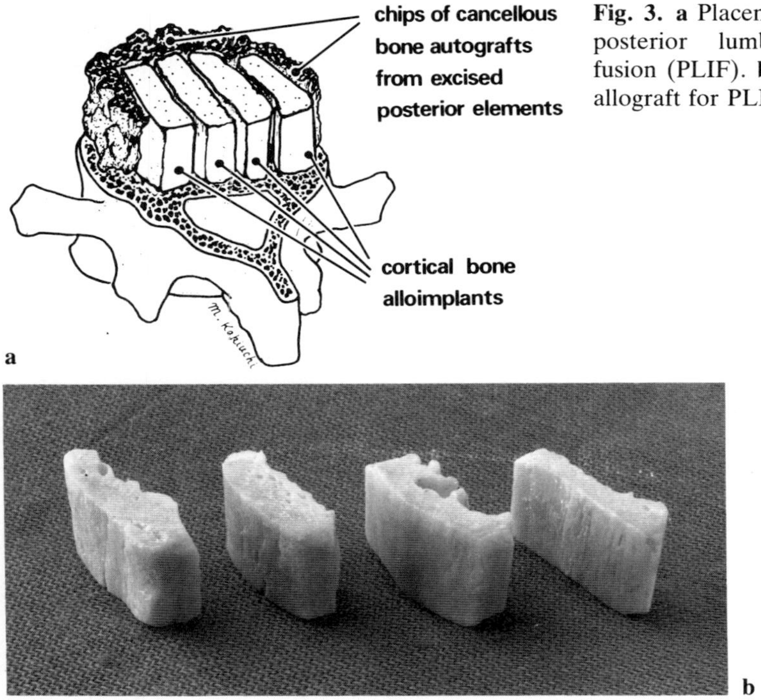

Fig. 3. **a** Placement of graft in posterior lumbar interbody fusion (PLIF). **b** Cortical bone allograft for PLIF

was obtained from excised posterior elements and that in ALIF was from the excised rib or the patient's own iliac crest. The patients were recumbent for a week after PLIF and for 2 weeks after ALIF. The cortical bone allograft was 5–15 mm in height at intervals of 1 mm and 20–30 mm in length. Thus, various bone sizes are available in the operating room (Fig. 3b).

PLIF was carried out using the following four methods:

1. Ordinary method. The allograft was driven into an intervertebral space which was expanded by a vertebra spreader. The height of the allograft should equal that of the expanded space.
2. Ordinary PLIF method reinforced with the hook and rod system of Kaneda's posterior device.
3. Distraction-compression fixation by allograft (Figs. 4 and 5). The allograft, which was higher than the expanded intervertebral space, was inserted sideways into the intervertebral space and twisted forcibly into a vertical position with a bone twister. The allograft produces a distraction force, which creates a taut annulus and ligament, resulting in distraction-compression fixation.
4. PLIF with a pedicle screw system (Figs. 6 and 7). A pedicle screw system was used for reduction of slip or correction of deformities. For correction

Fig. 4. a PLIF by distraction-compression fixation using cortical bone allograft. b Bone twisters

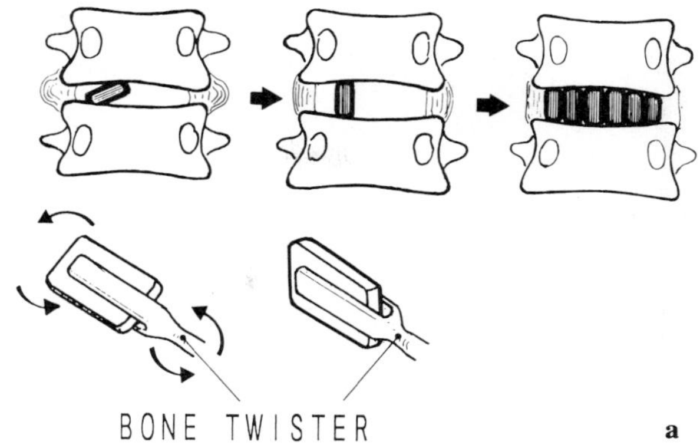

a

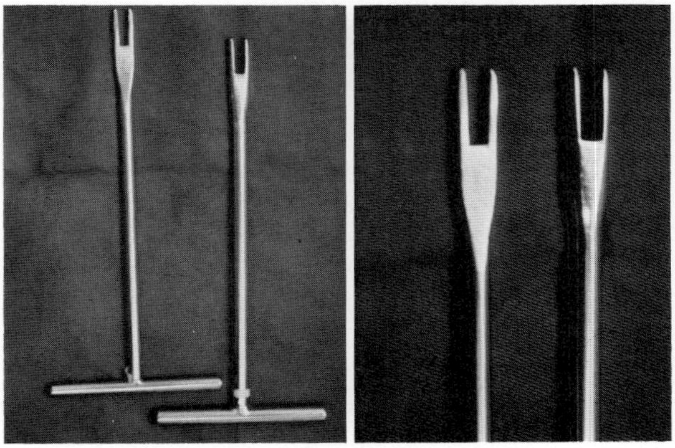

b

of kyphosis and degenerative scoliosis, cortical bone allograft expands the intervertebral space on one side and the pedicle screw system narrows the space on the opposite side.

Results

As shown in Table 1, the incidence of bony union in PLF and PF was extremely low, even though they were done for disk herniation only.

In PLIF, when distraction-compression fixation or pedicle screw fixation were utilized, there were no cases of non-union. Of the 21 cases which used the ordinary method with the hook and rod system, one showed non-union. Of the four cases in which the ordinary method was used without internal fixation, two showed non-union.

There was neither postoperative infection nor collapse or fracture of the allograft. Of the 14 cases of PF, 8 showed breakage of the wire, and of them 3 showed displacement of the allograft. In interbody fusions, the allograft was

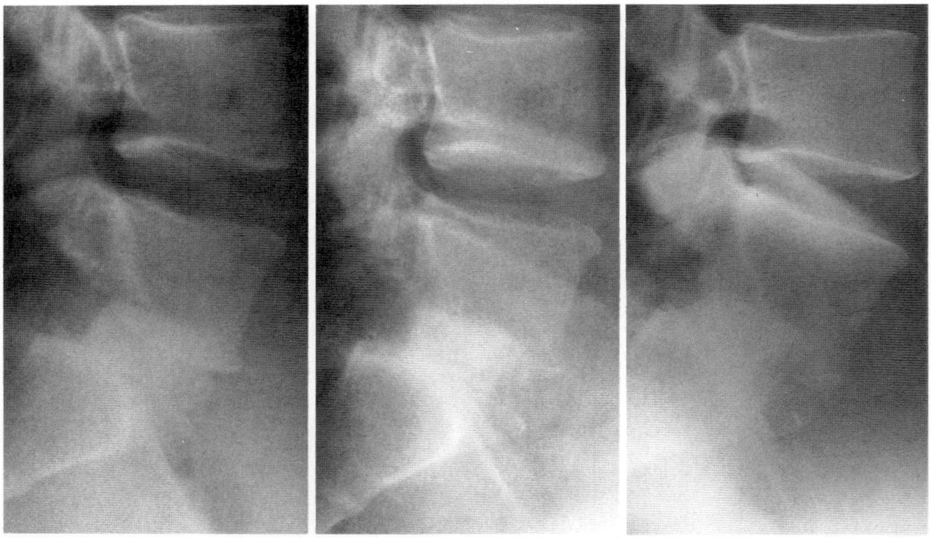

a, b c

Fig. 5a–c. PLIF by distraction-compression fixation for spondylolytic spondylolisthesis in a 26-year-old man. **a** One month after operation. **b** Six months after operation, bony union between cortical bone allograft and vertebrae was already achieved. **c** Two years after operation, the allograft was completely incorporated

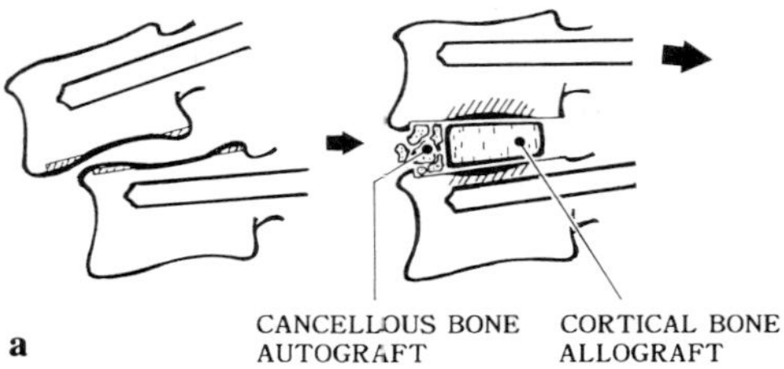

a

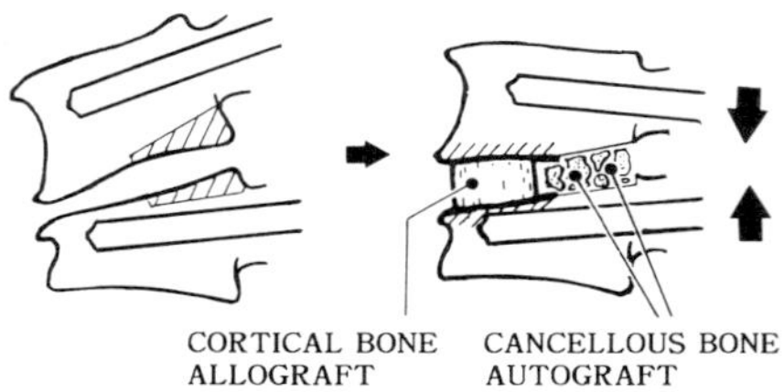

b

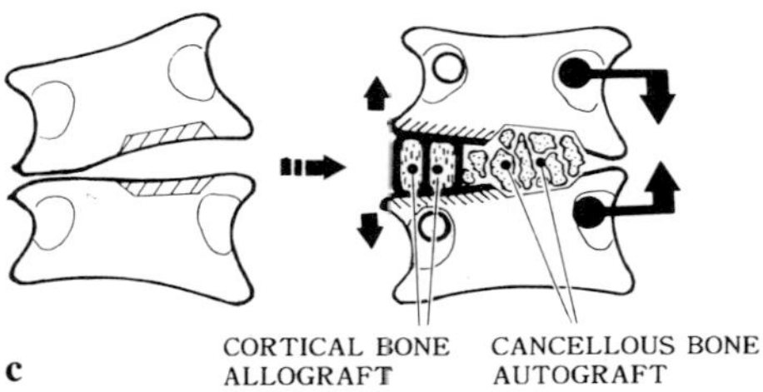

c

Fig. 6. **a** Reduction of slip in spondylolisthesis. **b** Correction of kyphosis. **c** Correction of degenerative scoliosis

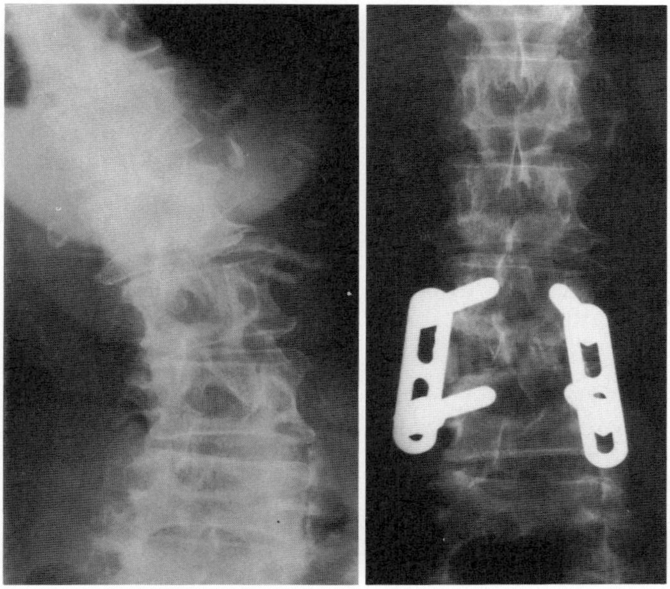

a b

Fig. 7a,b. Single-level PLIF with Steffee variable screw placement (VSP) system for correcting degenerative scoliosis with stenosis in a 70-year-old woman. **a** Before operation, the Cobb's angle was 28°. **b** After operation, the Cobb's angle was corrected to 0°

Table 1. Incidence of bony union.

	PLIF				ALIF	PLF	PF
	With pedicle screw system	Compression-distraction fixation	Ordinary method: With hook and rod	Ordinary method: Without hook and rod			
Incidence of bony union (%)	26/26 (100)	10/10 (100)	20/21 (95)	2/4 (50)	4/4 (100)	1/7 (14)	3/14 (21)
Spondylolisthesis							
Spondylolytic	10	4	–	1	–	–	–
Degenerative	7	6	4	–	–	–	–
Degenerative scoliosis	6	–	–	–	–	–	–
Post-traumatic kyphosis	3	–	–	–	2	–	–
Disk herniation	–	–	8	3	–	7	14
Failed back	–	–	9	–	2	–	–

PLIF, posterior lumbar interbody fusion; ALIF, anterior lumbar interbody fusion; PLF, posterolateral fusion; PF, posterior fusion

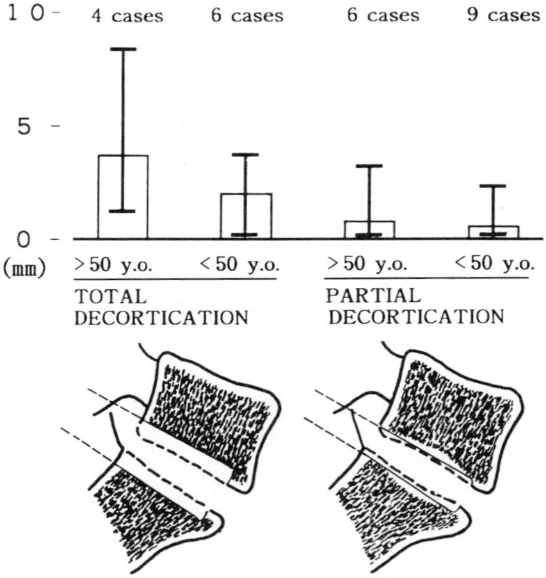

Fig. 8. Decrease in disk height by settlement of allograft into vertebral bodies. Values are means with maximums and minimums. *>50 y.o.*, 50 years old or more; *<50 y.o.*, less than 50 years old

never extruded, although in one case of PLIF using the ordinary method without internal fixation, there was slight movement of the allograft in the posterior direction. There was no instance of the pedicle screw breaking in PLIF.

The hard cortical bone allograft in interbody fusion, if pressed against the soft cancellous bone of the decorticated vertebra, may settle into the vertebral bodies and the height of the intervertebral space may decrease. The settlement may result in misalignment of the fused segment or loss of correction of deformities. Figure 8 shows the decrease in the height of the intervertebral space according to the patient's age and the extent of decortication of the cortical end-plates. Subjects had PLIF using the ordinary method with and without the hook and rod system. If the cortical end-plates were totally decorticated in patients aged 50 years or more, the allograft settled into the vertebral bodies.

Discussion

Cortical bone allograft is most effective for interbody fusions, especially when it is firmly fixed using compression-distraction fixation or pedicle screw fixation. However, it is less effective when used for posterior fusion or posterolateral fusion. In interbody fusions, decortication of cortical end-plates should not be total, but partial to prevent settlement of the allograft into the vertebrae.

In this situation, slowly resorbed cortical allograft acts as a biodegradable internal fixator and stabilizes the segment to be fused until union is achieved.

Cancellous bone autograft, under the protection of cortical bone allograft, facilitates new bone formation and then becomes a bony bridge uniting the two adjoining vertebral bodies. This bridge continues to stabilize the segment further until the allograft is replaced by new bone and remodelled. In this way, the two materials compensate for the other's deficiency.

References

1. Mikulski AJ, Urist MR (1975) An antigenic antimorphogenetic bone hydrophobic glycopeptide. Prep Biochem 5(1):21
2. Prolo DJ, Pedrotti MA, Burres KP, Oklund S (1982) Superior osteogenesis in transplanted allogeneic canine skull following chemical sterilization. Clin Orthop 168:230–242

5.3 A Titanium Implant for Interbody Fusion in Degenerative Lumbar Disk Disease

Julian W. Chang and Arthur C.M.C. Yau[1]

Introduction

Surgery is sometimes needed in the management of patients suffering from degenerative lumbar disk disease. Posterior diskectomy alone without stabilization of the motion segment often fails to relieve back pain. Scarring around and possible devascularization of the nerve root is sometimes responsible for recurrent and persistent symptoms. Posterolateral fusion has not been shown to control the motion segment effectively. On the other hand, anterior diskectomy with interbody fusion avoids these problems and effectively eliminates the motion segment in a high percentage of cases [1]. There are however inherent difficulties with anterior interbody fusion using autogenous iliac bone graft, including problems with harvesting enough good quality grafts, especially in cases involving revision, multi-level fusion, osteoporosis, and in ethnic groups such as the Chinese who often have thin pelvises. Donor site complications are common, such as pain, fracture, hematoma, and wound drainage. The quality of the graft can also cause problems with graft extrusion, nonunion, and early or delayed graft collapse. For these reasons, a search was begun for a graft substitute that would ideally be available in various sizes, be biocompatible, be strong enough to support the spine, have mechanical properties close to the normal lumbar motion segment, and preferrably allow biological fixation.

In 1979, Yau and co-workers [2] at the University of Hong Kong first reported using a single titanium block as a graft substitute based on the design by Gallante et al. [3]. However, the grafts were bulky, making insertion difficult, bone resection was considerable, and disk height restoration and therefore facet joint alignment was not ideal. Subsequently, the senior author of this paper redesigned the blocks, and we present here a report of the first 200 cases that were followed up for a minimum of 6 years. A previous paper was also presented at the 16th Annual Meeting of the International Society for the Study of Lumbar Spine in Kyoto [4].

[1] Suite 205, St. George's Building, 2, Ice House Street, Hong Kong

Materials and Methods

Of the 200 patients, 185 were followed up through office visits and X ray examination and the remaining 15 through written communication and X rays sent in for study. There were 125 male and 75 female patients, and 67% were Chinese, 38% Caucasian, and 5% from other ethnic groups, including Filipinos, Japanese, Indians, Malays, and Indonesians. At the time of operation the average age was 44.75 years and the average body weight was 150.9 lbs. The symptoms and signs of the disease were typically longstanding in an older age group. Frequently there was an interchangeable course between back pain and leg pain which was heavily dependent on posture. Not infrequently there was an absence of physical signs. Patients either presented with segmental instability and/or dural or nerve root irritation. In our study a good history and physical examination with a myelogram provided the best clue to the surgical level required. We have now had 3 years of experience with MRI, and find that its sensitivity as well as specificity is equal to the myelogram for the surgical level but it is perhaps more useful in picking out border-line levels above or below the intended surgical site. Together with a saline acceptant test at the time of surgery, we are able to avoid missing a hitherto undetected problem level. All the patients underwent adequate preoperative conservative treatment, and 90% had a positive myelogram and/or MRI.

The approach used was the standard left flank incision with wide retraction of the blood vessels especially at the L5–S1 level. A saline acceptant test was performed in all cases and at all the disk levels intended for surgery as well as the level above or below as appropriate. Disks not to be operated on that showed an abnormal saline acceptant test, i.e., more than 2 cm^3, were included in the procedure. Total diskectomy was carried out with thinning of the posterior annulus. Subchondral bone was preserved as much as possible and if there was evidence of leg pain, a close search for any possible sequestered fragment was carried out. The disk fragments were frequently dry and lumpy and occasionally a subligamentous herniation was found. The disk spaces were then distracted and the implants inserted making sure that there was no penetration of the implant posteriorly (Figs. 1,2). Closure was in the usual manner over a suction drain. Patients were kept on intravenous antibiotics for about 24 h. Usually we found that with a small incision of around 3 inches, bowel sounds returned rapidly within 24 h and sometimes as early as 8 h after operation. Patients were nursed in bed for about 4 days and mobilized on the 5th day without external support. Usually the average time for patients to be discharged from the hospital was after 7–12 days, with an average time of 10 days. Sedentary workers were allowed to go back to work as early as after 6–8 weeks, but manual labourers were not permitted to go back to work until after a minimum of 4–5 months.

The implant itself was made of commercially pure titanium wires sintered to form a rectangular block. Commercially pure titanium was preferred over Ti 6A14V because of reports of a more natural tissue reaction [5,6]. It has a

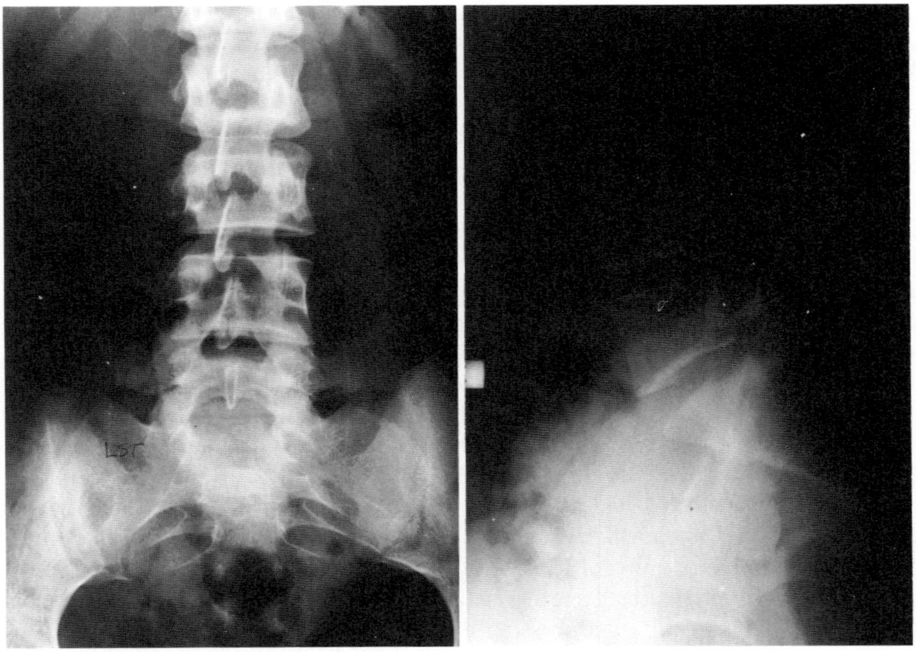

1

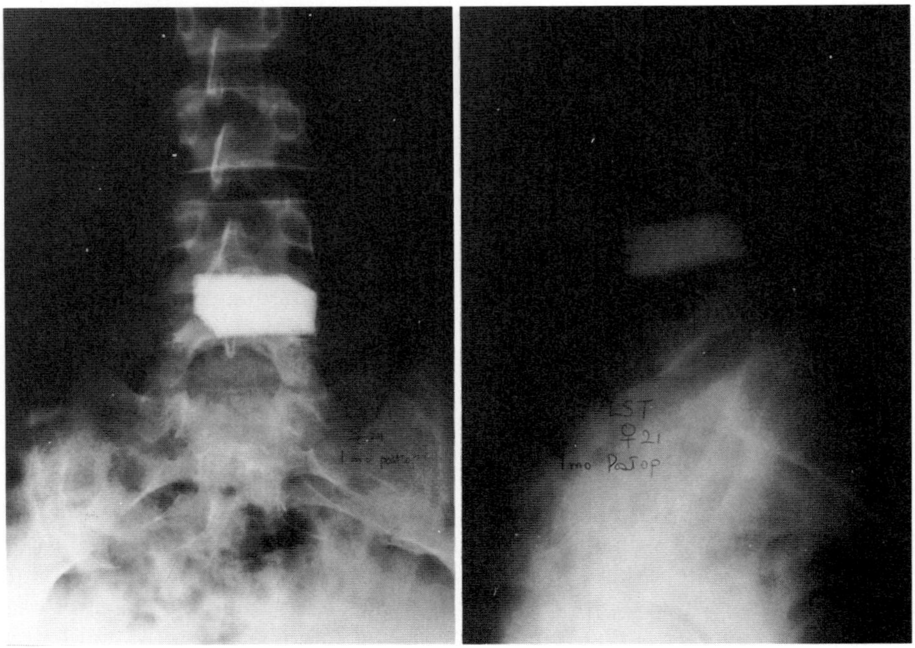

2

Fig. 1. Patient LST, a 21-year-old female, preoperation

Fig. 2. Patient LST, a 21-year-old female, 1 month postoperation

Table 1. The distribution of levels.

	Patients (*n*)		
	Total	Male	Female
One level	122	73	49
Two levels	76	50	26
Three levels	2	2	0
One level			
L3/4	4	2	2
L4/5	70	43	27
L5/S1	48	28	20
Two levels			
L3/4, L4/5	16	11	5
L4/5, L5/S1	60	39	21

Table 2. Clinical results symptomatic relief of back/leg pain.

	Cases with excellent/good results (%)	
	4 years	6 years
One level	95	98.3
Two levels	87	94.7
Three levels	50	50.0

density of 50% and a stiffness of 7,843 N/mm, a value higher than that of 1,400 N/mm reported for the lumbar vertebral motion segment. We feel that this value is desirable to provide sufficient support for the spine while avoiding a major transition in mechanical properties. Several modifications of the physical dimensions were made to allow a wider sizing. Use of the implant greatly reduced the operating time and intraoperative blood loss, with a one-level fusion having an average operating time of 45 min and blood loss of under 100 cm^3.

The distribution of different level operations performed is shown in Table 1.

Results

The results are divided into clinical and radiological considerations. The clinical results are summarized in Table 2.

Radiologic Results

Fusion was defined as lack of motion on lateral flexion extension X rays. Bone growth around the implant, if any, could not be seen until at least 3 years later and was observed in 10% of cases at 6 years. By this criteria, fusion occurred as early as 3 months postop (23%) or as late as 19 months (2%) in cases that

Table 3. Fusion rate.

	4 years	6 years
One level	100	100.0
Two levels	95 (L5/S1)	97.3
Three levels	66 (L3/4 L4/5)	83.3

Table 4. Complications.

Onset	Complication	Cases (*n*)	Remarts
Early	Infection	0	
	Deep venous thrombosis		All Chinese
	DVT	5	
	PE	2	
	Aggravated back/leg pain due to over distraction	11	
	Spinal canal intrusion by mesh	2	
Late	Deformed implant		These presented with transient back pain of less than 10 days duration.
	At 4 years	16	
	At 6 years	19	There was no correlation with weight, but the complication was seen more in male patients and in the 30- to 40-year-old age group
	Implant disintegration	2	Both cases were seen at 4 years and were asymptomatic

DVT, deep venous thrombosis; PE, pulmonary embolism

went on to fusion. Fusion was seen in 41% of cases at 6 months and in 85% of cases at lyear. The fusion rate is summarized in Table 3.

The complications encountered can be seen in Table 4. There were no instances of vertebral body penetration and no cases of protrusion at levels above or below the operated level. The latter is attributed to routine application of the saline acceptance test at the level above and below the level intended for operation. There were no toxic/allergic reactions seen.

Discussion

The main result of this study shows that the implant provide a good alternative to autogenous iliac graft in interbody fusion. The complications attributed to its use are all technical in nature, and the physical dimensions of the implant and the implantation technique have subsequently been modified to avoid a repeat of the same problems. Commercially pure titanium was chosen because of its biocompatibility, its mechanical properties close to those of vertebral bone, and its more natural tissue reaction as compared to that of Ti 6A14V [5,6]. In the majority of cases indirect evidence of biological fixation was seen: 10% of cases showed bone growth around the implant after years. In one case, the implant was re-explored and extracted to relieve symptoms due to over distraction. Histological evidence of osseointegration was found, although on X ray analysis no signs of bone growth were present. There was no evidence of vertebral penetration. This should be compared with a separate series we did using cobalt chrome blocks where seven out of ten cases resulted in symptomatic vertebral penetration. The cobalt chrome blocks had a stiffness value of 48,485 N/mm compared with that of 7,843 N/mm for the titanium block. According to experimental mechanical testing, various titanium blocks, modified in terms of wire size and block size and with stiffness values 1,815–2,585 N/mm, were found to be too deformable. No toxic reactions were seen, and tissue retrieved from around the implant showed no foreign body reaction. Incidentally, in the two cases explored posteriorly at 2 years, the facet joints were not spontaneously fused.

Conclusion

In the treatment of patients with symptomatic degenerated lumbar disks, diskectomy alone often fails to relieve back pain due to segmental instability. A total diskectomy, required to prevent recurrent herniation, can best be achieved via an anterior approach. Stabilization of the motion segment and facet joint is achieved by restoration of disk height through distraction and fusion with graft insertion. Autogenous iliac graft, whilst providing excellent osteoinduction and conduction also has numerous inherent problems. Graft availability, quality and donor site problems are frequently limiting factors towards achieving good results. Our experience with commercially pure titanium blocks followed up for 6 years shows that they produce equally good results with far fewer complications.

References

1. Chang J, Yau A (1987) Anterior lumbar interbody fusion. A review of 189 cases. Proceedings of the Western Pacific Orthopaedic Association 25th Annual Meeting, Dec, Manila, Philippines
2. Leong JCY, Chow SP, Yau ACMC, Rostoker W (1983) The use of porous titanium mesh implant after diskectomy in patients with prolapsed intervertebral disk. The 10-year results of a prospective trial. Proceedings of 3rd Congress of Spinal Section, Western Pacific Orthopaedic Association University of Hong Kong Press, Hong Kong, pp 114–115
3. Gallante J, Rostoker W, Lueck R (1971) Sintered fiber metal composites as a basis for attachments of implant to bone. J Bone Joint Surg [Am] 53:101–114
4. Chang J, Yau A (1990) Anterior lumbar diskectomy and interbody fusion using a titanium mesh implant. Orthop Trans 14:54, no. 1

5. Barth E, Ronningen H, Solheim FL (1985) Comparison of ceramic and titanium implant in cats. Acta Orthop Scand 56:491–495
6. Johansson C, Lausmaa J, Ask M, Hansson H-A, Albrektsson T (1989) Ultrastructural differences of the interface zone between bone and Ti 6A14V or commercially pure titanium. J Biomed Eng 11:3–8

5.4 Use of Hydroxyapatite Blocks in Posterior Interbody Fusion

Nobumasa Suzuki and Yasuhiko Iwamoto[1]

Introduction

When a patient is aged and osteoporotic, the collapse of the graft bone used in lumbar interbody fusion is a common problem [1] and occurs even if some type of spinal instrumentation such as a Zielke system or Steffee VSP plate is added. Before 1988, we performed posterior lumbar interbody fusion (PLIF), using only autograft with spinal instrumentation. Among 19 patients whose age was over 60.3 (16%) had graft bone collapse which resulted in pseudoarthrosis. Pain at the donor site is also a common complaint after surgery. To prevent these problems, we have used a hydroxyapatite (HA) block as the interbody spacer, and we will analyze the results here.

Materials and Methods

Between 1988 and 1991, 45 patients underwent PLIF using HA blocks and iliac bone grafts along with trans-pedicular spinal instrumentation. We analyzed 32 patients, 20 male and 12 female, ranging in age from 27 to 76 years, with an average of 58.9 years. The follow-up time ranges from 6 to 37 months with an average of 17.5 months. The Steffee VSP plate system was used in 28 cases, the Zielke system in 3 cases, and no instrumentation in 1 case. The indications for supplemental use of the HA block were when (1) the bone was osteoporotic, (2) multilevel interbody fusion was required, and (3) graft bone was difficult to harvest due to previous operations.

[1] Department of Orthopaedics, Saiseikai Central Hospital, 1-4-17 Mita, Minato-ku, Tokyo, 108 Japan

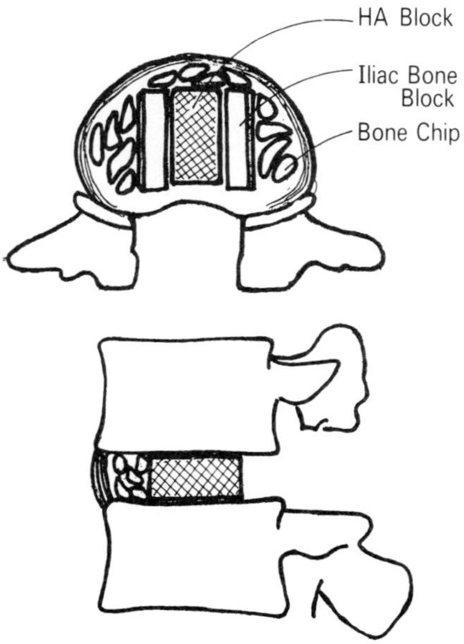

Fig. 1. Posterior lumbar interbody fusion (PLIF) with hydroxyapatite (HA) block. The sandwich method

Hydroxyapatite Materials

The HA utilised in this series was the porous hydroxyapatite Boneceram P (Sumitomo Cement Co., Osaka). This material is sintered at 1,150°C. The porosity is 35%–40%, and the pore size is 50–300 μm. The compressive strength is about 500 kg/cm, and the bending strength is about 165 kg/cm. The HA block is made in a range of sizes to suit the most frequent sizes of interbody space: 8, 10, 12, 15 mm. The size can be adjusted using either an airtome or a spinal rongeur.

Fusion Techniques

For interbody fusion two iliac bone blocks, with cortex on one side, and an HA block were grafted together into an interbody space as in a sandwich. Cancellous bone chips were grafted onto the front and side of the block (Fig. 1). In addition to this, posterolateral fusion was done in all cases for better fusion and stability. In the aged patients, the graft bone was minced and mixed with HA chips to increase the volume of the graft material, saving on the amount of the graft bone harvested [1] (Hamburger technique).

Clinical assessment of the surgical outcome used the Japanese Orthopaedics Association (JOA) Low Back Pain Score [2] and the pain at the donor site. X-ray assessment included bony union, interbody space height, and graft collapse. The interbody bony union was assessed as excellent, good, or poor. The criteria were disk space narrowing, collapse of the graft, a clear zone between

Table 1. Results from 32 cases.

		Remarks
JOA score		
Preoperative	10.1	
Postoperative	25.4	
Average % improvement	81.0%	
Pain at the donor site (*n*)	5	Disappeared within 6 months
Complications (*n*)		
Infection	4	Diabetic patients
Dislocation of graft leading to pseudoarthrosis and screw breakage	1	Postoperative delirium

the vertebral body and the HA block, screw breakage, instability, and incorporation of the HA block or autograft bone with vertebral body. An assessment of excellent was given when the incorporation of the graft with the vertebral body was obvious without other findings; good was when there was incorporation of the autograft bone, but a slight clear zone was visible between the HA block and the vertebral body without other findings; poor was when there was an obvious clear zone between the HA block and the vertebral body with one or more other findings.

Results

Excellent or good results were seen in 95% of the patients (Table 1). The average JOA score was 10.1 preoperatively and 25.4 postoperatively, with an average improvement of 81.0%. All patients had excellent bone union.

Although five patients suffered moderate pain at the donor site, it disappeared completely within 6 months. There have been no complications at all since 1989, but there were four cases of deep infection in 1988. This was found to be due to a malfunction of the ventilation system in the operating room and was not related to the surgical technique nor the HA material. In two cases infection was treated successfully by continuous irrigation without removal of the metal implant. In the other two cases, metal implant removal was required. In all cases of infection, the HA did not cause any unfavourable effects at all.

Pseudoarthrosis and screw breakage occurred in one case after dislocation of the graft due to severe postoperative delirium. However, this was extremely exceptional and was treated successfully by reoperation.

Interbody space height increased immediately by an average of 3.3 mm. It decreased slightly 2–4 weeks postoperatively and stabilized 6 weeks postoperatively. On average, 6 months postoperatively it was 2.1 mm wider than the preoperative height.

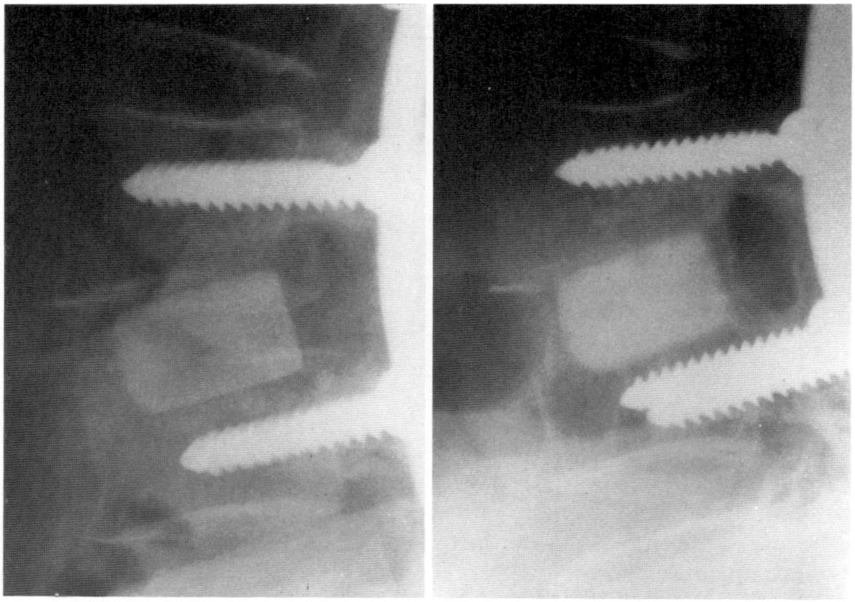

a b

Fig. 2. Final roentgenograms taken 3 months (**a**) and 15 months (**b**) postoperatively

Although a very slight sinking of the HA block into the vertebral body was common, problematic sinking did not occur in any of the patients. Final roentgenograms showed excellently stabilized spines (Fig. 2). Solid fusion can usually be seen 1 year postoperatively.

Case Studies

Case 1. A 66-year-old lady, with degenerative spondylolisthesis. PLIF was done at L4–L5, and a 94.4% improvement in the JOA score was seen (Fig. 3).

Case 2. A 70-year-old man who was confined to a wheelchair. The patient showed 92% improvement at follow-up, after four-segment fusion from L2 to S1 with a three-segment PLIF (Fig. 4). He resumed teaching aikido 8 months postoperatively.

Discussion

Hydroxyapatite is an excellent biomaterial as it is biocompatible and can bond to bone directly [3]. Bone growth into the pores of the HA blocks used here

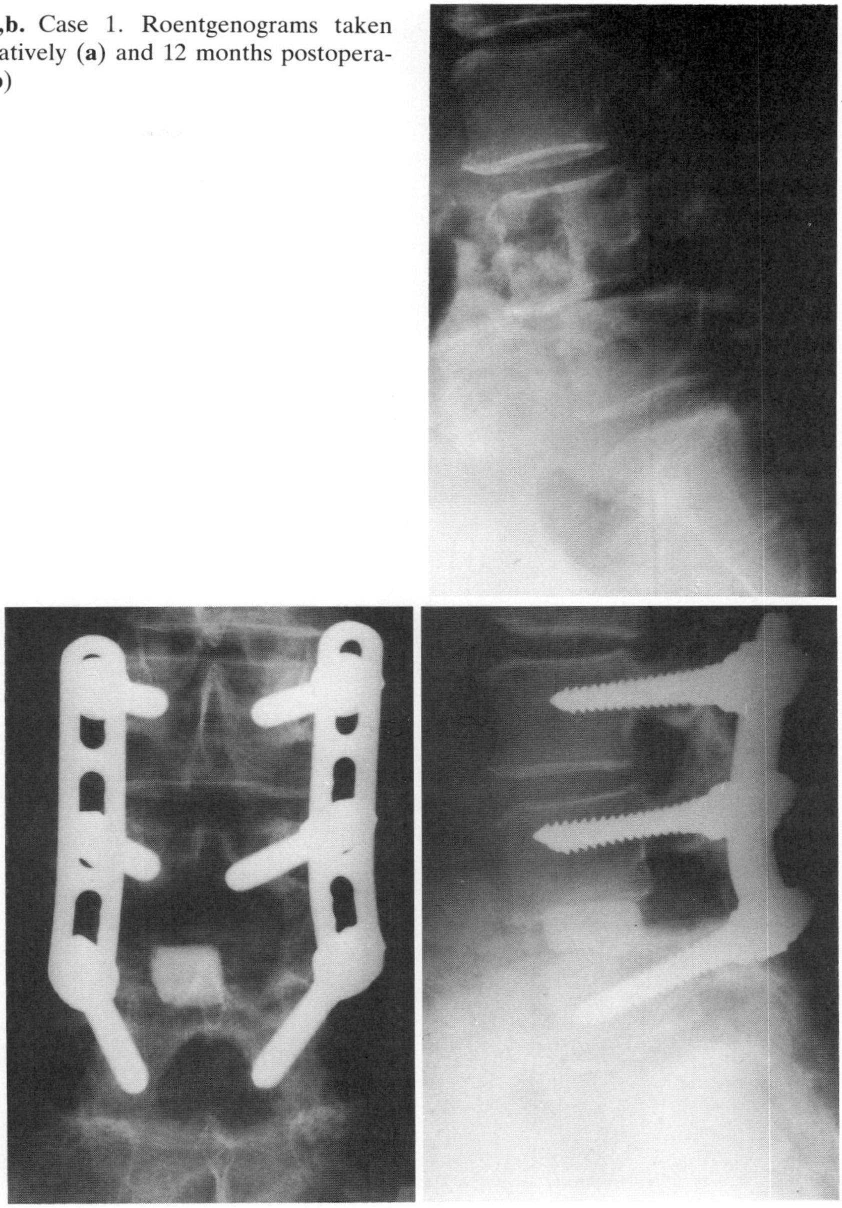

a

b

Fig. 3a,b. Case 1. Roentgenograms taken preoperatively (**a**) and 12 months postoperatively (**b**)

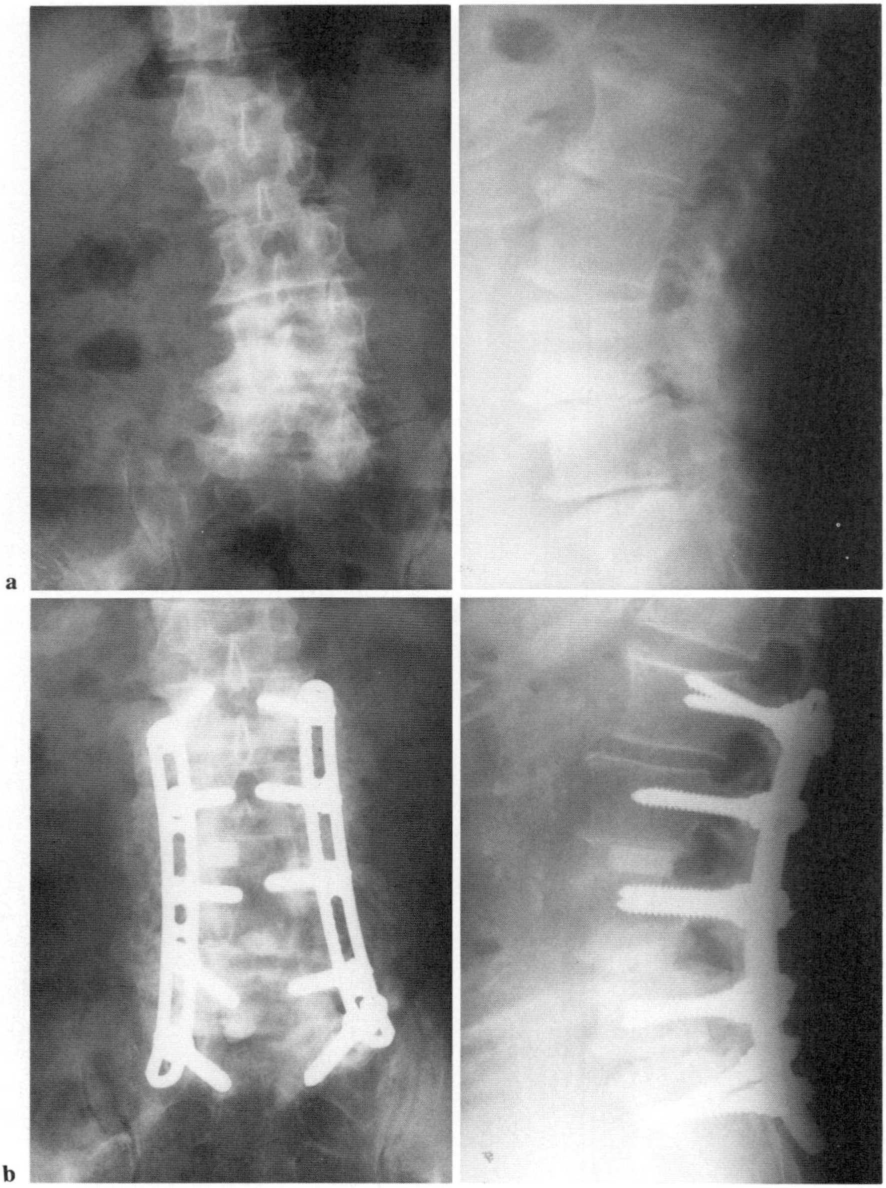

Fig. 4a,b. Case 2. Roentgenograms taken preoperatively (**a**) and 15 months postoperatively (**b**)

has already been confirmed histologically by many authors [4–7]. The HA blocks are superior in mechanical strength to other porous products [8]. In addition, the blocks are easy to form and machine, and also easy to sterilize because they can be autoclaved. Although the mechanical strength of an HA block is lower than that of alumina ceramics, there were no cases of block collapse with spinal instrumentation.

In our series a specimen was taken from the posterolateral fusion mass at the time of hardware removal 2 years after the initial operation. The specimen showed solid fusion and excellent bone ingrowth. It is important to note that the HA blocks or chips do not produce unfavorable effects where there is deep infection, even though they are foreign bodies. This is further evidence as to their excellent biocompatibility. Because of this and their bone conductivity, the HA blocks used here are an excellent scaffold for solid fusion.

The fusion technique itself is the most important aspect of PLIF. Adequate preparation of the graft bed and grafting of a sufficient amount of cancellous bone chips along with bicortical iliac bone are all essential to obtain solid fusion.

The HA block must be inserted gently to prevent breakage at the time of insertion. It is advisable to spread the interbody space using a bone spreader or lamina spreader when the block is inserted. The fusion technique shown here, if done properly, is extremely useful for multilevel interbody fusion in aged patients. We found no disadvantages in the supplemental use of HA. The advantages of its use are obvious: it prevents graft bone collapse; it makes multilevel fusion possible; it reduces the amount of autogenous graft bone required, thereby reducing pain at the donor site; and it helps to reduce the operation time.

In conclusion, the HA utilized here is superior to any other artificial fusion material. It is useful not only in aged patients but also in younger patients who require interbody fusion.

References

1. Suzuki N, Mitani T, Tezuka M, Suda H, Matsumoto H (1989) Application of hydroxyapatite (Boneceram-P) to spinal fusion. The Clinical Report 23:5263–5174
2. Japanese Orthopaedic Association (1986) Assessment of treatment for low back pain. J Jpn Orthop Assoc 60:1–4
3. Yamamuro T (1986) Classification of bioceramics and character of bioactive ceramics (in Japanese). Rinsho Seikei Geka 21:1221–1224
4. Hori M (1990) Basic studies of hydroxyapatite. Jpn Soc Biomaterials 8:11–22
5. Holmes RE, Bucholz RW, Hooney V (1986) Porous hydroxyapatite as a bone graft substitute in metaphyseal defects. J Bone Joint Surg [Am] 68:904–911
6. Flatley TJ, Lynch KL, Benson M (1983) Tissue response to implants of calcium phosphate ceramic in the rabbit spine. Clin Orthop 179:246–252

7. Robert WB, Carlton A, Ralph EH (1987) Hydroxyapatite and tricalcium phosphate bone graft substitutes. Orthop Clin North Am 18:323–335
8. Shibata O, Tsuruoka H (1990) A technique of hydroxyapatite implantation. Orthopedics 23:89–94

5.5 A Carbon Fiber Implant to Aid Interbody Lumbar Fusion: 1-year Clinical Results in the First 26 Patients

John W. Brantigan[1] and Arthur D. Steffee[2]

Introduction

Posterior lumbar interbody fusion (PLIF), pioneered by Ralph Cloward in the 1940's [1,2] is a biomechanically optimum fusion. A successful PLIF maintains the disk height, protects the nerve roots, restores weight bearing to anterior structures, restores the annulus to tension, and immobilizes the unstable degenerated intervertebral disk area. A successful PLIF restores every mechanical function of the functional spinal unit except motion. Problems with PLIF have included excessive bleeding (usually epidural), the need for donor bone (with risk of AIDS and hepatitis), prolonged healing time of donor bone, the difficulty of cutting precise bony channels, the difficulty of providing sterile donor bone of precise dimensions, the potential of instability, the risk of retropulsion of graft and consequent neural damage, and post-operative collapse of the donor bone and pseudarthrosis.

In 1985 Cloward [2] claimed 87%–92% clinical success and 92% fusion success in over 40 years of PLIF surgery. Lin [3,4] has reported 82% clinical success and 88% fusion success, and Ma [5] has reported 83% clinical success and 85% fusion success. Unfortunately, many other surgeons have had unsuccessful results with uninstrumented PLIF and have abandoned the procedure. In our practice, Arthur Steffee did an early series of 12 uninstrumented PLIF procedures many years ago and had a 100% failure rate due to continued instability of the surgical construct. This series was never published as both authors and editors dislike publishing unsuccessful studies. William Gazale, who developed a commercially produced PLIF chisel, has presented his surgical results of uninstrumented PLIF at several meetings, with about a 90% failure rate. This study also has not been published.

[1] Orthopaedic Surgery, Creighton University, 601 N. 30th St. Omaha, NE 68131, USA
[2] Cleveland Spine and Arthritis Center, 2709 Franklin Blvd. 6th Floor, Cleveland, OH 44113, USA

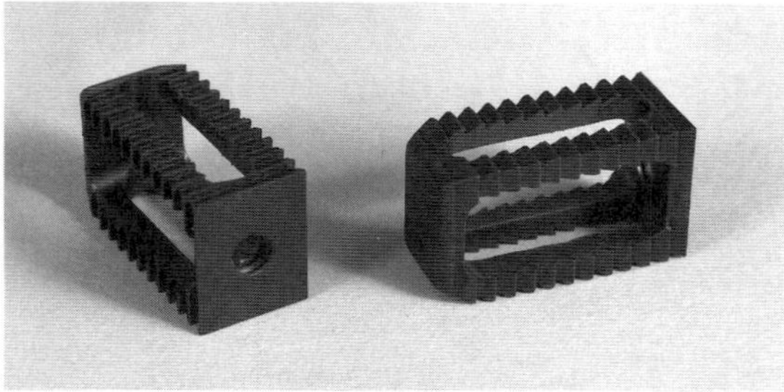

Fig. 1. Carbon fiber reinforced polymer implant

More recently, the use of pedicle screws and plates have allowed surgeons to reduce degenerative deformities of the lumbar spine and maintain absolute positional control of the motion segment in anatomic alignment and in normal sagittal and coronal plane balance [6,7]. Pedicle screws have not, however, eliminated the need for weight-bearing support in the anterior column. The likely result of lack of anterior column support is broken screws, a problem that is not solved by designing a stronger screw. If a deformity is corrected and disk space height is restored, physiologic anterior column support must be regained by use of interbody bone graft.

Of the first 697 pedicle screw/VSP cases done at the Cleveland Spine and Arthritis Center, PLIF was done in at least one level in 501 cases (71%). Our standard PLIF procedure [8] includes segmental fixation using pedicle screws and variable screw placement (VSP) plates, ethylene oxide (ETO) sterilized interbody allograft (most commonly two cancellous blocks 13 × 13 × 25 mm), and autologous posterolateral graft (often local bone from the posterior decompression). Generally satisfactory clinical results are achieved; however, the failure rate of the interbody graft remains at about 20%.

The current problem has been the quality of the bone graft, which is less than optimum both biologically and as a load bearing device. The donor bone of PLIF is expected to serve both a mechanical device function and a biologic bone-growth function. The PLIF bone must bear substantially all of the body's weight above the PLIF level while it is being incorporated by the erosive process of "creeping substitution." We explored the mechanical properties of allograft bone for PLIF in a previous study [9] and found the average bone to be inadequate for the required mechanical function.

We have developed a carbon fiber reinforced polymer implant to aid interbody fusion (Fig. 1). The implant has ridges or teeth to resist retropulsion, struts to support weight, and a hollow area to allow packing of autologous bone graft. The carbon structure is radiolucent to allow visualization of healing by normal radiographic techniques. The cage implant separates the device and biologic functions of PLIF by providing an actual device designed to meet the mechanical requirements of PLIF, and replacing the donor bone with autologous cancellous bone, the best possible bone for healing. Mechanical tests of the implant in isolated motion segments in cadaver spines have shown that cage

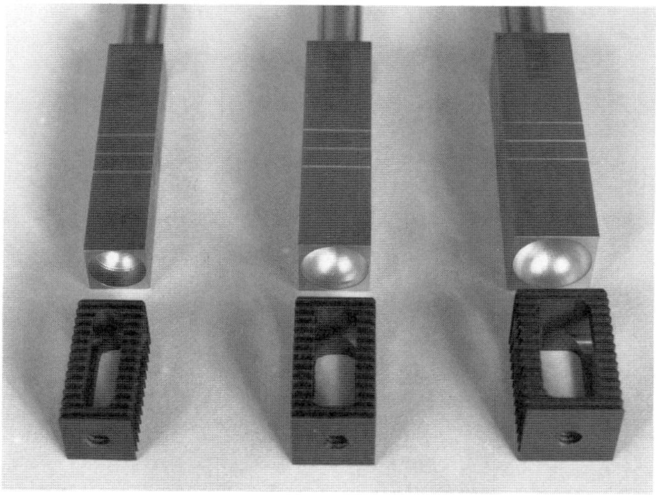

Fig. 2. Cage implants are sized to the 11-, 13-, and 15-mm finish broach of the ADS PLIF Broach System (AcroMed, Cleveland, Ohio)

struts support all anticipated compression loads and the ridges or teeth resist retropulsion with a measured resistance to pull-out three times greater than that of blocks of donor bone [10]. The carbon fiber material has a modulus of elasticity approximating that of cortical bone. The purpose of this paper is to report results on the first 26 patients treated with the carbon cage implant who have reached the 1-year follow-up interval.

Materials and Methods

Initial cages were machined from blocks of composite made of 68% long-fiber pyrolytic carbon fiber in PEEK (polyether ether ketone) (ICI Advanced Materials, Wilmington, DE). More recently, cages were fabricated from a composite made from long-fiber carbon in Ultrapek (polyether ketone ether ketone ketone) obtained from BASF Structural Materials, Anaheim, CA. Both materials demonstrate resistance to all solvents except sulfuric acid and appear equivalent in most biologic and mechanical properties.

The cage implants are implanted in horizontally opposed transverse channels prepared in the disk space using the ADS PLIF Broach System (AcroMed Corp., Cleveland). Figure 2 shows the three standard sizes of carbon fiber implants adjacent to the 11-mm, 13-mm, and 15-mm finish broaches, to which the implants are sized.

Between May, 1989 and July, 1990, 26 patients had surgery including interbody fusion with the carbon cages. Patients were selected for use of the carbon

Table 1. Outcome for pre-IDE use of Brantigan I/F cages.

Patient	Prior surgery (n)	Date of cage surgery	Surgical indication	Surgeon	Cage material	VSP levels	Cage levels	ETO levels	6 month clinical status	12 month clinical status	ETO fusion	Cage fusion	Re-op (Y/N)	Purpose of re-op
AP	2	5/09/89	Failed ETO PLIF	ADS	PEEK	L4–S1	L4–S1	none	E	E	–	5	N	
EC	6	7/21/89	Failed ETO PLIF	ADS	PEEK	L4–S1	L4–L5	L5–S1	G	F	2	5	Y	Failed ETO PLIF L5
EC*	7	1/02/91	Failed ETO PLIF	JWB	UPEK	L4–S1	L5–S1	none	G	–	–	4	N	
LD	2	8/08/89	Instability	JWB	PEEK	L4–S1	L4–L5	none	E	E	–	5	N	
GMP	0	8/09/89	Instability	ADS	PEEK	L3–S1	L3–L4	L4–L5	F	G	4	5	Y	Remove 1 plate
BA	1	8/11/89	Spondylolisthesis below HRI	ADS	PEEK	L4–S1	L4–L5	none	G	G	–	5	–	
PR	2	10/11/89	Failed ALIF	ADS	PEEK	L2–S1	L3–L4	L2–L3	F	P	2	5	Y	Repair burst fx
PR*	3	3/05/91	L1 burst fracture – instability	JWB	UPEK	T12–L2	T12–L2	none	–	–	–	–	N	
MSC	1	12/05/89	Failed PLIF	ADS	PEEK	L5–S1	L5–S1	none	G	F		5	N	
IWT	1	12/11/89	Gr III Spondylolisthesis	ADS	PEEK	L4–S1	L5–S1	none	G	G	–	5	N	
SRD	3	1/05/90	Failed PLIF	ADS	PEEK	L2–S1	L4–L5	L2–L4	G	G	4	5	N	
MK	2	1/08/90	Stenosis at fusion	ADS	PEEK	L4–S1	L5–S1	none	G	G	–	5	Y	Remove VSP
MS	0	1/15/90	Spondylolisthesis	ADS	PEEK	L2–S1	L2–L3	L4–L5	F	F	4	5	N	
JB	0	1/19/80	Dislocation L5–S1	ADS	PEEK	L4–S1	L5–S1	none	F	G	–	5	Y	Myelographic block
MJD	0	1/19/90	D-Spondylolisthesis	ADS	PEEK	L4–S1	L5–S1	L4–L5	E	E	1	5	N	
FA	5	1/31/90	Failed PLIF	ADS	PEEK	L4–S1	L5–S1	none	E	E	–	5	N	

EEH	0	2/21/90	L-Spondylolisthesis	ADS	PEEK	L4–S1	L5–S1	L4–L5	E	E	5	5	N
HF	0	3/07/90	D-Spondylolisthesis	ADS	PEEK	L4–L5	L4–L5	none	E	E	–	5	N
RJL	1	3/07/90	Post-diskectomy	ADS	PEEK	L4–S1	L4–S1	none	F	G	–	5	N
MP	1	3/13/90	Failed Perk	RSB	PEEK	None	L5–S1	none	–	E	–	5	N
LH	1	3/14/90	Post-diskectomy	RSB	PEEK	None	L5–S1	none	F	F	–	5	N
DER	1	3/19/90	Failed chymopapain treament	ADS	PEEK	L4–S1	L5–S1	L4–L5	E	E	4	5	N
AG	1	3/19/90	D-Spondylolisthesis	ADS	PEEK	L2–L5	L3–L4	L4–L5	E	E	5	5	N
DEL	2	3/30/90	Failed Zielke	ADS	PEEK	L2–L1	L4–L5	L3–L5	P	P	2	5	N
SED	2	4/18/90	Post-diskectomy	JWB	PEEK	L3–S1	L3–S1	none	E	E	–	5	N
DDD	0	4/25/90	D-Spondylolisthesis	JWB	PEEK	none	L4–L5	none	G	G	–	4	N
DC	3	7/09/90	Failed PLIF	ADS	PEEK	T12–S1	L5–S1	none	P	P	–	?	N
JC*	0	7/09/90	Burst fracture L1	JWB	UPEK	none	T12–L1	none	E	E	–	5	N

Patient*, anterior interbody fusion with large oval cage

Surgical indication: ETO, ethylene oxide; PLIF, posterior lumbar interbody fusion; HRI, Harrington rod instrumentation; ALIF, anterior lumbar interbody fusion; Gr III, Grade III; Perk, percutaneous suction diskectomy; Zielke, treatment with Zieike instrumentation

Surgeon: ADS, Arthur D. Steffee; JWB, John W. Brantigan; RSB, Robert S. Biscup

Cage material: PEEK, carbon fiber in PEEK; UPEK, carbon fiber in Ultrapek

Clinical status: E, excellent; G, good; F, fair; P, poor

Fusion result. 1, collapse of construct; 2, probable pseudarthrosis; 3, fusion status radiographically uncertain; 4, probable radiographic fusion; 5, radiographic fusion

VSP, variable screw placement instrumentation

cage device if they had failed PLIF with ETO bone, if they had high grade or traumatic spondylolisthesis, if they required strong anterior support due to technical difficulties with other devices at surgery, or if numerous other surgeries had failed. Several patients had cages as primary surgery.

Table 1 lists each patient, date of surgery, surgeon, cage material, VSP fixation levels, carbon cage levels, PLIF levels done with ETO sterilized bone, 6 and 12 month clinical status, fusion status for carbon cages and ETO PLIF levels, and information regarding re-operation. Clinical results are graded excellent, good, fair, or poor according to generally accepted criteria summarized in Table 2. Radiographic evidence of fusion was graded from 1 (obvious pseudarthrosis) to 5 (fusion radiographically solid) by criteria summarized in Table 3.

Results

In the 26 patients there were 63 total fusion levels: 32 levels had carbon cage interbody fusions, 11 levels had ETO donor bone PLIF's, and 20 levels had posterolateral fusion, using autologous bone with pedicle screw and plate support without interbody fusion. One-year follow-up X-rays were obtained on 31 cage levels and 11 allograft levels in 25 patients. There were no failed fusions with the carbon cage. In the same patients there were four established pseudarthroses with ETO bone for a pseudarthrosis rate of 36.3% for donor bone levels. The difference in fusion rates is significant at the $P = 0.0379$ level by the Mann-Whitney test. In 7 patients the carbon cage was used to treat pseudarthrosis from failed ETO donor bone PLIF or ALIF. In one patient (DC) we could not obtain a 1-year follow-up X-ray. The other 6 failed PLIFs treated with the carbon cage resulted in successful fusion.

At 1-year, 11/26 patients had excellent, 8/26 good, 4/26 fair, and 3/26 poor clinical results.

Of the poor clinical results, each had a clearly demonstrable reason for failure unrelated to the carbon cage. PR originally had a burst fracture at L1. She had previously undergone four procedures by other surgeons including interbody fusions at L4–5 and L5–S1 using bovine bone. She had a fifth operation, by ADS, to repair the two-level failed ALIF. This surgery included resection of pedicles at L5, osteotomy at L5 joining the bodies of L4 and L5, a carbon cage interbody fusion at L3–4, and an ETO allograft interbody fusion at L2–3. At follow-up she continued to have back pain, her allograft PLIF level was not healed, and her long fusion ended at two cephalad damaged disk levels. She subsequently had further surgery to reinforce the graft posterolaterally at L2–3 and to extend her fusion to T10. She is in the early postoperative period, and clinical expectations for her are limited.

DEL has a poor result, but has failure of an ETO PLIF level at L3–4, above the carbon cage level. DC had a previous 5-level PLIF (L1–S1) with ETO bone complicated by loss of bowel and bladder function and pseudarthrosis of

Table 2. Description of surgical results by reference.

Excellent and good results		
Reference	Excellent result	Good result
[11]	Returns to former occupation; no pain or minimal pain; sports or recreational activities unrestricted	Returns to former occupation; occasional pain not persisting more than 12 h; not restricted from "less strenuous sports"
[5]	Returns to original work; regular activities; minimal medication; occasional episodes of pain; no neurologic deficits, fusion solid by X-ray	Returns to original work; resumes regular activities; takes occasional medication for episodes of back or leg pain, no neurologic deficits, radiographic solid or questionable fusion
[12]	No complaints whatsoever and no residual ill effects	Relief of the major symptom of pain but with minor residual symptoms such as numbness, paresthesias, minor backache
[14]	(no excellent category acknowledged)	Relief of most (76%–100%) of back pain; able to return to previous work; minimal limitation of activities; minimal medication
[15]	Complete recovery; free of all limitations; never have pain greater than mild pain that the patient is aware of but not bothered by	Return to full activities, sports, the same job or prophylactic limitation to light work; 70% relief of pain; no daily habituating medication
[13]	Score 9 or 10: working at previous occupation; no pain except for rare episodes	Score 7 or 8: able to work, but not at previous occupation or full status; no pain or a low level of pain
Fair and poor results		
Reference	Fair result	Poor result
[11]	Restricted to lighter work; sports and recreational activities restricted; less pain than pre-op but pain still a problem	Unable to work; pain level no better than pre-operatively
[5]	Returns to original or lighter work; some limitation of activities; occasional medication; more frequent back or leg pain; minor neurologic deficit; fusion questionable or pseudarthrosis	Changes to lighter work or disabled; limitation of activities; frequent medication, incapacitating pain or neuro deficit; pseudarthrosis seen on X-ray examination
[12]	Improved; relief of the major pain symptom but with residual paresthesias, numbness, or backache requiring further treatment	failure; no relief
[14]	Partial relief of pain (26%–75%); able to return to previous work with limitations or lighter work; activities limited; medication used frequently	Little or no relief (0%–25%) of pain; disabled for work; activities greatly limited; strong analgesic or narcotic medication used frequently
[15]	Patient able to work but at lighter capacity; less than 70% pain relief; activities limited; occasional episodes of severe pain; or daily pain medication	No improvement or worsening; 25% or less subjective relief of pain, episodes of severe pain; disability; reoperation
[13]	Score 5 or 6: able to work but not at previous occupation; moderate continuing pain	Score 2, 3, or 4: no gainful occupation; moderate to severe pain

Table 3. Criteria for grading radiographic evidence of fusion.

Grade	Fusion result	Description
1	Obvious radiographic pseudarthrosis	Collapse of the construct, loss of disk height, vertebral slip, broken screws, displacement of the carbon cage implant, or resorption of the bone graft
2	Probable radiographic pseudarthrosis	Significant resorption of the bone graft, or a major lucency or gap visible in the fusion area (2 mm or more around the entire periphery of the graft or cage)
3	Radiographic status uncertain	Bone graft is visible in the fusion area at approximately the density originally achieved surgically. A small lucency or gap may be visible involving just a portion of the fusion area with at least half of the graft area showing no lucency between the graft bone and vertebral bone
4	Probable radiographic fusion	Bone bridges the entire fusion area with at least the density originally achieved at surgery. There should be no lucency between the donor bone and vertebral bone
5	Radiographic fusion	The bone in the fusion area is radiographically more dense and more mature than originally achieved in surgery. Optimally, there is no interface between the donor bone and the vertebral bone; however, a sclerotic line between the graft and vertebral bone indicates fusion. Other signs of solid fusion include mature bony trabeculae bridging the fusion area, resorption of anterior vertebral traction spurs, anterior progression of the graft within the disk space, fusion of facet joints, the "ring" phenomenon on CT, or 3D imaging evidence

one PLIF level. The pseudarthrosis was treated with a carbon cage PLIF. By telephone at 1-year, he reported that his main difficulty is recurrent urinary infections, episodes of septicemia, and bladder dysfunction. He lives in Montana, where he has no insurance and declines to provide a 12-month X-ray.

Of the fair results, MSC has collapse of the L4–5 disk above the cage fusion. MS is disabled by a previous stroke and residual neurologic pain that is most likely secondary to extensive cervical degenerative disease. EC had failure of an ETO PLIF at L5–S1. LH was examined after 1-year by his local orthopedist who reported significant improvement. He was included in the fair result group because he felt unable to return to work to manual labor.

Previous surgery had been done in 18 of the 26 patients; these patients had undergone a total of 37 previous operations. Of these 18 patients, 7 had excellent, 5, good, 2, fair, and 3, poor clinical results. Complications were minimal, and there were no surgical infections. One patient had post-operative numbness due to damage to sensory fibers of one nerve root. These were no cases of motor deficit or cauda equina syndrome. Incidental durotomy (i.e., "dural tears") occurred in several patients; however, there were no cases of post-operative cerebrospinal fluid (CSF) leakage, no requirement for secondary dural repair, and no prolongation of hospitalization. There were no cage-device-related complications, no removals of the cage or revisions of the cage interbody fusion. No retropulsion or change in position of any cage was noted in any patient.

Re-operations were done in 5 of the 26 patients. In EC, the second failed ETO PLIF level was further revised to a carbon cage. Six-month clinical status is good following the second cage surgery. GMP had removal of one VSP plate, then piriformis tendon release due to residual nerve pain. At 1 year she had some residual nerve discomfort but still had a good clinical result. PR had further surgery described above. MK had removal of pedicle screws and VSP plates and had nerve root foraminotomy. A fragment of bone from the posterolateral fusion was found to be compromising the neural foramen at the L5 root. JB was re-explored for a myelographic block at L4–5, one level higher than the L5–S1 cage fusion. She had been treated for a traumatic dislocation at L5–S1 and was found to have the cage fusion solidly healed in anatomic position but had bony arachnoiditis above the fusion. In retrospect, her myelogram before the cage surgery showed the bony arachnoiditis. Her clinical result was substantially improved by cage surgery.

Case Report

AP was a 54-year-old male at the time of carbon cage surgery. His first operation was a laminectomy and disk excision at L4–L5 in 1987. He experienced early recurrence of back and right leg pain with some right-sided weakness. In January, 1988, he complained of marked limitation of activity tolerance, continuous moderate pain, and frequent episodes of severe pain. X-ray demonstrated an unstable degenerative slip at L4–5 with complete loss of disk height (Fig. 3). A mild slip was also noted at L5–S1.

On 1/25/88 AP had a second operation, including reduction of disk height, reduction of the spondylolisthesis, segmental fixation using pedicle screws, and VSP plates with two-level PLIF using ETO allograft. X-rays taken on 2/25/88 are shown in Figs. 4 and 5. After initial satisfactory results, it was noted on 8/2/88 that one S1 screw had broken and there was collapse of the graft and foramenal closure. His activity level was decreasing with increasing pain. By 2/9/89, 1 year following his ETO PLIF procedure, all four grafts had collapsed, five of six screws had broken, slip had recurred, and disk space was again lost (Figs. 6,7). He had increasing pain and disability and urgently requested further treatment.

On 5/9/89 AP had further surgery including removal of broken screws and plates, restoration of alignment and disk height, and revision PLIF using carbon cages at L4–5 and L5–S1. During his office visit on 7/20/89, he reported moderate daily activity and no pain. Two month post-operative X-rays are shown in Figs. 8 and 9.

On 10/17/89 AP reported "absolutely no pain at all" and returned to work as a radio dispatcher for Columbia Gas of Ohio. At his 1-year follow-up visit on 6/19/90, he reported no pain, he was working full-time, and motor strength had

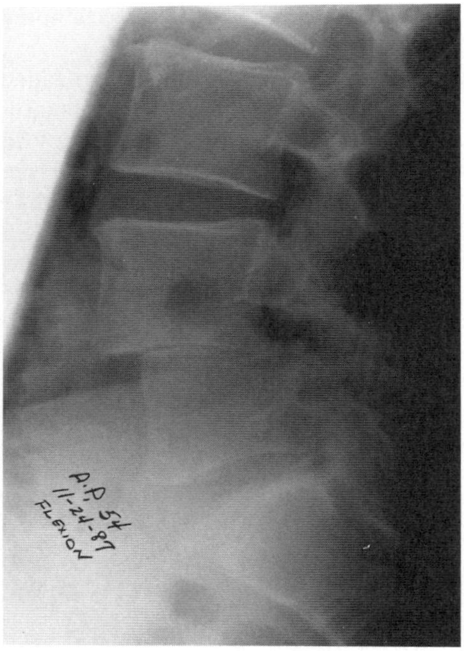

Fig. 3. Lateral X-ray on patient AP (taken 1/88) shows post-diskectomy segmental instability

returned to normal. X-rays showed solid bone bridging both interspace levels, (Figs. 10–12) no broken screws, intact implants, and normal alignment and disk height. He has continued to have excellent results at 2 years post-operation.

Discussion

Results in lumbar fusion surgery are usually evaluated by determining the rate of clinical success and rate of fusion success. While there are some variations in the definitions of excellent, good, fair, and poor surgical results, as summarized in Table 2, the parameters addressed include pain, occupational status, activity level, and use of medication [5,11–15].

We have compared our results with other reports in the literature. Reports of surgical treatment of failed diskectomies [3,16–21] have shown an average clinical success of 66.5% and an average fusion success of 85.1%. Reports of fusion success by number of levels [22–24] have shown an average fusion success of 90.0% at one-level attempts, 77.2% with two-level attempts, and 65.4% with three-level attempts. Our surgical results appear favorable when compared with these previous reports. Exact statistical comparisons, however, are difficult since most of our patients are post-surgical failed backs of varying etiologies. Certainly the results are sufficiently favorable to warrant a careful prospective study in which patients are divided into prognostically distinct groups by specific inclusion and exclusion criteria. Such a study is being initiated.

Pseudarthrosis rates have been studied as long as fusion surgeries have been done. During this century, most authors have agreed that the quoted fusion statistics are flawed by uncertainties of normal radiographic methods of determining fusion. Authors who have used more precise methods of assessing fusion have reported twice the pseudarthrosis rate as compared with authors using less precise criteria [20,25,26]. From Hibbs and Swift in 1929 [27] to Thompson et al. in 1974 [28] to Brodsky et al. in 1991 [29], many authors have stated that only direct surgical exploration will differentiate fusion and pseudarthrosis.

We have outlined standard radiographic criteria in Table 3 and have defined a 5-point numeric scale for interpreting success or failure of radiographic fusion. The ETO allograft pseudarthrosis in Figs. 6 and 7 is clearly evidenced by crushing of the PLIF graft and collapse of the surgical construct indicated by broken screws and vertebral displacement. Cage fusions consistently met the highest descriptive category. For example, the successful carbon cage fusion in Figs. 11 and 12 is indicated by mature trabecular bone bridging the vertebral interspaces with no lucencies in the fusion areas. The numeric format will be useful in database comparisons of larger patient study groups.

Interpretation of successful interbody fusion, both for donor bone and for the carbon composite cages, requires that the X-ray projection be parallel to the endplates. Any obliquity obscures the essential view of the interface between graft and vertebra. This is particularly true in the coronal plane. Figure 10 shows a straight AP view in which the projection is not parallel to either L4–5 or L5–S1. These interspaces appear somewhat amorphous. The up-angled projection in Fig. 11 is parallel to the L4–5 interspace and clearly shows detail not apparent in the straight AP view. Optimum visualization of L5–S1 would require a greater projection angle.

Relative radiodensities of carbon composite and bone provide an interesting index of arthrodesis for the cage PLIF. The carbon composite cage is radiolucent, not radiotransparent. In the 2-month post-operative view in Fig. 8, the details of the cages are indistinct since the cages have approximately the same radiographic density as the cancellous autograft. In Fig. 11, at 1-year post-op the autograft bone has become relatively more dense in the interspace, and the cage is now relatively more lucent, showing the visible rectangular pattern of cage struts as a sign of maturing arthrodesis.

Our experience of 31/31 (100%) apparently successful interbody fusion using the carbon cage is a remarkable improvement in surgical results for the PLIF procedure as compared with donor bone. The fusion success rate of 7/11 (64%) with ETO-sterilized allograft is typical of our experience in PLIF procedures in patients with this degree of clinical complexity. The fusion success rate is also consistent with the results of our histologic study of interbody fusions in goats. In goats sacrificed at 1 year, we have achieved 100% fusion with the carbon

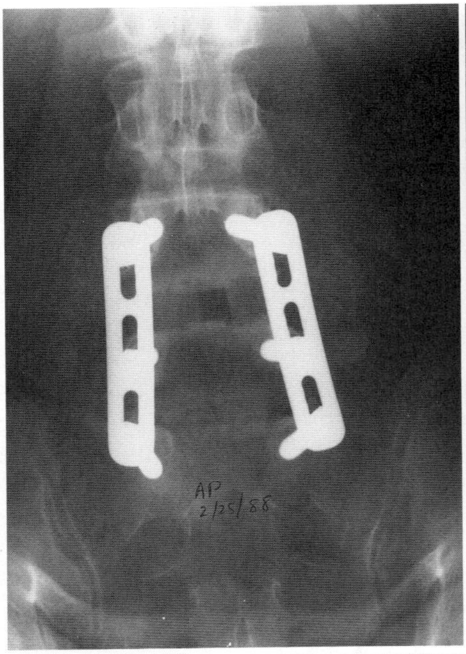

4

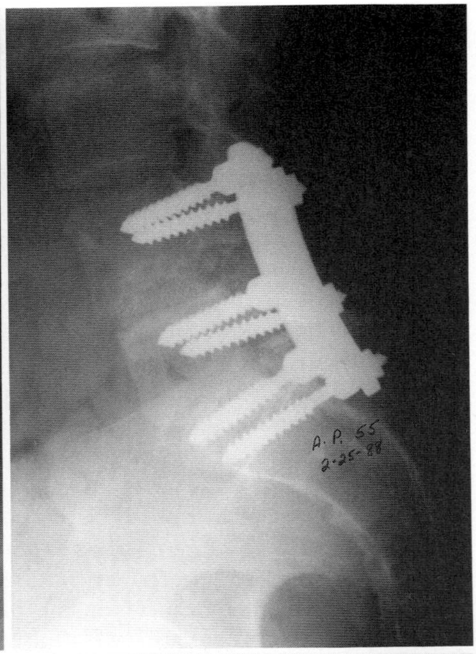

5

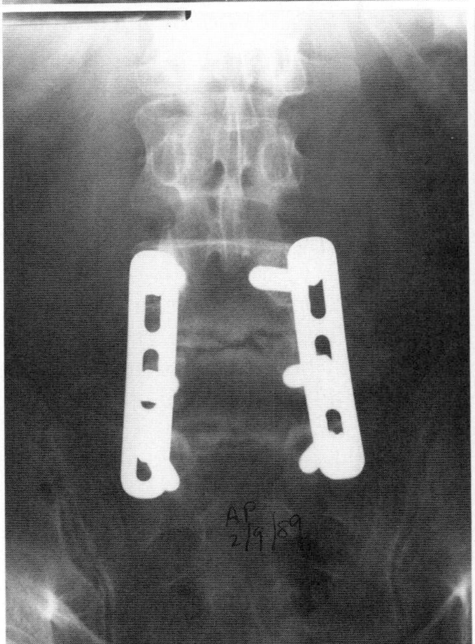

6

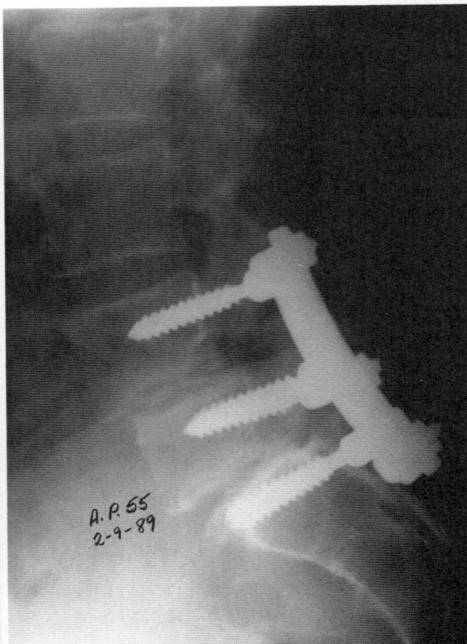

7

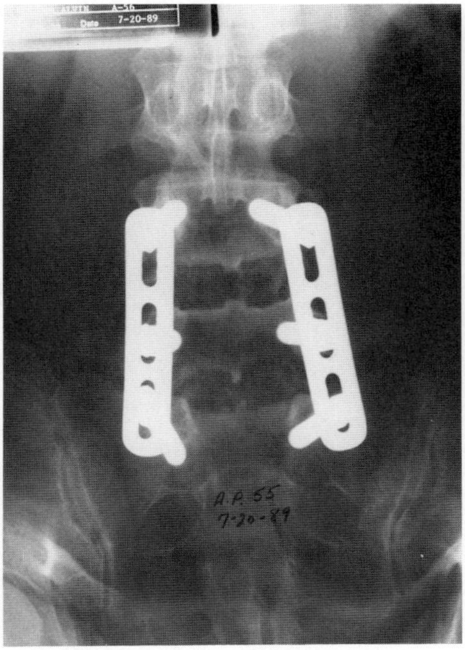

8

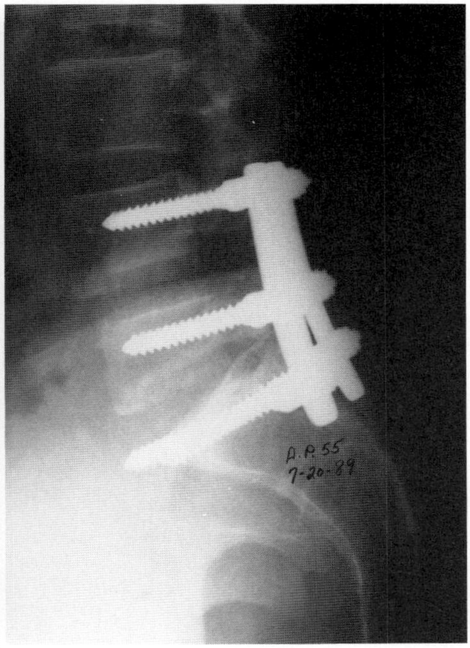

9

Fig. 8. Up-angled anteroposterior X-ray taken 7/20/89, Two-months post-operation. Revision PLIF with the carbon implants shows early appearance of the cage PLIF

Fig. 9. Lateral X-ray taken 7/20/89 shows restoration of disk height and alignment with early appearance of cage PLIF

Fig. 4. Up-angled anteroposterior view taken 2/25/88 One-month post-operation. Two-level PLIF using ETO-sterilized allograft bone shows good restoration of disk height and placement of grafts

Fig. 5. Lateral X-ray taken 2/25/88 shows good correction of spondylolisthesis

Fig. 6. Anteroposterior X-ray taken 2/9/89 One-year post-operation. Allograft PLIF shows that the allograft has collapsed, several screws are broken, and the disk height has been lost

Fig. 7. Lateral X-ray taken 2/9/89 shows loss of disk height and recurrence of slip deformity

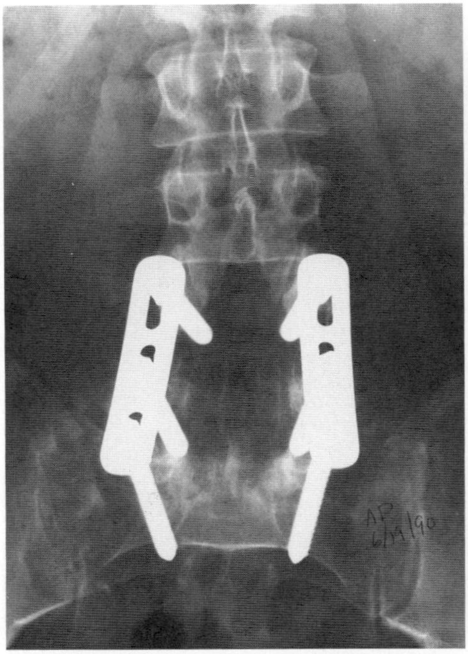

10

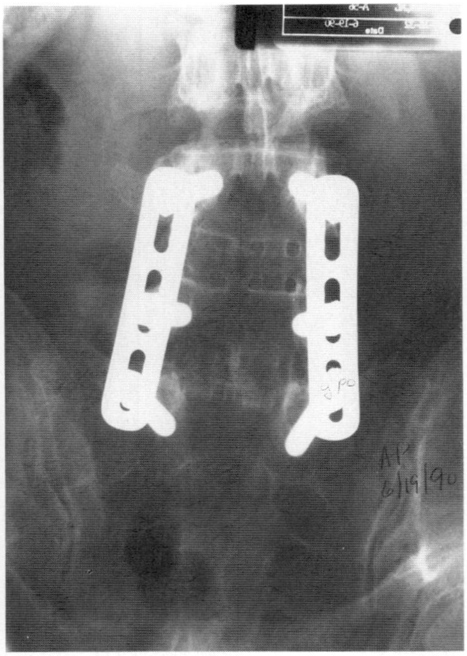

11

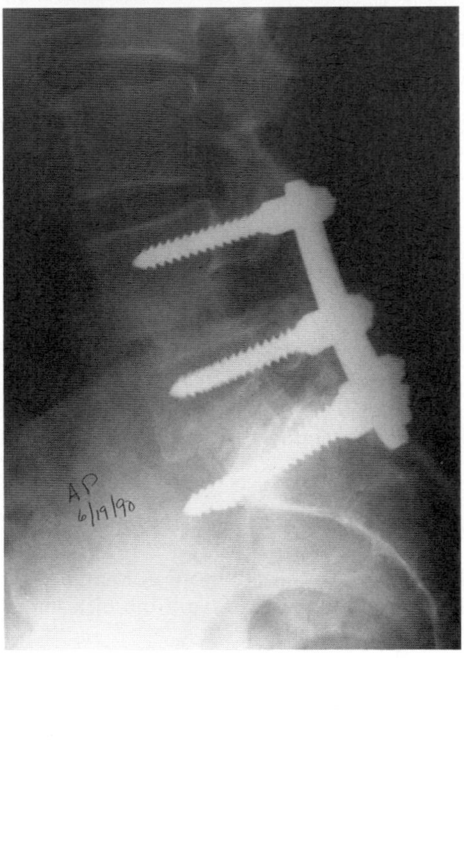

12

Fig. 10. Anteroposterior X-ray taken 6/19/90, One-year post-operation. The carbon cage PLIF does not show the cages or interbody graft because the projection does not parallel the disk space

Fig. 11. Up-angled anteroposterior X-ray taken 6/19/90 shows mature bone within the cages and increasing relative lucency of cage structs due to increasing density of the graft bone

Fig. 12. Lateral X-ray taken 6/19/90 shows mature healed PLIF with the carbon cages

cages, and 67% fusion with the ETO-sterilized allograft [30]. In our clinical series we probably should have used the carbon cages in all PLIF levels in patients in this study. Because our supply of carbon cages was limited, we often used carbon cages only in the most unstable level and used allograft at other levels.

Many surgeons have abandoned the PLIF procedure bacause their fusion rates have been considerably lower than reported by Cloward [2], Lin [3,4], and Ma [5]. Additionally, it is widely believed that a failed PLIF has a far worse clinical result than failure of other fusion procedures. We are not aware of any reports of successful treatments of failed PLIF's anywhere in the literature. Wetzel and LaRocca recently reported evaluation and treatment of 12 failed PLIF's and concluded "we are unable to recommend any successful salvage for the failed PLIF" [31]. Our treatment of 6 failed interbody fusions appears to have achieved 100% fusion success, albeit with lower clinical success (2 excellent, 0 good, 2 fair, and 2 poor results).

Although we have had few complications in the indexed surgery in this series, we must point out that any PLIF procedure is more difficult and dangerous than many other types of lumbar surgery and should not be undertaken casually. For an experienced surgeon, each PLIF level will add 1 h to the surgical procedure and one unit of blood loss on the average.

The five-level ETO allograft PLIF done prior to this series on DC was complicated by neurogenic bowel and bladder in spite of somatosensory evoked potential monitoring during the surgery. We believe that this distressing complication was due to a traction injury of the cauda equina caused by restoration of disk height at the five levels. Four- and five-level PLIF procedures are dangerous and should generally be avoided. PLIF at L1–L2 should be avoided because of potential spinal cord damage from the required retraction.

Degenerative lumbar deformities represent an unsolved clinical problem requiring new techniques and implants. No study has reported satisfactory fusion success in multiple-level fusions without internal fixation. Traditional systems using hooks and distraction rods are unsuited to the degenerative lumbar spine as they produce a painful flat-back deformity when used over multiple segments, and hook sites are often unavailable due to surgical decompression. Pedicle screw systems have provided secure segmental fixation and absolute positional and angular control. We recommend that the surgeon evaluate the mechanical integrity of each element of the motion segment and repair these elements as necessary. This approach requires reduction of deformity, restoration of disk space height to relieve foramenal stenosis, restoration of weight-bearing support to the anterior column using interbody fusion where required, and restoration of normal spinal alignment in sagittal and coronal plane balance. Patients who have failed multiple previous surgical attempts can often be given meaningful surgical improvement if there is a specific mechanical abnormality that can be addressed.

Conclusions

1. A carbon fiber cage-like implant separates the mechanical and biologic functions of PLIF.
2. In 1-year follow-up of the first 26 consecutive patients having interbody fusion with the carbon cage, 31/31 (100%) cage levels show radiographic fusion.
3. In the same patients 7/11 (63%) ETO allograft PLIF levels achieved radiographic fusion.
4. The cage implant achieved successful fusion in 6/6 (100%) of followed patients treated for a failed ETO allograft interbody fusion.
5. Clinical results were excellent in 11/26, good in 8/26, fair in 4/26, and poor in 3/26.
6. Determination of the exact fusion success, rate of clinical success, and nature and frequency of complications will require completion of the multicentered prospective study that is being initiated.

Acknowledgments. The authors would like to thank Mrs. Janet Brantigan, RPT, who coordinated patient follow-up visits, maintained patient data, and provided other technical assistance without which adequate clinical data on these patients could not have been obtained.

References

1. Cloward RB (1953) The treatment of ruptured lumbar intervertebral disks by vertebral body fusion. J Neurosurg 10:154
2. Cloward RB (1985) Posterior lumbar interbody fusion updated. Clin Orthop 193: 16–19
3. Lin PM, Cautilli RA, Joyce MF (1983) Posterior lumbar interbody fusion. Clin Orthop 180:154–168
4. Lin PM (1985) Posterior lumbar interbody fusion technique: Complications and pitfalls. Clin Orthop 183:90–102
5. Ma GW (1985) Posterior lumbar interbody fusion with specialized instruments. Clin Orthop 193:57–63
6. Steffee AD, Sitkowski DJ (1988) Reduction and stabilization of grade IV spondylolisthesis. Clin Orthop 227:82–89
7. Steffee AD, Biscup RS, Sitkowski DJ (1986) Segmental spine plates with pedicle screw fixation. Clin Orthop 203:45–53
8. Steffee AD (1989) The variable screw placement system with posterior lumbar interbody fusion. In: Lin PM, Gill K (eds) Lumbar interbody fusion: Principles and techniques in spine surgery. Aspen, Rockville, MD, pp 81–93
9. Brantigan JW, Cunningham BW, Warden K, McAfee PC, Steffee AD (in press) Compression strength of allograft bone for PLIF. Spine
10. Brantigan JW, Steffee AD, Geiger JM (1991) A carbon fiber implant to aid interbody lumbar fusion: Mechanical testing. Spine 16:S277–282
11. Henderson ED (1966) Results of the surgical treatment of spondylolisthesis. J Bone Joint Surg [Am] 48:619–642

12. Naylor A (1974) The late results of laminectomy for lumbar disk prolapse: A review after 10–25 years. J Bone Joint Surg [Br] 56:17–29
13. Prolo DJ, Oklund SA, Butcher M (1986) Toward uniformity in evaluating results of lumbar spine operations: A paradigm applied to posterior lumbar interbody fusions. Spine 11:601–606
14. Spengler DM, Ouellette EA, Battie M (1990) Elective diskectomy for herniation of a lumbar disk. J Bone Joint Surg [Am] 72:230–237
15. White AH, Von Rogov P, Zucherman J, Heiden D (1987) Lumbar laminectomy for herniated disk: a prospective controlled comparison with internal fixation fusion. Spine 12:305–307
16. Finnegan WJ, Fenlin JM, Marvel JP, Rothman RH (1979) Results of surgical intervention in the symptomatic multiply-operated back patient. J Bone Joint Surg [Am] 61:1077–1082
17. Flynn JC, Hoque MA (1979) Anterior fusion of the lumbar spine. J Bone Joint Surg [Am] 61:1143–1150
18. Hutter CG (1983) Posterior intervertebral body fusion: A 25-year study. Clin Orthop 179:86–96
19. Quimjian JD, Matrka PJ (1988) Decompresion laminectomy and lateral spinal fusion in patients with previously failed lumbar spine surgery. Orthopedics 11: 563–659
20. Stauffer RN, Coventry MB (1972) Anterior interbody lumbar spine fusion: Analysis of Mayo Clinic series. J Bone Joint Surg [Am] 54:756–768
21. Waddell G, Kummel EG, Lotto WN, Graham JD (1979) Failed lumbar disk surgery and repeat surgery following industrial injuries. J Bone Joint Surg 61: 201–207
22. Chow SP, Leong JCY, Ma A, Yau ACMC (1980) Anterior spinal fusion for deranged lumbar intervertebral disks: A review of 97 cases. Spine 5:452–458
23. Goldner JL, Urbaniak JR, McCollum DE (1971) Anterior disk excision and interbody spinal fusion for chronic low back pain. Orthop Clin North Am 2:543–568
24. Prothero SR, Parkes JC, Stinchfield FE (1966) Complications after low-back fusion in 1,000 patients. J Bone Joint Surg [Am] 48:57–65
25. Cleveland M, Bosworth DM, Thompson FR (1948) Pseudarthrosis in the lumbosacral spine. J Bone Joint Surg [Am] 30:302–312
26. Zinreich SJ, Long DM, Davis R, Quinn CB, McAfee PC, Wang H (1990) Three-dimensional CT imaging in postsurgical "failed back" syndrome. J Comput Assist Tomogr 14:574–580
27. Hibbs RA, Swift WE (1929) Developmental abnormalities at the lumbosacral juncture causing paint and disability. Surg Gynecol Obstet 48:604–612
28. Thompson WAL, Gristina AG, Healy WA (1974) Lumbosacral spine fusion: A method of bilateral posterolateral fusion combined with a Hibbs fusion. J Bone Joint Surg 56:1643–1647
29. Brodsky AE, Kovalsky ES, Khalil MA (1991) Correlation of radiologic assessment of lumbar spine fusions with surgical exploration. Spine 16:S261–265
30. Brantigan JW, Cunningham BW, Warden K, McAfee PC, Steffee AD (1992) Interbody lumbar fusion using a carbon fiber cage implant vs. allograft bone: An investigational study in the Spanish goat. Orthopaedic Surgical Research Society Meeting, February 18, Washington D.C.
31. Wetzel FT, LaRocca H (1991) The failed posterior lumbar interbody fusion. Spine 16:839–845

Keyword Index

Allograft 19, 170, 200, 205, 211, 349, 354, 380
  cortical bone 362
  ethylene oxide sterilized 354, 380
  indications 216
  preparation 355
Anterior column 4, 271
Anterior interbody fusion 10, 63, 70, 76, 172, 221, 365; *see also* Posterior lumbar interbody fusion
  complications 224
  interspinous block 221
  long-term results 72
  non-union 220
AO screw
  cancellous 289
  cortex 289
AO fixateur 279
Apex 109
Arthrodesis, *see* Fusion
Autogenic bone, *see* Autograft
Autograft 19, 170, 205
Autoimmune mechanism to disk material 43

Banked bone 205, 345
  survey 349
Bending bilm 13
Biomechanical study 66
  interbody fusion 70
  lumbar fusion 3–8
  pedicle screw system 288
Bone graft 169–170, 199
  allogeneic, *see* Allograft
  autogenous, *see* Autograft
  collapse 208
  defatted 355
  donor site 218
  gas-sterilized 353
  homogenous 171
  interbody fusions 357
  procurement 354
  sterilization 355
  substitute
    hydroxyapatite block 371
    titanium 364
  tricortical 200
  viral infection 356
Bone morphogenic protein 199, 205
Bony union 170
  roentgenography 212

C-D iliosacral screw 261
C-D method 123
Carbon fiber implant 380
Complications 386
  anterior interbody fusion 224
  donor site 364
  external fixation 30
  neurological, pedicle screw fixation 321
  PLIF 132
  reduction of spondylolisthesis 245
  translaminar pedicle screw fixation 238
  transpedicular fixation 338
Computerized axial tomography (CT) 14, 20
  3-D 14
Concavity 109
Criteria, surgical results 301

Cruneal nerves 218

Degenerative changes
  adjacent to fusion 84, 132
  grades 100
Degenerative disk disease, bone marrow changes 40
Diapason screw 289
Disc, intervertebral
  neutrition 43
  degeneration above a fusion 71; *see also* Degenerative changes
  prolapse 5
Diskectomy 254
  total 200
Diskogenic pain 179
Diskography 25, 32, 64, 180, 228, 301
  provocative 25
Distraction 64
Donor site complications 364
Dysplasia index 245

Ethylene oxide 355, 380
  allograft 393; *see also* Allograft
  residual 356
External fixation 25
  complications 30

Facet
  hypertrophy 109
  joints 6
Facetectomy 6, 254
Failed back 388
Flat-back
  deformity 393
  syndrome 87
    surgical results 150
Freeze-dried bone 350
Frontier zone 251
Functional unit 249
Fusion 16
  biomechanical consideration 3–8
  criteria for a successful outcome 93
  evaluation 13, 16
  heave labor work 78, 83
  indications 278, 299
  L4–L5 disk 83
  long 63, 65
  long-term effect 54
  lumbosacral 278, 297
    indications 299
  reontgenographic feature 18, 386, 389
  role of 345
  success rate 205, 379

Gill procedure 180
Grafted bone collapse 371

Hamburger technique 372
Harrington distraction instrumentation 261
Hartshill system 312
Healing of injury 7
Heavy labor 78
Hepatitis 342
Hinge torque index 244
Hydroxyapatite 374
Hypermobility 71

Implant
  carbon fiber 379
  hydroxyapatite 365
  titanium 365
    roentgenographic feature 367
Incorporation, *see* Fusion
Infection 340, 373
Injury 4
  adaptation 7
  healing 7
Instability 3
  biomechanical study 249
  in vivo measurement 45
  magnetic resonance 35
  measurement 45
  multiple-level 126
  roentgenographic examination 40
  segmental 40
instability clinical 6
Interbody fusion 63, 76, 171; *see also* Anterior and Posterior interbody fusion
Internal fixation 278
  biomechanics 279
  computer assisted design 332
  spinal fusion 227
Interspinous block 221
Interspinous ligament 254
Intervertebral disk 4; *see also* Disc

Intraforaminal stenosis 131
ISOLA
  Galveston technique 261
  iliac screw 261

Jackson's criteria 99

Kluger fixateur 279
Kyphosis
  degenerative 88, 113, 135, 150
    etiology 144
    indications 150
    manifestation 136
    myelography 136
    roentgenography 136
    surgery 158
  fusion 147
  stage 146
  thoracolumbar 145

Laminectomy
  extensive 164
  indications 163
Lateral recess stenosis 131
Lateral translation 109, 121
Ligament
  anterior longitudinal 248
  interspinous 254
  posterior longitudinal 248
  supraspinous 254
Ligamentotaxis 132
Lin's classification 203
Lordosis 87, 132, 193
Lumbar spinal canal stenosis 76, 90, 124
Lumbosacral flxation
  biomechanics 259
Lumbosacral junction 259
Luque method 123
Luque rectangular rods 261

Magnetic resonance imaging (MRI) 20, 40
Maximum angulation at failure 265
Maximum strain 265
Middle column 4, 271
Motion segment 31
  adjacent to fusion 62
  adjacent to the lumbosacral fusion 84
Multi-segmented spondylosis 86
Muscle 7
Myelography 109

Neural injury 341, 344
Neurological complications, *see* Complications
Neutral zone of Panjabi 251, 280
Non-union 13
  rates 389
  roentgenography 18
Nut loosening 342

Operative time 344
Osteoporosis 149

Pars defect 179
Pedicle breakout 342
Pedicle screw
  fatigue test 294
  translaminar 277; *see also* Translaminar pedicle screw fixation
Pedicle screw fixation
  indications 192, 195
  neurological complications 321
  spondylolisthesis 195
  technical problems 341
Pedicle screw purchase 87
Pedicle screw system
  advantages 321
  biomechanical study 278, 288
    comparative study 278, 288
  mechanical tests 293
  VSP System 127
Pedicular screw plating 297
Post-decompression olisthesis 131
Posterior column 4
Posterior fusion 63, 171
Posterior lumbar interbody fusion (PLIF) 127, 188, 197
  allograft 208
  bone union 193
  complications 87, 132
  grafting technique 183
  indications 192
  lordosis 193
  non-union 195
  postoperative care 183
  roentgenography 16, 211
  spondylolisthesis 181, 193

surigical intervention 192
Posterolateral fusion 10, 63, 171
Problem back 32
Pseudarthrosis, *see* Non-union
rates
roentgenography
Psychological problem 83

Radicular pain 180
Radicular sign 119
Radioactive bone scans 19
Technetium bone scan 19
Rate of improvement 189
Rigid body spring model 173
Rigid fixation system 64, 174, 294
Rods and plates bending test 291
Roentgenography
biplanar 14
stressed film 19

Saline acceptance tests 64, 365
Schanz screw 289
Scoliosis
adult idiopathic 106
degenerative 89, 98, 106, 113, 118
curvature 111
instrumentation 111
nerve root compression 109
surgery 111, 122
treatment 99
choice of operative procedures 122
pathomechanism of neurological 118
roentgenographic feature 115
disk degeneration 109
Score system of treatment for back pain, the Japanese Orthopaedic Association 35
Screw
breakage 171, 343
entrance point 299
fatigue test 290
placement 342
purchase, sacrum 273
tapered 289
Segmental instability, *see* Instability
Semirigid fixation system 175, 294
Simmons plating system 303
Slipping index 245
SOCON fixateur 279
Spinal canal stenosis 63, 170
Spinal column 4
Spinal instability, *see* Instability
Spinal instrumentation 171, 338
C-D method 123
Diapason screw 289
evaluation 279
Harrington distraction system 261
Hartshill system 312
ISOLA 261
Luque method 123
mechanism of failure 267
modular segmental spinal system (MOSS) 316
pedicular screw plating 297
Simmons plating system 303
SOCON fixateur 279
Steffee plate system 261
variable screw placement (VSP) system 127
Zielke screw 289
Spondylolisthesis 178, 312
congenital 313
degenerative 76, 126, 130, 178, 183
iatrogenic 178
lytic 178
indications 184
mechanism of pain 179
multisegmental 92
reduction 241, 313
complicaitons 245, 314
roentgenographic evaluation 244
traumatic 178
Stabilizing capacity of implant 281
Stauffer and Coventry criteria 301
Steffee plate system 261
Sterilization bone graft 355
Stiffness 46, 265
motion segment 45, 51
Stress unfused segment 70
Stress study 38
Supraspinous ligament 254

Tapered screw 289
Technetium bone scan 19
Tension band wiring 172–174

Titanium 368
Tomogram, lateral 19
Transfusion 342
Translaminar pedicle screw fixation
  complications 238
  indications 228
  technique 229
Translaminar screw fixation
  spondylolisthesis 237
Translation 254
Transpedicular fixation 321; *see also* Pedicle screw fixation
  complications 338

Vertebral rotation 121
Viscoelastic effects of the spine 5

X-ray, biplanar 14

Zielke screw 289